Adolescent Medicine

Editors

WILLIAM B. SHORE
FRANCESCO LEANZA
NICOLE CHAISSON

PRIMARY CARE:
CLINICS IN OFFICE PRACTICE

www.primarycare.theclinics.com

Consulting Editor
JOEL J. HEIDELBAUGH

September 2014 • Volume 41 • Number 3

ELSEVIER

1600 John F. Kennedy Boulevard • Suite 1800 • Philadelphia, Pennsylvania, 19103-2899

http://www.theclinics.com

PRIMARY CARE: CLINICS IN OFFICE PRACTICE Volume 41, Number 3
September 2014 ISSN 0095-4543, ISBN-13: 978-0-323-32339-0

Editor: Jessica McCool
Developmental Editor: Yonah Korngold

Primary Care: Clinics in Office Practice (ISSN: 0095–4543) is published quarterly by Elsevier Inc., 360 Park Avenue South, New York, NY 10010-1710. Months of issue are March, June, September, and December. Periodicals postage paid at New York, NY and additional mailing offices. Subscription prices are $225.00 per year (US individuals), $392.00 (US institutions), $115.00 (US students), $275.00 (Canadian individuals), $444.00 (Canadian institutions), $175.00 (Canadian students), $345.00 (international individuals), $444.00 (international institutions), and $175.00 (international students). Foreign air speed delivery is included in all *Clinics* subscription prices. All prices are subject to change without notice. POSTMASTER: Send address changes to *Primary Care: Clinics in Office Practice*, Elsevier Periodicals Customer Service, 11830 Westline Industrial Drive, St. Louis, MO 63146. Customer Service Health Sciences Division, Subscription Customer Service, 3251 Riverport Lane, Maryland Heights, MO 63043. **Customer Service: 1-800-654-2452 (U.S. and Canada); 314-447-8871 (outside U.S. and Canada). Fax: 314-447-8029. E-mail: journalscustomerservice-usa@elsevier.com (for print support); journalsonlinesupport-usa@elsevier.com (for online support).**

Reprints. For copies of 100 or more, of articles in this publication, please contact the Commercial Reprints Department, Elsevier Inc., 360 Park Avenue South, New York, NY 10010-1710. Tel. 212-633-3874; Fax: 212-633-3820; E-mail: reprints@elsevier.com.

Primary Care: Clinics in Office Practice is covered in *MEDLINE/PubMed (Index Medicus)* and *EMBASE/Excerpta Medica, Current Contents/Clinical Medicine, and ISI/BIOMED.*

Contributors

CONSULTING EDITOR

JOEL J. HEIDELBAUGH, MD, FAAFP, FACG
Clinical Associate Professor, Departments of Family Medicine and Urology; Clerkship Director, Department of Family Medicine, University of Michigan Medical School, Ann Arbor, Michigan; Ypsilanti Health Center, Ypsilanti, Michigan

EDITORS

WILLIAM B. SHORE, MD, FAAFP
Professor, Department of Family and Community Medicine, University of California, San Francisco, San Francisco, California

FRANCESCO LEANZA, MD
Associate Professor, Department of Family Medicine and Community Health, Icahn School of Medicine at Mount Sinai; Institute for Family Health, New York, New York

NICOLE CHAISSON, MD, MPH
Assistant Professor, Department of Family and Community Health, University of Minnesota Medical Center, Minneapolis, Minnesota

AUTHORS

MICHELE ALLEN, MD, MS
Investigator, Program in Health Disparities Research; Assistant Professor, Department of Family Medicine and Community Health, University of Minnesota Medical School, Minneapolis, Minnesota

DAVID L. BELL, MD, MPH
Associate Professor, Department of Pediatrics and Department of Population and Family Health, Columbia University Medical Center, New York Presbyterian Hospital, New York, New York

IRIS WAGMAN BOROWSKY, MD, PhD
Associate Professor and Division Director, Division of General Pediatrics and Adolescent Health, Department of Pediatrics, University of Minnesota, Minneapolis, Minnesota

JENSENA CARLSON, MD
Academic Fellow, Department of Family Medicine, University of Wisconsin School of Medicine and Public Health, Madison, Wisconsin

NICOLE CHAISSON, MD, MPH
Assistant Professor, Department of Family and Community Health, University of Minnesota Medical Center, Minneapolis, Minnesota

VEENOD L. CHULANI, MD, MSEd, FSAHM
Director, Division of Adolescent Medicine, Arnold Palmer Hospital for Children, Orlando, Florida; Clinical Associate Professor of Pediatrics, Florida State University College of Medicine, Tallahassee, Florida

JESSICA DALBY, MD
Assistant Professor, Department of Family Medicine, University of Wisconsin School of Medicine and Public Health, Madison, Wisconsin

NAOMI NICHELE DUKE, MD, MPH
Assistant Professor, Division of General Pediatrics and Adolescent Health, Department of Pediatrics, University of Minnesota, Minneapolis, Minnesota

JENNY FRANCIS, MD
Department of Pediatrics, Mount Sinai Adolescent Health Center, Icahn School of Medicine at Mount Sinai, New York, New York

DIEGO GARCIA-HUIDOBRO, MD
Associate Professor, Departments of Family Medicine and Community Health, Minneapolis, Minnesota; Graduate Student, Department of Family Social Science, University of Minnesota Medical School, St Paul, Minnesota; Faculty, Department of Family Medicine, School of Medicine, Pontificia Universidad Catolica de Chile, Santiago, Región Metropolitana, Chile

ERICA J. GIBSON, MD
Assistant Professor, Department of Pediatrics and Department of Population and Family Health, Columbia University Medical Center, New York Presbyterian Hospital, New York, New York

LONNA P. GORDON, MD, PharmD
Clinical Fellow in Adolescent Medicine, Department of Pediatrics, Mount Sinai Adolescent Health Center, Icahn School of Medicine at Mount Sinai, New York, New York

DIANE HAUSER, MPA
Department of Family Medicine and Community Health, Icahn School of Medicine at Mount Sinai; Institute for Family Health, New York, New York

RONNI HAYON, MD
Assistant Professor, Department of Family Medicine, University of Wisconsin School of Medicine and Public Health, Madison, Wisconsin

BLAIR HEINKE, MD
Team Physician, Associate Professor, Medstar Georgetown University Hospital, Georgetown University, Washington, DC

CAROLYN BRADNER JASIK, MD
Assistant Professor of Pediatrics, University of California, San Francisco, San Francisco, California

CLARISSA CALLIOPE KRIPKE, MD, FAAP
Health Services Clinical Professor; Director of Developmental Primary Care; Family and Community Medicine, University of California, San Francisco, San Francisco, California

FRANCESCO LEANZA, MD
Associate Professor, Department of Family Medicine and Community Health, Icahn School of Medicine at Mount Sinai; Institute for Family Health, New York, New York

JANET LEE, MD
Department of Pediatrics, Mount Sinai Adolescent Health Center, Icahn School of Medicine at Mount Sinai, New York, New York

ERICA B. MONASTERIO, MN, FNP-BC
Clinical Professor and Director, Family Nurse Practitioner Program, Department of Family Health Care Nursing; Nurse Faculty, Division of Adolescent and Young Adult Medicine, Department of Pediatrics, University of California, San Francisco, San Francisco, California

ROBERT E. MORRIS, MD
Professor Emeritus, General Pediatrics, Department of Pediatrics, University of California at Los Angeles, Los Angeles, California

JUSTIN MULLNER, MD
Sports Medicine Fellow, Atlantic Health Sports Medicine, Morristown, New Jersey

MARILIA G. NEVES, PsyD
Assistant Professor, Harlem Residency in Family Medicine, Department of Family Medicine and Community Health; Director of Behavioral Science for the Institute for Family Health, The Institute for Family Health, Icahn School of Medicine at Mount Sinai, New York, New York

RAYMOND C.W. PERRY, MD, MS
Medical Director, Department of Health Services, Los Angeles County Juvenile Court Health Services, Los Angeles, California

SHERINE A. POWERFUL
MPH Candidate, Department of Population and Family Health, Columbia University Medical Center, New York, New York

WILLIAM B. SHORE, MD, FAAFP
Professor, Department of Family and Community Medicine, University of California, San Francisco, San Francisco, California

JOHN STEEVER, MD
Assistant Professor, Department of Pediatrics, Mount Sinai Adolescent Health Center, Icahn School of Medicine at Mount Sinai, New York, New York

MARÍA VERÓNICA SVETAZ, MD, MPH
Medical Director, Aqui Para Ti/Here for You Clinic for Latino Youth; Faculty, Department of Family and Community Medicine, Hennepin County Medical Center, Minneapolis, Minnesota

Contents

Adolescent Health Care Maintenance in a Teen-Friendly Clinic 451

Nicole Chaisson and William B. Shore

> Adolescence is marked by complex physical, cognitive, social, and emotional development, which can be stressful for families and adolescents. Before the onset of puberty, providers should clearly lay the groundwork for clinical care and office visits during the adolescent years. This article addresses the guidelines and current legal standards for confidentiality in adolescent care, the most frequently used psychosocial screening tools, and current recommendations for preventive health services and immunizations. Through the creation of teen-friendly clinics, primary care providers are well positioned to offer guidance and support to teens and their parents during this time of transition and growth.

Adolescent Growth and Development 465

Veenod L. Chulani and Lonna P. Gordon

> Adolescence is a developmental stage defined by physical and psychosocial maturation. This article reviews normal pubertal development and the evaluation and management of adolescents with suspected pubertal abnormalities and provides an overview of adolescent psychosocial development.

Home

Parents and Family Matter: Strategies for Developing Family-Centered Adolescent Care Within Primary Care Practices 489

María Verónica Svetaz, Diego Garcia-Huidobro, and Michele Allen

> Healthy adolescent development and successful transition to adulthood begins in the family. Supporting families in their communities and cultures ultimately makes this support system stronger. Parenting adolescents is described as the most challenging life stage for parents. Primary care providers are in an ideal position to support families with teens. This article reviews stressors, recommends strength-based strategies, describes how health care delivery systems can be organized to address the needs of adolescents and their families, shares a case study of a family-oriented, youth-friendly primary care clinic, and provides practical strategies for developing family-centered adolescent care within primary care practices.

Education

Clarissa Calliope Kripke

> Disability is a natural part of the human experience. To maximize potential, adolescents with disabilities require multidisciplinary transition planning and life-skill training. Health care professionals can reduce barriers to accessing health care. They can encourage self-determination and connect patients to self-advocacy organizations. They can facilitate smooth transitions to adult health care services. Careful descriptions of a patient's baseline traits and function are critical, not only to assist in person centered planning processes, but to ensure that new caregivers and clinicians have the information they need to recognize changes in function or behavior that can signal illness.

Eating

Carolyn Bradner Jasik

> Eating behavior in adolescents can be as high risk as other behaviors that arise during this period and can have serious health consequences. This article presents a framework for screening and treatment of abnormal adolescent eating behavior by the primary care provider. A review of the types of disordered eating is presented along with suggested ways to screen. Indications for subspecialty eating disorder referrals and key aspects of screening and intervention in adolescent obesity and eating disorders are also reviewed. Specific attention is paid to the aspects of care that can be provided in primary care and multidisciplinary care.

Activity

Blair Heinke and Justin Mullner

> Participation in athletic activities among children and adolescents is on the rise in the United States. Approximately 35 million children ages 5 to 18 play organized sports each year. High school athletes suffer approximately 2 million injuries per year, resulting in 500,000 doctor visits and 30,000 hospitalizations. In addition, early specialization in sports has led to increased incidence of overuse injury in adolescents. Head injuries among adolescents are also on the rise. Primary care providers are called on to complete preparticipation evaluations and to see adolescents with acute injuries. The goal of this article is to discuss these issues common to adolescent athletes.

Francesco Leanza and Diane Hauser

> Teens are avid users of new technologies and social media. Nearly 95% of US adolescents are online at least occasionally. Health care professionals

and organizations that work with teens should identify online health information that is both accurate and teen friendly. Early studies indicate that some of the new health technology tools are acceptable to teens, particularly texting, computer-based psychosocial screening, and online interventions. Technology is being used to provide sexual health education, medication reminders for contraception, and information on locally available health care services. This article reviews early and emerging studies of technology use to promote teen health.

Drugs (Substance Use/Abuse)

Substance use in adolescence is common, but not all use indicates a substance use disorder. The primary care provider has an essential role in screening for substance involvement, assessing the level of substance use and its impact on function, and engaging in a brief intervention to encourage and support behavioral change related to substance use. This article summarizes the literature on adolescent vulnerability to substance use disorders and their impact on adolescent health and well-being. Practical concrete suggestions for approaches to screening, brief interventions, and referral to treatment provide a stepwise approach to adolescent substance use assessment and intervention.

Depression (Mental Health)

The primary care setting is considered the entry point of adolescents with mental illness in the health care system. This article informs primary care providers about the diagnostic features and differential of mood disorders in adolescents, screening and assessment, as well as evidence-based psychosocial and psychopharmacologic therapies. The article also provides a framework for decision making regarding initiating treatment in the primary care setting and referral to mental health services. Furthermore, the article highlights the importance of the collaboration between primary care and mental health providers to facilitate engagement of adolescents with mood disorders and adherence to treatment.

Sex (Sexuality/Reproductive Health)

7% of US teen women became pregnant in 2008, totaling 750,000 pregnancies nationwide. For women ages 15 to 19, 82% of pregnancies are unintended. Adolescents have a disproportionate risk of medical complications in pregnancy. Furthermore, adolescent parents and their infants both tend to suffer poor psychosocial outcomes. Preventing unintended and adolescent pregnancies are key public health objectives for Healthy

health services in correctional settings can help health care providers who work in youth detention facilities and those who see youth for follow-up care after incarceration. Several challenges exist to providing care in detention facilities, but overcoming these barriers to optimally serve youth is critical. When youth are released to their homes, community providers must understand the extent of care offered in detention facilities, the unique considerations for youth on probation, and the aspects of follow-up care that should be addressed.

PRIMARY CARE:
CLINICS IN OFFICE PRACTICE

RELATED INTEREST

Pediatric Clinics of North America, February 2014 (Vol. 61, Issue 1)
Adolescent Cardiac Issues
Pooja Gupta and Richard Humes, *Editors*
Available at: http://www.pediatric.theclinics.com/

Foreword
Know Your Audience

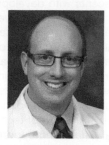

Joel J. Heidelbaugh, MD, FAAFP, FACG
Consulting Editor

Clinicians in primary care practices encounter adolescent patients on a daily to weekly basis for a variety of reasons, ranging from acute to chronic conditions, well examinations, and reasons for which their parents or guardians have brought or sent them in. As the years pass by and my expertise theoretically grows, I find it increasingly challenging to adequately address all of the appropriate acute and screening provisions necessary for adolescents in a single office visit. Even if an adolescent presents for an acute issue, due diligence tells me that I should ask him or her about 20-odd questions to assess their safety and promote the best health status for them that I can offer. Then, I have to hope that the adolescent can believe, understand, remember, and integrate the information. So, I often reflect upon some great advice that my medical school advisor once gave me relative to patient encounters: *know your audience!*

Do you remember going to the doctor when you were an adolescent? Odds were, that you didn't want to be there, conversed and interacted with the clinician very little, and freaked out over the prospect of any form of a "sensitive" examination. This is likely the typical response from most teenagers. Was the visit for a sports physical? To catch up on immunizations? For birth control or sexually transmitted disease testing that you didn't want your parents to find out about?

Clinicians are left with asking: "How many adolescents actually seek out health care clinicians on their own, without any pressure or guidance from an adult, to simply ask their doctor for help?" Of those, how many actually feel comfortable discussing their fears, embarrassments, and nightmares with their clinician? Every day, the lay press is riddled with accounts of children being bullied for being obese or gay, teenagers engaging in homicidal and suicidal behavior, and overdosing on illicit drugs. Rates of drug use among adolescents are skyrocketing due to increased availability of both prescription and narcotic substances. It seems as if attempts to "win the war on drugs" have not only failed, but have also left the doors wide open to our country's middle schools, high schools, and neighborhoods.

Prim Care Clin Office Pract 41 (2014) xiii–xiv
http://dx.doi.org/10.1016/j.pop.2014.06.003
0095-4543/14/$ – see front matter © 2014 Elsevier Inc. All rights reserved.

This issue of *Primary Care: Clinics in Office Practice* provides an outstanding compendium of articles dedicated to adolescent medicine for primary care clinicians. This edition commences with the blueprints for health maintenance in adolescents, predicated upon normal growth and developmental parameters including psychosocial development, and highlights strategies to care for adolescents with developmental delay. The article entitled, "Parents and Family Matter: Strategies for Developing Family-Centered Adolescent Care Within Primary Care Practices," provides key strategies on how to talk with adolescents and, more importantly, how to listen to them. Expert clinician authors provide current data-rich articles on how to approach the adolescent with suspected or documented eating disorders and body dysmorphism, caring for incarcerated adolescents, how to conduct a preparticipation sports physical, and how to evaluate and treat adolescents with substance dependence and mental illness. A provocative article takes an in-depth look at the role of technology in the daily life of the adolescent, surveying both potential pitfalls and opportunities for proactive health engagement. Articles highlighting teen violence, bullying prevention, and sexuality provide informative constructs for clinicians to engage adolescents and offer appropriate support, resources, and acceptance. The common thread in all of these articles allows for enhancement of communication between clinicians and their adolescent patients, perhaps the most important tenet in promoting health care in this group.

I would like to compliment and thank Drs Shore, Leanza, and Chaisson for their extensive efforts in creating this unique and densely informative volume of articles dedicated to improving the health care of adolescents. This is truly an invaluable reference that has the potential to substantially improve outcomes in adolescent health care. I hope that the readers of *Primary Care: Clinics in Office Practice* will find this volume to be as engaging and didactic as I have.

Joel J. Heidelbaugh, MD, FAAFP, FACG
Departments of Family Medicine and Urology
University of Michigan Medical School
Ann Arbor, MI, USA

Ypsilanti Health Center
200 Arnet Suite 200
Ypsilanti, MI 48198, USA

E-mail address:
jheidel@umich.edu

Preface

Adolescent Medicine

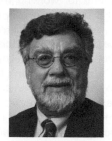 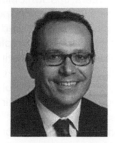 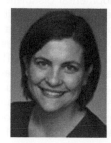

William B. Shore, MD, FAAFP   Francesco Leanza, MD   Nicole Chaisson, MD, MPH

Editors

We delight in the beauty of the butterfly, but rarely admit the changes it has gone through to achieve that beauty.

—*Maya Angelou*

Adolescence is a normal developmental stage, and the changes that accompany this developmental journey may be exciting, challenging, and even frightening for teens, their families, and their health care providers. It is a period of complex physical, cognitive, social, and emotional development that spans the transition from childhood to adulthood. Adolescence typically begins with the physical changes of puberty that occur during the preteen years and ends with the successful adoption of adult roles and responsibilities by the early to mid-twenties. During these years, teens often establish habits and refine beliefs that remain with them throughout much of their adult lives. These habits and beliefs are influenced by parents, peers, religious and ethnic communities, and society at large. Parents and physicians often worry about negative influences during the adolescent years. Nevertheless, healthy and supportive relationships between youth, their family, friends, and other caring adults can provide a framework for developing positive social behaviors and maintaining resiliency in the face of personal or social stress.

This issue of *Primary Care: Clinics in Office Practice* focuses on common diagnoses and health issues that often first present in primary care offices along with guidelines to create the supportive environment that is fundamental to the care of adolescents and their families. The first two articles focus on more "routine" aspects of the typical primary care adolescent office visit. The first article reviews health care maintenance and screening recommendations, describes confidentiality standards for working with adolescents, and provides suggestions for creating a teen-friendly clinic. The second article describes normal adolescent growth and development followed by a description of the approach to patients who vary in their development.

The subsequent articles are organized in a format that resembles the HEEADSS Screen, a well-known adolescent psychosocial screening tool. In the Home section,

Prim Care Clin Office Pract 41 (2014) xv–xvii
http://dx.doi.org/10.1016/j.pop.2014.06.002
0095-4543/14/$ – see front matter © 2014 Published by Elsevier Inc.

primarycare.theclinics.com

the authors focus on the parent/teen relationship, describe strategies to keep families positively involved in their teenager's lives, and present a case study of a youth-friendly clinic that promotes that involvement. Under the Education section, the author presents a comprehensive description of the challenges of working with adolescents with developmental disabilities and offers tips for office etiquette for working with these patients and their families. The Eating section includes a thorough review of disordered eating behaviors commonly encountered with adolescent patients, including obesity, and provides clear strategies for the role of the primary care clinician working with these patients. The first article in the Activity section includes guidelines for completing the sports preparticipation evaluation, current recommendations for screening adolescent athletes for potential cardiac problems to minimize sudden cardiac death, and current recommendations for evaluating when teens can return to sports following concussion or musculoskeletal injury. This is followed by a brief review of the emerging use of technology as a tool for providing innovative health care to teens.

In the Drugs section, the author describes strategies and screening tools for the primary care clinician to identify adolescents who are at risk for or are using drugs or other substances inappropriately, including guidelines for intervention and resources for teens and their families. The section on Depression is a comprehensive review of mood disorders in adolescents and the role of the primary care provider to identify mood disorders, assess risk for suicide, and access resources for integrative behavioral health intervention. There are three articles linked to the Sexuality/Reproductive Health section of this issue. In the first article, the authors open with a dialogue about teen pregnancy and pregnancy options counseling followed by a comprehensive review of the current methods of contraception available to adolescents with a focus on the most effective methods for adolescents. The next article in this section reviews the most common sexually transmitted infections among adolescents along with current recommendations for treatment and prevention. In the third article of this section, the authors provide important definitions, descriptions, and guidance for providers working with LGBT-identified youth. The Safety section focuses on bullying and interpersonal violence. The authors describe strategies to identify high-risk situations and approaches that can be helpful in primary care offices. Finally, the article on incarcerated youth focuses on the care of this special population of adolescents, by addressing the health risks of teens and young adults who are incarcerated, and provides guidelines for primary care providers to continue their medical care after their release from incarceration.

These articles describe several ways in which primary care providers may interact with adolescent patients and their families. Although there is limited research dedicated to the quality of the youth/health care provider relationship and its correlation with adolescent health outcomes, national guidelines suggest that the quality of that relationship may be just as important as the content of the health care services provided.[1] The benefits of these relationships are particularly enhanced when a longitudinal relationship is established over many years. Access to comprehensive, youth-friendly primary care services is important for improving the health of adolescents. Primary care has the capacity to provide high-quality screening, assessment, and care management for teens in a confidential and supportive environment. Creating that environment is fundamental.

The editors would like to thank all of the authors for their expertise and commitment to supporting high-quality care for adolescents by their primary care clinicians. We are also grateful for the assistance of Yonah Korngold and Jessica McCool from Elsevier—particularly when we were reaching the deadline! And we are all indebted to and thankful for our families, who have supported us even when they haven't seen much of us lately. Finally, we want to thank our adolescent patients and their families, who inspire us and keep us humble.

William B. Shore, MD, FAAFP
Department of Family and Community Medicine
University of California, San Francisco
995 Potrero, Building 80, Ward 83
San Francisco, CA 94110, USA

Francesco Leanza, MD
Department of Family Medicine and Community Health
Icahn School of Medicine at Mount Sinai
New York, NY, USA

Nicole Chaisson, MD, MPH
Department of Family and Community Health
University of Minnesota Medical Center
Family Medicine Residency
2020 East 28th Street
Minneapolis, MN 55407, USA

E-mail addresses:
shorew@fcm.ucsf.edu (W.B. Shore)
fleanza@institute2000.org (F. Leanza)
chai0027@umn.edu (N. Chaisson)

REFERENCE

1. National Research Council and Institute of Medicine. Adolescent health services: missing opportunities. Committee on Adolescent Health Care Services and Models of Care for Treatment, Prevention, and Healthy Development. In: Lawrence RS, Appleton Gootman J, Sim LJ, editors. Board on Children, Youth, and Families. Division of Behavioral and Social Sciences and Education. Washington, DC: The National Academies Press; 2009.

Adolescent Health Care Maintenance in a Teen-Friendly Clinic

Nicole Chaisson, MD, MPH[a], William B. Shore, MD[b],*

KEYWORDS

- Confidentiality • Psychosocial screening tools • Screening and prevention
- Health maintenance • Teen-friendly clinic • Immunizations

KEY POINTS

- Primary care providers should be knowledgeable of confidentiality laws in their state and communities.
- Confidentiality practice guidelines should be reviewed with parents and adolescents.
- Adolescent psychosocial screening tools are effective in identifying adolescent strengths and high-risk behaviors.
- Every clinical encounter with adolescents is an opportunity to address screening and prevention.

CARING FOR TEENS IN THE PRIMARY CARE SETTING

Although access to primary care services is important for improving the health of adolescents, several decades of research within the United States and across the globe have documented the barriers that adolescents and young adults experience when trying to access these services.[1] Both the World Health Organization and the Institute of Medicine have developed frameworks for the development of youth-friendly services to call attention to the need for improved access to adolescent health services.[2,3] Primary care has the capacity to provide high-quality screening, assessment, and care management for teens in a confidential and supportive environment. Creating that environment is fundamental.

Communication with Teens and Their Families

The role of families and caregivers is important in adolescent care. Families can be an asset through providing a thorough medical history, supporting teen development and

Disclosures: None.
[a] Department of Family and Community Medicine, University of Minnesota Medical Center, Family Medicine Residency, 2020 East 28th Street, Minneapolis, MN 55407, USA;
[b] Department of Family and Community Medicine, University of California, San Francisco, 995 Potrero, Building 80, Ward 83, San Francisco, CA 94110, USA
* Corresponding author.
E-mail address: shorew@fcm.ucsf.edu

Prim Care Clin Office Pract 41 (2014) 451–464
http://dx.doi.org/10.1016/j.pop.2014.05.001
0095-4543/14/$ – see front matter © 2014 Elsevier Inc. All rights reserved.
primarycare.theclinics.com

independence, clarifying expectations and setting limits, and ensuring ongoing access to care. Although limited research has been performed on partnerships between parents of teens and health care professionals, recent qualitative data describe both direct and indirect strategies to strengthen parent/provider relationships to influence adolescent health outcomes.[4] Direct strategies include efforts that create improved communication and partnership between the provider and the parent, and indirect strategies increase the provider's influence on parent/teen communication within the context of clinic visits.[4] This research is built on the concept of triadic relationships; a third person can often stabilize and improve the relationship between the other 2 people. These strategies could be particularly useful for family medicine clinics, where providers are seeing both adolescents and their parents as patients, creating an opportunity for growth of a strong triadic relationship.[5]

Before the onset of puberty, primary care providers should clearly lay the groundwork for health care visits during the adolescent years. Parents and their preteen children should be informed that issues discussed individually, with adolescents or parents, are confidential, and that adolescents may be examined without the parents present.[6] It is important for providers to acknowledge that the adolescent is the patient; they should greet the adolescent first and then ask to be introduced to the family. Providers should take time to talk with both parents and teens to build trust, develop rapport, and support their relationship, but consider noting that it is "clinic policy" to talk with teens alone for some of the visit to allow for more open conversation. A qualitative study using focus groups with mother/son dyads showed that regular, routine inclusion of time alone during adolescent visits starting in early adolescence could lead to greater parental comfort with this process and increased disclosure by the adolescent.[7]

During the interview, providers should practice listening more than speaking; open-ended questions should be used to probe deeper, especially when asking about difficult subjects. If concerns arise, refrain from lecturing—teens do not need another parent—rather, practitioners should be open and honest and criticize the activity, not the adolescent.[8,9] When performing the physical examination, providers should remember to wash their hands within the view of the adolescent; previous research noted that teens ranked providers washing hands as the most important item that affects their decision to seek health care.[10] During the physical examination, providers should also respect their patients' privacy and modesty by making sure they are appropriately gowned, discussing and explaining each part of the physical examination, and asking about any discomfort with the examination.

Systems/Structure

A clinic does not have to be a "teen clinic" to be teen-friendly; this goal can be accomplished in many ways. The Adolescent Health Working Group (www.ahwg.net) developed a Provider Toolkit Series that provides guidelines for teen-friendly services.[11] First and foremost, providers and staff should enjoy working with adolescents. Structurally, it can be useful to create a space in the waiting area or another part of the clinic that includes posters, educational resources, and magazines geared toward teens. If financially possible, providing access to a computer space or guest wireless access may be appreciated by the more tech-savvy teens.

When registering for clinic services, adolescents and their family should be presented with brochures describing the clinic's policies regarding minor consent and access to confidential care. Clinics that care for adolescents should also advocate within their sponsoring institutions to ensure confidentiality is maintained after the clinic visit is complete. A qualitative study of clinician perspectives on adolescent care in urban primary care clinics found that, although clinicians were committed to offering preventive care during adolescents visits, systems issues must be developed that enhance consistency of delivery of confidential services that meet the recommended guidelines.[8] Failure to meet those guidelines may contribute to skepticism among adolescent patients and their parents. Explanation of benefits notifications, patient satisfaction surveys, billing statements, or other forms of communication about the adolescent visits are often inadvertently sent to parents.[12] Protection from these lapses should be paramount in teen care.

MINOR CONSENT AND CONFIDENTIALITY

When working with adolescents in clinic, it is important to understand the state laws regarding minor consent for treatment and access to confidential care. The laws related to adolescent consent and confidentiality vary by state. Most states have up to 10 different minor consent rules and an equal number of potentially different confidentiality laws.[13,14] Because of this complexity and the potential changes in these laws because of shifting political climates, it is important for providers to stay up to date. National organizations exist that monitor minor consent and confidentiality laws. The Center for Adolescent Health & the Law (www.cahl.org)[13] and the Guttmacher Institute (www.guttmacher.org)[14] are organizations that regularly monitor state laws regarding minor consent and access to confidential services. Both organizations provide updated state-by-state information.

Generally, parental consent is required to provide medical care for patients younger than 18 years. However, many states allow for exceptions to parental consent. These exceptions may be defined by the status of the minor or the category of care that is needed. Teens living separately from their parents and managing their own financial affairs and those who are married and/or have borne a child are often considered emancipated minors and are given the legal status to consent for their own care.[15] Some states also define *mature minors* as teens 15 years of age or older and allow them to assent to care and treatment for minor, low-risk illnesses such as evaluation of strep throat or a rash. Most states also allow for minors to consent for certain services related to pregnancy, sexually transmitted infections, contraceptive services, alcohol and drug treatment, emergency care (including evaluation for sexual assault), and mental health evaluation.[15] These minor consent laws allow adolescents to access important medical services in circumstances in which they might otherwise forego care if a parent had to be involved.[16,17]

When providing health care to teens, confidentiality must be assured to gain their trust and allow space for them to be honest and feel safe disclosing personal information, especially information related to the sensitive topics noted within minor consent laws. Confidentiality laws ensure that care allowed by minor consent laws may only be accessed or released by the teen patient, giving control of certain aspects of the medical record to the adolescent. Studies have shown that for certain conditions, such as mental health problems or pregnancy, many minors will delay or not seek care if they think their parents may find out.[16,17] Of course, if the teen is potentially at risk for harm to oneself or another, these laws do allow for parental notification to assure safety. Unfortunately, although states allow for protected rights to confidentiality of certain services, this is not always demonstrated in the real world. Providers should be aware of potential breaches of confidentiality, especially along administrative channels, including insurance notification of services (explanation of benefits), billing statements, and routine request of release of records to other health care providers or academic institutions.[12] This area has been especially tricky with the new electronic health records, wherein advancements in technology have not always allowed for protected information to remain separate within the medical record. Ultimately, clinics and health organizations should develop policies and procedures to protect against these breaches in confidentiality, which are considered violations of the Health Insurance Portability and Accountability Act (HIPAA).[18,19] As advocates for youth, providers can encourage teens to request alternate forms of communication (eg, personal cell phone numbers), promote efforts to allow teens to restrict access to their medical chart, and inform teens about their right to file complaints with health care organizations if they feel their rights are violated.[18]

STRENGTHS AND RESILIENCY

Recognizing a patient's strengths can identify areas of resilience in teens. Several experts recommend that providers identify an adolescent's strengths first to balance the rest of the behavioral screening.[20,21] Studies confirm that the following can be protective factors for adolescents regardless of race, class, or gender:

- An authoritative parenting style with consistent limit-setting
- A sense of connectedness with one caring adult
- Involvement with parents
- A positive body image
- Participation in extracurricular supervised activities
- Nonusing peer group
- Strong school affiliation[22–24]

Successful transition to adulthood is often bolstered by the connections that youth have with prosocial peers, schools, adult mentors, and the wider community. Much research in the past 3 decades has supported this idea that connectedness with others and within communities has been protective against several risky behaviors and supportive of healthy youth development. Identifying an adolescent's strengths and interests and supporting prosocial connections may help families support their teen's successful growth and development.[22–24]

ASSESSING RISK FACTORS

The leading causes of morbidity and mortality in adolescents continue to be the result of risky behaviors and poor decisions; these will be the health issues that physicians encounter in adolescent patients.[25] Risk-taking behaviors (eg, alcohol, drugs, unsafe driving) and unhealthy decisions (eg, diet, inactivity) can have a dramatic and lasting impact on these teens and their future health. For this reason, adolescence is a prime time for clinicians to promote healthy behaviors with adolescent patients and to provide guidance for their families to intervene before the behaviors result in life long negative outcomes. Realizing that behaviors affect the health of teens and that those behaviors may change over the course of several months, many professional organizations have established guidelines for adolescent preventive care (Table 1). These guidelines include appropriate screening tools for asking adolescents about risk and protective factors in their lives.

PSYCHOSOCIAL SCREENING TOOLS

Although discussing sensitive issues may be challenging for primary care providers, studies consistently confirm that adolescents and their parents want these sensitive issues to be addressed during both acute and preventive care visits.[26,27] Several psychosocial screening tools have been developed to identify adolescent risks and strengths and to provide a nonthreatening mechanism to discuss sensitive issues with adolescents. The HEADSSS assessment is the most frequently used and effective screening tool to identify adolescent psychosocial risks, and has recently been updated to incorporate screening for eating behaviors and diet (HEEADSSS: *Home, Education/Employment, Eating, Activities, Drugs, Sexuality, Suicide/Depression, and Safety*) (**Table 2**).[28–30] During health maintenance visits, asking open-ended questions pertinent to each area can be helpful for identifying red flags in the history that can be further assessed with appropriate assessment tools and referred for additional care if necessary. Alternatively, the SSHADESS screen (*Strengths, School, Home, Activities, Drugs/substance use, Emotions/depression, Sexuality, and Safety*) was more recently developed to include inquiry about adolescent strengths and indentify features of resiliency.[30] Regardless of the screening tool used, the following questions are essential to ask at every adolescent visit[31]:

- Have there been any significant changes/losses in your home/family/community?
- Do you have someone who you can turn to if you are having a problem, worry, or bad day?

These brief questions help identify the ways that a teen is connected to others, or not. Assessing for family conflict or stress and addressing family dysfunction play an important role in preventing high-risk behaviors in adolescence. Youth who have recently lost support or who cannot identify connections to others in their family or community may require further guidance and support from the clinical environment.

HEALTH MAINTENANCE AND SCREENING

Health screening is the cornerstone of primary care. The wellness visit or preventive health checkup has become less about the actual physical examination and more about the conversation and guidance regarding healthy behaviors and screening for preventable or treatable illness. Although opinions differ regarding the frequency of adolescent wellness visits, The American Academy of Pediatrics' *Bright Futures* guidelines and the American Medical Association's Guidelines for Adolescent Preventive Services recommend annual preventive care services for patients aged 11 to 21 years, whereas the U.S. Preventive Services Task Force (USPSTF) and American Academy of Family Physicians recommend an individualized schedule (see **Table 1**).[32–35] But what happens if the patients do not have these visits? Studies indicate that a minority, 38% or less, of adolescent patients have annual preventive care visits.[36] and 70% have preventive visits an average of every 4 years.[37] In these studies, the rates for preventive services were lower for patients from lower socioeconomic status and those who were uninsured. Additionally, providing anticipatory guidance was low during these visits, as low as 31% in some groups. Because adolescents visit primary care offices more often for nonpreventive care, these studies recommended that every contact with adolescent patients should be an opportunity to address preventive care and anticipatory guidance (or patient education). Clearly, screening must occur outside the traditional "well-teen visit" or it may not get done at all.

Because of a lack of evidence-based research regarding preventive services, evidence-based guidelines that are universally accepted are difficult to develop. However, data are increasing from the field of public health that addresses social determinants of health in conjunction with Adolescent Health, focusing on a more holistic view

Table 1
Comparing guidelines for adolescent preventive care

	GAPS[33]	Bright Futures/AAP[32]	USPSTF[34]	AAFP[35]
Frequency of Visit	Annually	Annually	One every 1–3 y as necessary	One every 1–3 y as necessary
Target Age Range	11–21 y	11–21 y	11–24 y	13–21 y
Vaccination	Follow ACIP schedule			
Parental Involvement	At least once during early and middle adolescence	Three times during adolescence	No recommendation	Three times during adolescence
Health Guidance for Teens				
Normal Development	Screen at each visit		No recommendation	Screen at each visit
Injury Prevention	Screen/discuss at each visit		Insufficient evidence	
Nutrition	Screen/discuss at each visit		Consider selective counseling for at-risk youth	
Dental Health	No recommendation	Screen at each visit/no recommendation	No recommendation	
Skin Protection	Discuss at each visit	Discuss at each visit	Counsel individuals with fair skin to minimize exposure to ultraviolet radiation	
Testicular Self-Examination	No recommendation	Teach to patients after age 20 y	Recommends against testicular cancer self-screening	Recommends against testicular cancer self-screening
Screening and Counseling				
Obesity	Screen at each visit, discuss nutrition and exercise recommendations	Screen at each visit, discuss nutrition and exercise	Screen at each visit, discuss nutrition and exercise and offer referral to comprehensive behavioral interventions to improve weight	
Contraception		Assess risk and discuss at each visit		
Tobacco Use	Ask/counsel at each visit		Unclear benefit to screening; insufficient evidence	Ask/counsel at each visit
Alcohol Use				Recommend avoiding alcohol
Substance Abuse				No recommendation
Hypertension	Screen at each visit			Insufficient evidence to screen ages <18 y

Depression/Suicide	Assess annually		Screen annually when systems are in place to ensure diagnosis and therapy; No recommendation
Eating Disorders			
School Problems			
Abuse	No recommendation		Screen for family violence; No recommendation
Hearing	No recommendation	At age 12 y and as indicated/ vision testing at ages 12, 15, and 18 y and as indicated	No recommendation
Vision	No recommendation	Hearing testing as indicated	No recommendation
Testing Recommendations			
Tuberculosis	Screen if exposed or lives/works in high-risk area	Screen if at risk	Screen at clinician's discretion Screen if at high risk
		Every 3 y at 21 y of age; recommends against screening if age <21 y	Every 3 y at 21 y of age; recommends against screening if age <21 y
HIV	Offer test to high-risk patients	Screen if at-risk because of behaviors	Age <15 y, screen those with risk factors; Age $\geq$15 y, screen all individuals
Sexually Transmitted Infections	Screen any teen annually if sexually active	Screen all sexually active	Screen all sexually active females annually; Insufficient evidence for boys
Cholesterol	Screen once if family has early cardiovascular disease or hyperlipidemia	Assess risk and screen (test fasting lipid profile at age 20 y)	Insufficient evidence No recommendation
Urinalysis	No recommendation	Perform at least once during adolescence	Do not test asymptomatic patients
Hematocrit		Annually for all menstruating patients	No recommendation
Health Guidance for Teens			
Normal Development	Screen at each visit	Screen at each visit	No recommendation Screen at each visit
Injury Prevention	Screen/discuss at each visit		Insufficient evidence
Nutrition	Screen/discuss at each visit		Consider selective counseling for at-risk youth
Dental Health	No recommendation	Screen at each visit	No recommendation

Abbreviations: AAFP, American Academy of Family Physicians; AAP, American Academy of Pediatrics; GAPS, Guidelines for Adolescent Preventive Services; USPSTF, U.S. Preventive Services Task Force.
Data from Refs.[32–35]

Table 2
The psychosocial history using HEEADSS screening questions

H	**Home** Who do you live with? Where do you live? What are relationships like at home? Who can you talk to at home when you are having trouble?
E	**Education/employment** How are you doing in school (or at work)? Any recent changes? How are your relationships with teachers and classmates (or coworkers if employed)? What do you like and dislike about school/work? What are your future education/employment plans/goals?
E	**Eating** Does your weight or body shape cause you any stress? If so, tell me about it. Have there been any recent changes in your weight? Have you dieted in the last year? How? How often?
A	**Activities** What do you do with your friends for fun? What activities (sports, clubs, groups) do you participate in? What are your favorite hobbies, books, music, etc?
D	**Drugs** Have you or your friends ever tried cigarettes, alcohol, or other drugs? What have you tried? How often have you used them, and how much at one time? Do you ever drive or ride in a car when you have been using alcohol or drugs? Does anyone at home use tobacco, alcohol, or other drugs?
S	**Sexuality** Have you ever had a sexual relationship with anyone? With boys, girls, or both? How many partners have you had? Have you ever been pregnant or had a sexually transmitted infection? Have you used anything to prevent pregnancy or sexually transmitted infections? Have you ever been forced to have sex against your will
S	**Suicide/depression** What do you do when you are feeling sad/angry/hurt? Have you ever felt so sad/angry/hurt that you have wanted to hurt or kill yourself? Have you had any trouble with sleeping, or sleeping too much? Have you had any changes in appetite or concerns about eating?
S	**Safety** Do you feel safe at home and at school? In your neighborhood? Are there guns or other weapons in your home? How often do you wear a seatbelt when in a car? Do you wear a helmet when bike riding, skateboarding, and snowboarding or skiing?

Adapted from Reif CJ, Elster AB. Adolescent preventive services. Prim Care 1998;25(1):1–21 and Klein DA, Goldenring JM, Adelman WP. HEEADDSSS 3.0; the psychosocial interview for adolescents updated for a new century fueled by media. Contemp Pediatr 2014;31(1):16–28.

of the lifecourse.[38,39] All expert groups recommend that behavior screening in youth should focus on identifying both positive and risky behaviors so that providers can reinforce the positive while discouraging the negative. Risk factors for chronic diseases, such as those cause by alcohol and tobacco use, sedentary behaviors, and poor diet, begin in adolescence; thus, providing anticipatory guidance about these behaviors and encouraging ongoing dialogue between parents and their teens can change these behaviors. Ideally, several priorities to evaluate and address during teen visits can contribute to improved health (**Table 3**). Although this may be too

Table 3 Ideal teen visit prevention priorities	
Physical Growth & Development	Body image Oral health Physical activity
Social & Academic Competence	Connectedness School performance Interpersonal skills
Emotional Well-being	Coping Mood regulation Sexuality
Risk Reduction	Substance use Pregnancy prevention Sexually transmitted infection prevention
Violence & Injury Prevention	Seat belts Helmet use Access to guns Bullying

much for one visit, primary care providers should assess these issues longitudinally, across several visits.

Several national organizations provide recommendations about clinical preventive services for teens and young adults. Overall, the recommendations from these groups are more similar than different. The USPSTF recommendations for screening and counseling in adolescents (**Tables 4** and **5**)[34] are evidence-based and regularly updated as new data are reported; therefore, they remain the most current, evidence-based guidelines available. Current USPSTF recommendations for adolescent screening and counseling include[34]

- Cervical screening every 3 years beginning at 21 years of age. The USPSTF recommends against screening adolescents younger than 21 years.
- There is insufficient evidence to screen for primary hypertension in asymptomatic children and adolescents ages less than 18 years. Evidence does support blood pressure screening at every visit for individuals 18 years of age and older.
- Screening of adolescents 12 to 18 years of age for major depression if adequate treatment and follow-up can be provided.
- Screening for chlamydia and gonorrhea in sexually active girls younger than 25 years, and HIV screening for adolescents older than 15 years. Individuals younger than 15 years should be screened if they are at increased risk.

IMMUNIZATIONS

The most recent recommendations for children and adolescents from the Centers for Disease Control and Prevention and the Advisory Committee on Immunization Practices (ACIP) include changes for adolescents.[40,41] The ACIP recommends that preteens receive 1 dose of tetanus, diphtheria, and acellular pertussis (Tdap) vaccine at ages 11 to 12 years. At the same age, the ACIP also recommends 1 dose of meningococcal conjugate (MenACWY-CRM) vaccine with a booster at age 16 years. Human papillomavirus (HPV) vaccination is also recommended for both boys and girls before the onset of sexual activity. Data indicate a decrease in warts and abnormal Papanicolau smear results for patients receiving HPV vaccine; unfortunately, the rates for

Table 4
U.S. Preventative Services Task Force recommendations for screening/counseling in teens

Screening Test	Recommendations	Rating*
Cervical Cancer	Screening is not recommended for women age <21 y	D
Skin Cancer	Recommends counseling children, adolescents and young adults aged 10–24 y with fair skin about minimizing exposure to ultraviolet radiation	B
Testicular Cancer	Screening is not recommended	D
Blood Pressure	Age <18 y: insufficient evidence to screen asymptomatic teens Age ≥18 y: routine screening (per adult recommendations)	I
Lipids	Insufficient evidence	I
Obesity	Screen with body mass index annually and offer behaviorally based interventions	B
Scoliosis	Routine screening is not recommended	D
Depression	Screen teens age 12–18 y for major depression if adequate treatment and follow-up can be provided	B
Suicide Risk	Insufficient evidence	I
Chlamydia	Women: screen if sexually active (age <25 y) Men: insufficient evidence to screen	A
Gonorrhea	Women: screen if sexually active (age <25 y) Men: insufficient evidence to screen	B I
Herpes Simplex Virus	Routine serologic screening is not recommended	D
HIV	Age <15 y: screen if risk factors are present Age ≥15 y: screening recommended for all	A
Counseling on Injury Prevention	Insufficient evidence	I
Screening and Counseling on Substance Abuse	Age >18 y: screen for alcohol misuse Insufficient evidence for screening or counseling youth age <18 y for substance abuse	B I
Tobacco Use	Provide education and counseling to prevent initiation of tobacco use in adolescents	B
Counseling on Sexually Transmitted Infections	For sexually active adolescents; insufficient evidence for adolescents who are not sexually active	B

* see **Table 5**.
Data from U.S. Preventative Services Task Force. Available at: http://www.uspreventive servicestaskforce.org/. Accessed April 7, 2014.

completing the series of 3 vaccines are low.[42] The ACIP recommends 3 doses of quadrivalent HPV vaccine for girls aged 11 to 12 years (may start at age 9 years) and continuing for unvaccinated young women until age 26 years. The ACIP also recommends that boys receive 3 doses of HPV vaccine starting at aged 11 to 12 years, and continuing for young men aged 13 to 21 years who have not been vaccinated.[43] All of the age appropriate vaccines can be given in a single visit. The ACIP also recommends that preteens and older adolescents receive an annual influenza vaccine and any other overdue vaccines. Providers should use every health care visit as an opportunity to review adolescents' immunization histories, add any "catch up" vaccines, and ensure that every adolescent is fully vaccinated.[41]

Table 5
U.S. Preventative Services Task Force grading scale

Grade	Definition	Suggestions for Practice
A	The USPSTF recommends the service High certainty exists that the net benefit is substantial	Offer or provide this service
B	The USPSTF recommends the service High certainty exists that the net benefit is moderate, or moderate certainty exists that the net benefit is moderate to substantial	Offer or provide this service
C	The USPSTF recommends selectively offering or providing this service to individual patients based on professional judgment and patient preferences At least moderate certainty exists that the net benefit is small	Offer or provide this service for selected patients depending on individual circumstances
D	The USPSTF recommends against the service Moderate or high certainty exists that the service has no net benefit or that the harms outweigh the benefits	Discourage the use of this service
I Statement	The USPSTF concludes that the current evidence is insufficient to assess the balance of benefits and harms of the service Evidence is lacking, of poor quality, or conflicting, and the balance of benefits and harms cannot be determined	Read the clinical considerations section of USPSTF Recommendation Statement If the service is offered, patients should understand the uncertainty about the balance of benefits and harms

Abbreviation: USPSTF, U.S. Preventative Services Task Force.
Data from U.S. Preventative Services Task Force. Available at: http://www.uspreventive servicestaskforce.org/. Accessed April 7, 2014.

SUMMARY

Primary care clinicians treating adolescent patients are well positioned to have significant influence in minimizing poor future health outcomes for this population. Through using recommended psychosocial screening tools at all visits with teens, providers can identify adolescents' strengths and discover possible risky behaviors while providing support and guidance for healthy development.

Providing the best care for teens requires maintaining knowledge of state and local confidentiality laws, remaining up to date with the most current USPSTF guidelines for screening and prevention, and keeping updated on recommendations for immunization. Every clinical contact with an adolescent patient is an opportunity to address and update on health promotion and disease prevention strategies.

Creating teen-friendly services that appropriately include parents, while respecting the confidentiality and autonomy of the adolescent patient, can help promote a healthy transition to adulthood. Identifying strategies to work with parents or other caregivers to maximize adolescent potential is paramount to future research on adolescent health outcomes.

REFERENCES

1. Tylee A, Haller DM, Graham T, et al. Youth-friendly primary-care services: how are we doing and what more needs to be done? Lancet 2007;369:1565–73.
2. World Health Organization. Adolescent friendly health services: an agenda for change. Geneva (Switzerland): World Health Organization; 2002. Available at: http://www.who.int/maternal_child_adolescent/documents/fch_cah_02_14/en/. Accessed June 15, 2014.
3. National Research Council and Institute of Medicine. Adolescent health services: missing opportunities. In: Committee on Adolescent Health Care Services and Models of Care for Treatment, Prevention, and Healthy Development, Lawrence RS, Gootman JA, et al, editors. Board on children, youth, and families. Division of behavioral and social sciences and education. Washington, DC: The National Academies Press; 2009.
4. Ford CA, Davenport AF, Meier A, et al. Partnerships between parents and healthcare professionals to improve adolescent health. J Adolesc Health 2011;49(1):53–7.
5. Shore WB. The family physician's role in keeping parents involved in their adolescents' lives. Am Fam Physician 1994;49:327–8.
6. Ford CA, English A, Sigman G. Confidential health care for adolescents: position paper of the Society for Adolescent Medicine. J Adolesc Health 2004;35(2):160–7.
7. Rubin SE, McKee MD, Campos G, et al. Delivery of confidential care to adolescent males. J Am Board Fam Med 2010;23(6):728–35.
8. McKee MD, Rubin SE, Campos G, et al. Challenges in providing confidential care to adolescents in urban primary care: clinician perspectives. Ann Fam Med 2011;9:37–43.
9. Ginsburg KR, Forke CM, Cnaan A, et al. Important health provider characteristics: the perspective of urban ninth graders. J Dev Behav Pediatr 2002;23:237–43.
10. Ginsburg KR, Menapace AS, Slap GB. Factors affecting the decision to seek health care: the voice of adolescents. Pediatrics 1997;100(6):922–30.
11. Adolescent Health Working Group. AHWG's Provider toolkit series. Available at: www.ahwg.net. Accessed January 31, 2014.
12. Gold RB. Unintended consequences: how insurance processes inadvertently abrogate patient confidentiality. Guttmacher Policy Review 2009;12(4):12–6.
13. Center for Adolescent Health & the Law: Consent and Confidentiality Protection. Available at: http://www.cahl.org/publications/consent-confidentiality-protection. Accessed June 23, 2014.
14. Guttmacher Institute, State Policies in Brief. An Overview of Minor's Consent Laws. June 1, 2014. Available at: http://www.guttmacher.org/statecenter/spibs/spib_OMCL.pdf. Accessed June 10, 2014.
15. English A, Bass L, Boyle AD, et al. State minor consent laws: a summary. 3rd edition. Chapel Hill (NC): Center for Adolescent Health and the Law; 2010.
16. Ford CA, English A. Limiting confidentiality of adolescent health services: what are the risks? JAMA 2002;288:752–3.
17. Morreale MC, Kappahahn CJ, Elster AB, et al. Position paper on access to health care for adolescents and young adults. J Adolesc Health 2004;35:342–4.
18. English A, Ford CA. The HIPAA privacy rule and adolescents: legal questions and clinical challenges. Perspect Sex Reprod Health 2004;36:80–6.
19. Office for Civil Rights, HHS. Standards for privacy of individually identifiable health information. Final rule. Fed Regist 2002;67(157):53181–273.

20. Resnick MD, Bearman PS, Blum RW, et al. Protecting adolescents from harm. Findings from the National Longitudinal Study on Adolescent Health. JAMA 1997;278:823–32.
21. Ginsburg KR. Viewing our adolescent patients through a positive lens. Contemp Pediatr 2007;24(1):65–76.
22. Blum RW, Beuhring T, Shew ML, et al. The effects of race/ethnicity, income and family structure on adolescent risk behaviors. Am J Public Health 2000;90(12): 1879–84.
23. Blum RW, Rinehart PM. Reducing the risk: connections that make a difference in the lives of youth (No. 40). Minneapolis (MN): University of Minnesota, Division of Pediatrics and Adolescent Health; 1997.
24. Resnick MD, Harris LJ, Blum RW. The impact of caring and connectedness on adolescent health and well-being. J Paediatr Child Health 1993;29:S3–9.
25. Centers for Disease Control and Prevention. CDC releases 2013 youth risk behavior survey (YRBS) results. Available at: www.cdc.gov/Features/YRBS. Accessed March 8, 2014.
26. Brown JD, Wissow LS. Discussions of sensitive topics with youth during primary care visits: relation to youth perspectives of care. J Adolesc Health 2009;44(1):48–54.
27. Ford CA, Davenport AF, Meier A, et al. Parents and health care professionals working together to improve adolescent health: the perspectives of parents. J Adolesc Health 2009;44(2):191–4.
28. Goldenring JM, Cohen E. Getting into adolescent heads. Contemp Pediatr 1988; 5(7):75–90.
29. Goldenring JM, Rosen DS. Getting into adolescent heads: an essential update. Contemp Pediatr 2004;21(1):64–79.
30. Klein DA, Goldenring JM, Adelman WP. HEEADSSS 3.0: the psychosocial interview for adolescents updated for a new century fueled by media. Contemp Pediatr 2014;31(1):16–28.
31. Shalwitz J, Sang T, Combs N, et al. Behavioral health: an adolescent provider toolkit. San Francisco (CA): Adolescent Health Working Group; 2007. p. D-9-10. Available at: http://www.ahwg.net/resources-for-providers.html.
32. Hagen JF, Shaw JS, Duncan PM. Bright futures: guidelines for health supervision of infants, children, and adolescents. 3rd edition. Elk Grove Village (IL): American Academy of Pediatrics; 2008.
33. Elster AB, Kuznets NJ. Guidelines for Adolescent Preventive Services (GAPS): recommendations monograph. Baltimore (MD): Lippincott Williams and Wilkins; 1997.
34. U.S. Preventive Services Task Force. Child and adolescent recommendations. Available at: http://www.uspreventiveservicestaskforce.org/tfchildcat.htm. Accessed February 14, 2014.
35. Summary of recommendations for clinical preventive services. Leawood (KS): American Academy of Family Physicians; 2014. Available at: http://www.aafp.org/dam/AAFP/documents/patient_care/clinical_recommendations/cpsrecommendations.pdf.
36. Irwin CE, Adams SH, Park MJ, et al. Preventive care for adolescents: few get visits and fewer get services. Pediatrics 2009;123(4):e565–72. http://dx.doi.org/10.1542/peds.2008-2601.
37. Nordin JF, Solberg LI, Parker ED. Adolescent primary care visit patterns. Ann Fam Med 2010;8:511–6.
38. Resnick MD, Catalano RF, Sawyer SM, et al. Seizing the opportunities of adolescent health. Lancet 2012;379(9826):1564–7.

39. Viner RM, Ozer EM, Denny S, et al. Adolescence and the social determinants of health. Lancet 2012;379:1641–52.
40. Advisory Committee on Immunization Practices Recommended Immunization Schedules for Persons Aged 0 Through 18 Years — United States, 2014. MMWR February 7, 2014. Available at: www.cdc.gov/vaccines/schedules/hcp/child-adolescent.html#mmwr.
41. Loehr J. ACIP Releases 2014 Child and Adolescent Immunizations Schedules. Am Fam Physician 2014;89(4):302.
42. Centers for Disease Control and Prevention (CDC). FDA licensure of bivalent human papillomavirus vaccine (HPV2, Cervarix) for use in females and updated HPV vaccination recommendations from the Advisory Committee on Immunization Practices (ACIP). MMWR Morb Mortal Wkly Rep 2010;59(20):626–9.
43. Centers for Disease Control and Prevention (CDC). Recommendations on the use of quadrivalent human papillomavirus vaccine in males—Advisory Committee on Immunization Practices (ACIP), 2011. MMWR Morb Mortal Wkly Rep 2011;60(50):1705–8.

Adolescent Growth and Development

Veenod L. Chulani, MD, MSEd, FSAHM[a,b,*], Lonna P. Gordon, MD, PharmD[c]

KEYWORDS

- Adolescence • Puberty • Precocious puberty • Delayed puberty
- Psychosocial development

KEY POINTS

- Adolescence is a developmental stage defined by physical and psychosocial maturation.
- Pubertal growth and development is mediated by dynamic, physiologic changes in the neuroendocrine system.
- Although variability in the timing of attainment of pubertal milestones is common and most adolescents who display patterns of development outside of defined norms have no underlying pathology, abnormal patterns of development may be owing to underlying pathology and requires evaluation.
- The dynamic psychosocial changes of adolescence incrementally prepare youth to assume adult status and fulfill adult societal roles and expectations.

INTRODUCTION

Adolescence is a developmental stage defined by physical and psychosocial maturation. This stage encompasses puberty, a complex series of events mediated by genetic, hormonal, and environmental factors culminating in somatic maturity and the achievement of reproductive capacity. It is also accompanied by expanding cognitive abilities, the development of identity, and dynamic social transitions through which youth achieve adult status. Providers caring for adolescents require a sound knowledge of the physical and psychosocial changes of adolescence. This article reviews the neuroendocrine basis of puberty, normal pubertal development, and the evaluation and management of adolescents with suspected pubertal abnormalities. An overview of adolescent psychosocial development and the developmental tasks of adolescence is included.

Funding Sources: None.
Conflict of Interest: None.
[a] Division of Adolescent Medicine, Arnold Palmer Hospital for Children, 86 West Underwood Street, Suite 202, Orlando, FL 32806, USA; [b] Florida State University College of Medicine, 1115 West Call Street, Tallahassee, FL 32304, USA; [c] Icahn School of Medicine, Mount Sinai Adolescent Health Center, 320 East 94th Street, New York, NY 10128, USA
* Corresponding author. 86 West Underwood Street, Suite 202, Orlando, FL 32806.
E-mail address: veenod.chulani@orlandohealth.com

Prim Care Clin Office Pract 41 (2014) 465–487
http://dx.doi.org/10.1016/j.pop.2014.05.002
0095-4543/14/$ – see front matter © 2014 Elsevier Inc. All rights reserved.

primarycare.theclinics.com

PHYSICAL GROWTH AND DEVELOPMENT
Neuroendocrine Basis of Puberty

The neuroendocrine basis of puberty has been the subject of extensive investigation and the identification of the exact trigger of puberty onset has drawn considerable attention. Mediated by a complex interplay of inhibiting and activating factors, pubertal growth and development can be viewed as the result of physiologic changes in the hypothalamic-pituitary-gonadal (HPG), adrenal, and growth hormone axes.[1–4] The various axes are depicted in **Fig. 1.**

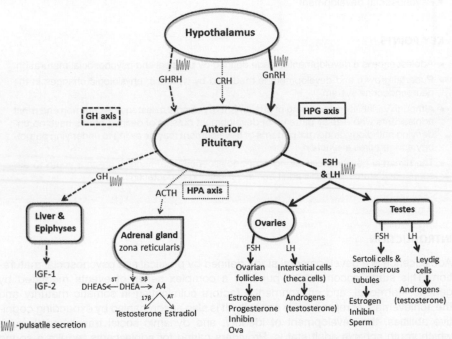

Fig. 1. Simplified diagram of the hypothalamic-pituitary-gonadal (HPG) axes, hypothalamic-pituitary-adrenal (HPA) axes, and growth hormone (GH) axes. The hypothalamus releases gonadotropin-releasing hormone (GnRH), corticotropin-releasing hormone (CRH), and growth hormone–releasing hormone (GHRH), which stimulate the anterior pituitary gland to release follicle-stimulating hormone (FSH) and luteinizing hormone (LH), adrenocorticotropic hormone (ACTH), and growth hormone (GH), respectively. GnRH, LH, GHRH, and GH are released in a pulsatile fashion that varies with pubertal stage. In the HPG axis, FSH stimulates the ovarian follicles to produce estrogen (from androgenic precursors produced from theca cells), inhibin, progesterone, and ova. Estrogen provides both a positive and negative feedback on GnRH. In females, a critical amount of estrogen is needed to produce a positive feedback to stimulate the LH surge that leads to ovulation. In males, FSH stimulates Sertoli cells and seminiferous tubules to produce estrogen, inhibin, and sperm. LH stimulates theca cells in females and Leydig cells in males to produce androgens. On the HPA axis, ACTH stimulates the zona reticularis of the adrenal gland to secrete dihydroepiandrosterone (DHEA). DHEA is then converted to dihydroepiandrosterone sulfate (DHEAS) via sulfotransferase (ST), and to androstenedione (A4) via 3 β-hydroxysteroid dehydrogenase (3β). A4 is then converted to testosterone via 17β-hydroxysteroid dehydrogenase (17β) and estradiol via aromatase (AT). In the GH axis, GH stimulates the liver and epiphyses of bone to produce insulin-like growth factor 1 (IGF-1) and insulin-like growth factor 2 (IGF-2).

Hypothalamic Pituitary-Gonadal Axis

The HPG axis is functional by 10 weeks' gestation and remains active until early infancy when it enters into a relatively quiescent phase.[5] The onset of puberty is marked the by the reemergence of pulsatile gonadotropin-releasing hormone (GnRH) secretion. Although the exact signals for the pulsatile release of GnRH remain undetermined, the role of hormones associated with nutritional status such as leptin, kisspeptin, and insulin-like growth factor-1 has been suggested.[6–9] GnRH stimulates the secretion of luteinizing hormone (LH) and follicle-stimulating hormone (FSH) by gonadotrophs in the anterior pituitary that promote gonadal maturation and the production of sex steroids or gonadarche. In females, mature HPG axis activity is also characterized by the development of positive feedback loop where a critical level of estrogen triggers a large release in GnRH and the subsequent LH surge resulting in ovulation.[10]

Adrenal Gland Changes

The adrenal cortex is divided into 3 zones, with the zona reticularis predominantly responsible for the secretion of the adrenal androgens, dehydroepiandrosterone (DHEA), DHEA sulfate, and androstenedione. The zona reticularis involutes shortly after birth and secretes only small amounts of DHEA and androstenedione.[11–13] Activation of the zona reticularis with increased secretion of adrenal androgens or adrenarche occurs between 6 and 8 years of age.[12,14] Adrenarche is independent from and precedes activation of the HPG axis by approximately 2 years.[11]

Growth Hormone Axes

During puberty, elevated sex steroid concentrations stimulate the activation of the GH axis characterized by an increase in the amplitude in the pulsatile release of GH. Circulating insulin-like growth factor-1 mediates the anabolic somatic effects of GH and increases correspondingly during puberty, with levels correlating with SMR stages and sex steroid levels.[12,14]

PHYSICAL CHANGES OF PUBERTY
Development of Secondary Sexual Characteristics

The development of secondary sexual characteristics is a hallmark of puberty. Sexual maturity ratings (SMR) scales developed by Marshall and Tanner provide for the staging of genital development in males and breast and pubic hair development in females (**Figs. 2** and **3**).[15–17] These scales allow monitoring of the development of secondary sexual characteristics. They also provide better correlation for the timing of pubertal events than does chronologic age owing to variability in the timing and tempo of pubertal development. Although variability in the timing and tempo is commonly observed, the sequence of pubertal events in males and females is highly predictable and is illustrated in **Figs. 4** and **5**.

The estimated age range of normal variation of pubertal development in US adolescent females is controversial in light of evidence of racial and ethnic differences and decreasing age onset of pubertal changes overall.[18–20] The normal age range of puberty is 7 to 13 years for white girls and 6 to 13 years in African-American girls.[5,21] Current estimates on the timing of attainment of various SMR stages in females is presented in **Table 1**. Female puberty generally begins with thelarche (B2), which commonly precedes pubarche (PH2) by about 1 to 1.5 years, although the latter may occur first or simultaneously.[22] Despite the earlier onset of breast and pubic hair development, the mean age at menarche of 12.9 (±1.20) years in white girls and 12.1 (±1.21) years in African-American girls[20,23] is not significantly younger than previously reported. Menarche most commonly occur during PH4 and usually occurs 2 to 2.5 years after thelarche.[17,24]

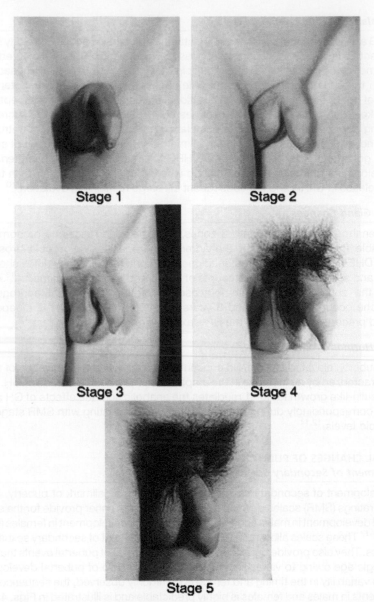

Fig. 2. Sexual maturity rating (SMR) stages in males. Stage 1 is prepubertal, with no pubic hair and childlike phallus and a testicular volume of ≤1.6 mL. Stage 2 shows sparse, straight pubic hair along the base of the penis with testicular enlargement and reddening and thinning of the scrotum, and a testicular volume of 1.6 to 6 mL. In stage 3, the hair is darker, coarser, and curlier, extending over the mid-pubis. Further testicular and scrotal enlargement and increase in phallic length. Testicular volume is 6 to 12 mL. In stage 4, hair is adult-like in appearance but does not extend to inner thighs. Further testicular and scrotal enlargement and increased phallic length and circumference; testicular volume is 12 to 20 mL. In stage 5, hair is adult in appearance, extending to the inner thigh. There is an adult scrotum and phallus. Testicular volume is ≥20 mL. (*From* Roede MJ, van Wieringen JC. Growth diagrams 1980: Netherlands third nation-wide survey. Tijdschr Soc Gezondheids 1985;63:1–34.)

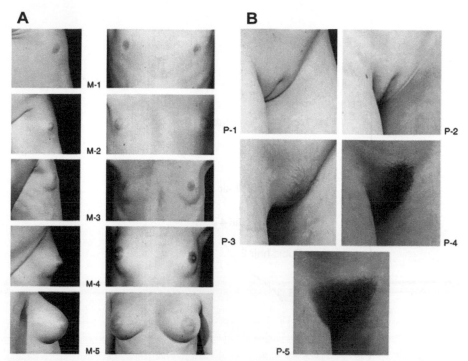

Fig. 3. (*A*) Sexual maturity rating (SMR) of breast development in girls. Stage 1 is prepubertal, with no palpable breast tissue. In stage 2, a breast bud develops, with elevation of the papilla and enlargement of the areolar diameter. In stage 3, the breast enlarges, without separation of areolar contour from the breast. In stage 4, the areola and papilla project above the breast, forming a secondary mound. In stage 5, the areola recesses to match the contour of the breast; the papilla projects beyond the contour of the areola and breast. (*B*) Sexual maturity rating (SMR) stages of pubic hair development in girls. Stage 1 is prepubertal, with no pubic hair. In stage 2, there is sparse, lightly pigmented straight hair along the medial border of the labia. In stage 3, there is a moderate amount of darker, coarser, and curlier and extends over the mid-pubis. Stage 4 hair resembles adult hair in coarseness and curliness, but does not extend to the inner thighs. Stage 5 hair is adult in appearance and extends to the inner thighs. (*From* Roede MJ, van Wieringen JC. Growth diagrams 1980: Netherlands third nation-wide survey. Tijdschr Soc Gezondheids 1985;63:1–34.)

The mean age of onset of male pubertal development is 11 years, with a normal range of variation of 9 to 14 years.[25] Estimates on the timing of attainment of various SMR stages in males are presented in **Table 2**. Male pubertal development typically begins with testicular enlargement (G2). Pubertal testicular enlargement is characterized by a longitudinal testicular measurement of >2.5 cm or testicular volume of >4 mL.[16,26,27] Pubarche (PH2) generally follows closely and correlates with penile growth under the common influence of androgens. Additional pubertal events include spermarche between G3 and G4 and the appearance of facial hair and voice change in SMR stage G4.[28]

Height Growth

Height growth averages approximately 5 to 6 cm per year throughout childhood,[6,29] with a slight deceleration in height growth immediately preceding puberty. During puberty, height velocity increases sharply and peaks during the adolescent growth spurt to ultimately account for about 20% of final adult height. In females, height velocity

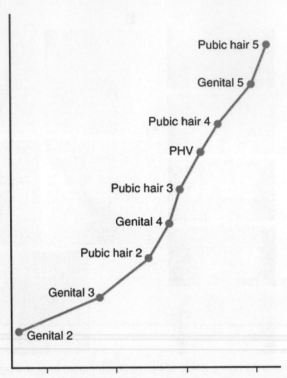

Fig. 4. Sequence of pubertal events in males. PHV, peak height velocity. (*From* Root AW. Endocrinology of puberty. J Pediatr 1973;83(1):1–19.)

accelerates at a mean age of 9 years and peak height velocity of approximately 8.3 cm per year is attained at a mean age of 11.5 years between SMR stages 2 and 3.[30] Height growth rates generally decelerate significantly and there is limited growth potential after menarche. In males, height growth accelerates at a mean age of 11 years and reaches a peak height velocity of approximately 9.5 cm per year at the mean age of 13.5 years during SMR stages 3 to 4.[30] Height growth rate decreases thereafter and is generally complete by SMR 5. The 12- to 13-cm male height advantage over females is best explained by the 2 additional years of prepubertal growth and greater peak height velocity rate.[29]

Prediction of adult height is useful in the monitoring of pubertal development. A commonly used method is based on the calculation of mid-parental height. Most individuals have an adult height that is within 10 cm or 4 inches (2 SD) of the mid-parental height as calculated below[31]:

$$\text{For girls} = \frac{(\text{fathers height} - 13\ \text{cm or 5 inches}) + \text{mothers height}}{2}$$

$$\text{For boys} = \frac{(\text{fathers height} + 13\ \text{cm or 5 inches}) + \text{mothers height}}{2}$$

Additional methods of height prediction are often employed in the specialty referral setting, including the Bayley Pinneau method,[32] which uses a combination of chronologic age, height, and skeletal age matched to standards.

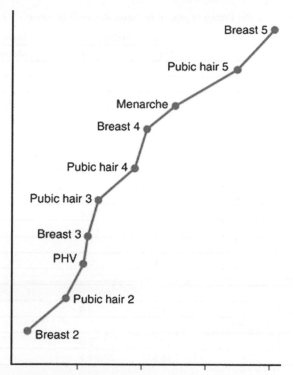

Fig. 5. Sequence of pubertal events in females. PHV, peak height velocity. (*From* Root AW. Endocrinology of puberty. J Pediatr 1973;83(1):1–19.)

Differential linear growth in upper and lower extremities results in changes to the upper/lower (U/L) segment ratio during puberty. With greater linear growth in the lower extremities, the U/L segment ratio decreases from about 1.4 in the prepubertal period to a mean of 0.92 in white and 0.85 in African-American adults.[33]

Body Composition

Despite an overall increase in lean body mass, the percentage of lean body mass in females decreases from about 80% of body weight in early puberty to about 75% at maturity owing to a greater rate of increase in adipose mass.[34] The percentage of body fat increases in females during puberty and is related to menstrual function, with 17% required for the initiation and 22% for maintenance of menstruation.[35] In males, lean body mass increases from 80% to 85% in early puberty to about 90% at maturity, reflecting increasing muscle mass and decreasing adiposity.[34]

Approach to Normal Pubertal Variations and Abnormal Pubertal Growth and Development

Clinicians caring for adolescents are tasked with monitoring the timing and progression of puberty and identifying abnormal patterns of growth and development. It should be noted that the majority of adolescents who display patterns of development outside of statistical norms have no pathology and simply lie within the extremes of normal variation. Definitions between normal and abnormal are purely arbitrary and are based on the assumption that pubertal events assume a normal distribution in the population, with a range of 2 standard deviations (SD) above and below the

Table 1
Descriptive statistics for the timing of sexual maturity stages in females

Stage	Onset of Stage		Mean Age for Stage	
	Mean	SD	Mean	SD
Breast stages				
Stage 2				
Roche et al (Ohio)	11.2	0.7	11.3	1.1
Herman-Giddens et al (USA)				
African American	8.9	1.9		
White	10.0	1.8		
Stage 3				
Roche et al (Ohio)	12.0	1.0	12.5	1.5
Herman-Giddens et al (USA)				
African American	10.2	1.4		
White	11.3	1.4		
Stage 4				
Roche et al (Ohio)	12.4	0.9		
Tanner pubic hair				
Tanner Stage 2				
Roche et al (Ohio)	11.0	0.5		
Herman-Giddens et al (USA)				
African American	8.8	2.0		
White	10.5	1.7		
Tanner Stage 3				
Roche et al (Ohio)	11.8	1.0		
Herman-Giddens et al (USA)				
African-American	10.4	1.6		
White	11.5	1.2		
Tanner Stage 4				
Roche et al (Ohio)	12.4	0.8		
Menarche				
Herman-Giddes et al (USA)				
African American	12.2	1.2		
White	12.9	1.2		
Percent menstruating	At Age 11		At Age 12	
African American	27.9%[a]		62.1%	
White	13.4%[a]		35.2%	
Onset of axillary hair (stage 2)				
African American	10.1 ± 2.0			
White	11.8 ± 1.9			

Mean age for stage 2, 11.3 ± 1.1; mean age for stage 3, 12.5 ± 1.5.

[a] African-American girls enter puberty approximately 1 to 1 1/2 years earlier than white girls and begin menses 8 1/2 months earlier.

Data from Roche AF, Weilens R, Attie KM, et al. The timing of sexual maturation in a group of U.S. white youths. J Pediatr Endocrinol 1995;8:11–8; Herman-Giddens ME, Slora EJ, Wasserman RC, et al. Secondary sexual characteristics and menses in young girls seen in office practice: a study from the Pediatric Research in Office Settings network. Pediatrics 1997;99:505–12; and *From* Melmed S, Polonsky K, Larsen PR, et al. Williams textbook of endocrinology. 12th edition. Philadelphia: Saunders; 2011. p. 1061. Table 25-2.

Table 2
Descriptive statistics for the timing of sexual maturity stages in males

| | | | Time Between Stages (y) | | |
| | | | | Percentile | |
Stage	Mean Age of Onset ±2 SD (y)	Stage	Mean	5th	95th
G2	11.6 ± 2.1	G2–3	1.1	0.4	2.2
G3	12.9 ± 2.1	PH2–3	0.5	0.1	1.0
PH2	13.4 ± 2.2[a]	G3–4	0.8	0.2	1.6
G4	13.8 ± 2.0	PH3–4	0.4	0.3	0.5
PH3	13.9 ± 2.1	G4–5	1.0	0.4	1.9
PH4	14.4 ± 2.2	PH4–5	0.7	0.2	1.5
G5	14.9 ± 2.2	G2–5	3.0	1.9	4.7
PH5	15.2 ± 2.1	PH2–5	1.6	0.8	2.7

[a] Mean is probably too high owing to experimental method.
From Barnes HV. Physical growth and development during puberty. Med Clin North Am 1975;59:1305.

mean used to define the limits of normal variability.[1,2,36] A proportion of adolescents, however, display abnormal patterns of development owing to underlying pathology, which makes the clinical evaluation of development outside statistical norms necessary. An approach in the evaluation of adolescents with abnormal development is presented.

History

- A comprehensive history pertaining to general health and growth, including a review of growth charts and the calculation of growth velocity.[37–40]
- Timing of observed pubertal changes, including whether pubertal changes are completely absent or if earlier pubertal noted changes have failed to progress.[23,40]
- General health conditions in the family, heights and growth patterns of parents and siblings, and their timing of attainment of pubertal milestones.[41–44]
- Nutritional history and review of eating habits.[39,40,45]
- Review of systems to rule out chronic illnesses, including a thorough review of the gastrointestinal, endocrine, and central nervous (CNS) systems.[39]

Physical Examination

- Determination of height and calculation of height velocity in the prior 6 to 12 months. A 6- to 12-month period is recommended to minimize the effect of observed seasonal variation in height growth.[41,42,46,47]
- Determination of weight and body mass index. HPG axis suppression with delay or disruption of puberty is observed at <80% of ideal body weight as in the case of chronic illness, malnutrition, and anorexia.[48] Obesity is a feature of a number of chromosomal syndromes associated with hypogonadism and delayed puberty such as the Prader-Willi and Laurence–Moon syndromes. Endocrine causes of short stature such as hypothyroidism and glucocorticoid excess commonly present with increasing weight and body mass index.[45]
- Examination of the endocrine system, including the thyroid for evidence of goiter, the breast for galactorrhea, and the skin for acne and hirsutism.
- Assessment of signs of puberty and determination of SMR stages. The assessment includes staging of pubic hair and genital development and measurement

of testicular volume in males and the staging of breast and pubic hair development in females.

- Neurologic examination, including examination of the optic discs and visual field examination.

Additional Physical Examination Points

- Although a pelvic examination can provide important information in the evaluation of females presenting with amenorrhea, the need for a pelvic examination should be individualized; imaging modalities such as ultrasonography, computed tomography, and magnetic resonance imaging (MRI) can serve to verify anatomy in the young female.[49]
- Measurement of arm span and U/L body segment ratios in patients with suspected hypogonadism. Hypogonadal patients generally present with increased arm span and decreased U/L segment ratios known as a eunuchoid habitus as a result of delayed epiphyseal fusion and continued growth of the extremities.

Laboratory and Diagnostic Testing in the Primary Care Setting

- Determination of serum levels of FSH, LH, estradiol, testosterone, and key hormones of the adrenal gland, and GH axes correlated with chronologic age and pubertal stage.
- Bone age studies are essential in the evaluation of short stature and delayed and precocious puberty.[50]
- Additional diagnostic testing may be indicated to establish diagnoses and rule out chronic conditions based on clinical information, review of systems, and physical examination findings.

Laboratory and Diagnostic Testing in the Referral Setting

- Stimulation testing performed in consultation with endocrinologists are especially useful in differentiating prepubertal versus pubertal patterns of HPG, adrenal, and growth hormone axes activity, evaluating pituitary and end-organ responsiveness, and in determining the activity of hormones with significant diurnal variation or where random testing lends limited information.[39,40,48,51]
- Karyotyping to exclude chromosomal conditions such as Turners and Klinefelter syndrome.[39]
- Brain computed tomography and MRI to exclude CNS abnormalities.[52]
- Ultrasonography, computed tomography, and MRI to rule out ovarian and adrenal pathology and genital tract abnormalities.[49]

NORMAL PUBERTAL VARIATIONS
Premature Adrenarche and Premature Thelarche

Premature adrenarche and premature thelarche are common, benign variants of normal puberty.[53–55]

Premature adrenarche refers to the appearance of isolated pubic and/or axillary hair before age 6 in African-American girls, age 7 in white girls, and age 9 in boys,[6] and is the result of the premature activation of the adrenal gland. It occurs more frequently in females, with a female:male ratio of around 9:1.[56] Children are often slightly taller than average for age and may have slightly advanced bone age relative to chronologic age, but maintain normal prepubertal growth velocity. DHEA sulfate and androstenedione levels may be elevated for chronologic age, but are normal for pubic hair stage. In males, testosterone levels are in the prepubertal range. The finding of markedly elevated androgen levels or significant androgen exposure such as virilization in females or development beyond SMR Stage G2 in males should prompt consideration of adrenal or gonadal pathology.[57] An algorithm for the evaluation of premature adrenarche in females is presented in **Fig. 6**. Premature adrenarche requires no specific treatment, but warrants observation for progression of puberty.

Premature thelarche refers to isolated breast development before age 6 in African-American and Mexican-American girls or age 7 in white girls.[6] It is most common in patients under age 4 and typically resolves during childhood, but may last until puberty.[58] Patients demonstrate a basal prepubertal growth pattern and normal bone age and other signs of pubertal development are absent. Reassurance and observation for pubertal development every to 4 to 6 months is recommended because progression to complete precocious puberty can occur in ≤20% of

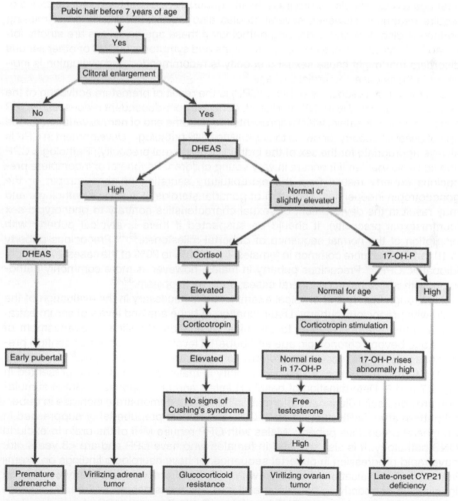

Fig. 6. Flowchart for the evaluation of pubic hair in normal phenotypic girls before 7 years of age. (*From* Melmed S, Polonsky K, Larsen PR, et al. Williams textbook of endocrinology. 12th edition. Philadelphia: Saunders; 2011. p. 1173.)

cases.[59,60] Progression of secondary sexual development, advanced bone age, and accelerated growth velocity warrant referral to a pediatric endocrinologist.[61]

ABNORMAL GROWTH AND DEVELOPMENT
Precocious Puberty

Precocious puberty is the appearance of signs of pubertal development at an abnormally early age. In boys, testicular enlargement before 9 years of age is precocious. Breast development before age 7 in white girls and 6 in black girls is considered precocious[6,21]; however, a high index of suspicion for underlying pathology should be maintained in any girl with thelarche before age 8.[48] The redefined lower age limits for pubertal development in girls is in light of evidence that many children previously considered to have mild sexual precocity may now be considered to have development at the extreme end of normal variation and that pubertal development occurring after age 6 is usually slowly progressive and generally does not have serious cause or require treatment. However, several studies also indicate the likelihood of missing endocrine disorders and underlying pathology if these age guidelines are strictly followed.[62–64] As such, close evaluation for signs and symptoms of CNS or other serious disorders that might cause sexual precocity is recommended and evaluation is indicated in those cases regardless of age.[5]

Central or true precocious puberty (CPP) is the result of premature activation of the normal HPG axis and is a CNS-mediated, gonadotropin-dependent processes.[40] CPP can be benign idiopathic, which represents the extreme end of normal variation for the age of onset of puberty, or owing to underlying CNS pathology. Development in CPP is always appropriate for the sex of the individual (isosexual precocity). Pathologic CPP should be suspected if it occurs in very young children. Peripheral or incomplete precocious puberty results from the extrapituitary secretion of gonadotropin or the gonadotropin independent secretion of gonadal steroids. It is always pathologic and may result in the development of sexual characteristics contrary to phenotypic sex (contrasexual precocity). It should be suspected if there is atypical puberty with disruption of the normal sequence of pubertal milestones.[39,48] Precocious puberty is 10 to 15 times more common in females[51] and 50% to 90% of the cases are benign, idiopathic CPP.[39] Precocious puberty in males, however, is more commonly pathologic, with >50% being peripheral cases, such as neoplasm.[39,48]

A thorough history and physical examination is necessary in the evaluation of the child with precocious puberty. Determination of bone age and levels of serum estradiol and testosterone are key to the initial evaluation. Significant advancement of bone age beyond chronologic age and pubertal levels of sex hormones confirm precocious puberty and necessitate referral to a pediatric endocrinologist.[50] Algorithms for the further evaluation of sexual precocity in males and females are presented in **Figs. 7** and **8**. Determination of basal LH levels and LH response to GnRH stimulation provide useful diagnostic information. LH levels demonstrate increase in pubertal pattern after GnRH stimulation in CPP and remain prepubertal or suppressed in peripheral precocious puberty. Males with CPP require MRI of the brain to exclude CNS pathology. It is also required in females who have CPP and are <3 years old, have rapid progression in pubertal sequence, or have neurologic findings on examination.[49] The evaluation of children with peripheral precocious puberty centers on localization of underlying pathology and includes measurement of free T4, thyroid-stimulating hormone, serum DHEA sulfate, 17-OH-P, and β-HCG. Adrenal, pelvic, and testicular ultrasounds are useful in identifying hormonally active cysts and tumors.

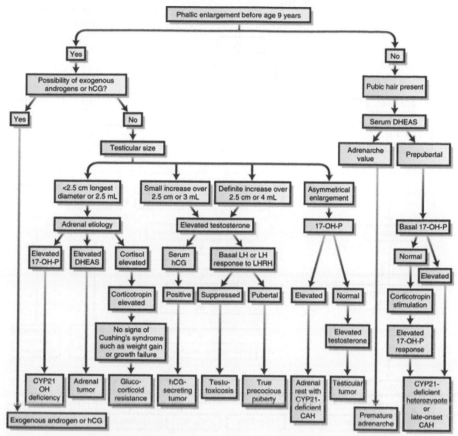

Fig. 7. Flowchart for diagnosing sexual precocity in a phenotypic male. CAH, congenital adrenal hyperplasia; DHEAS, dehydroepiandrosterone sulfate; hCG, human chorionic gonadotropin; 17-OH-P, 17-hydroxyprogesterone. (*From* Melmed S, Polonsky K, Larsen PR, et al. Williams textbook of endocrinology. 12th edition. Philadelphia: Saunders; 2011. p. 1174.)

The treatment of CPP with slowly progressive pubertal development consists of observation and reassurance that premature development is an extreme variation of normal. GnRH agonists are the treatment of choice for rapidly progressive CPP that can result in premature epiphyseal closure and adversely affect height potential. Treatment with GnRH agonists serves to reverse or suspend puberty development until a more appropriate age for it to proceed.[65] Treatment of peripheral precocious puberty is directed at the underlying cause and may include thyroxine, glucocorticoids, glucocorticoids, anti-androgens, and surgery. Children may have pseudo-precocious puberty owing to exogenous exposure to sex steroids and present with secondary sexual development and suppressed FSH and LH.[66] Removal of exposure abates pubertal development.[39,40,48]

Delayed Puberty

Delayed puberty is defined as absence of signs of pubertal development by age of 13 in females or 14 in males. Adolescent females who fail to achieve menarche by age 15 or within 5 years after the onset of puberty and males who fail to complete secondary

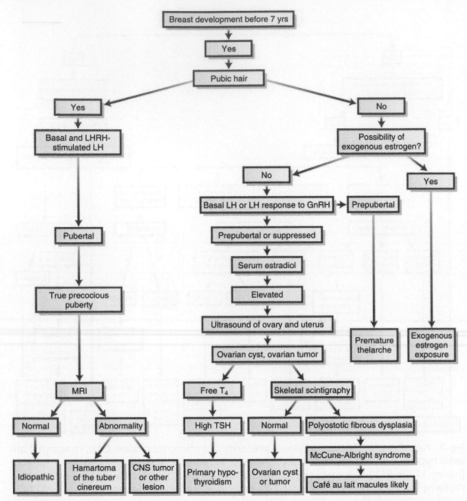

Fig. 8. Flowchart for diagnosing sexual precocity in girls. CNS, central nervous system; FSH, follicle-stimulating hormone; LH, luteinizing hormone; T_4, thyroxine; TSH, thyroid-stimulating hormone. (*From* Melmed S, Polonsky K, Larsen PR, et al. Williams textbook of endocrinology. 12th edition. Philadelphia: Saunders; 2011. p. 1172.)

sexual development within 4.5 years from attaining SMR stage G2 are also considered to have delayed puberty and require evaluation.[36] The primary considerations in pubertal delay include hypothalamic, pituitary, or gonadal disorders and constitutional delay of growth and puberty. The approach to males and females with delayed puberty is presented in **Figs. 9** and **10**. Constitutional delay of growth and puberty is the most common cause of delayed puberty and represents the extreme variant in the timing of normal puberty with delayed activation of the HPG axis. It is much more frequently encountered in boys and is characterized by height that is consistently short and typically between the 3rd and 25th percentiles for chronologic age with normal growth velocity of 5 to 6 cm per year. Bone age is delayed compared with chronologic age and consistent with height age. Family history of similar delay in pubertal development is common. The findings of subnormal growth velocity or the lack of an observed growth

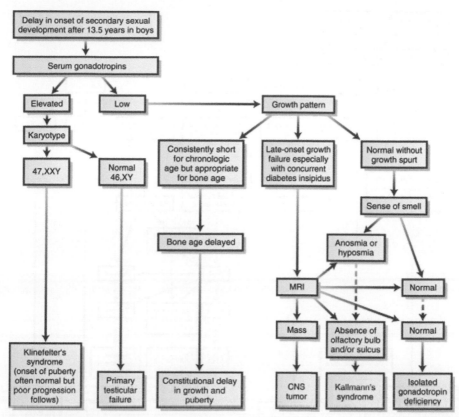

Fig. 9. Flowchart for the evaluation of delayed puberty in boys. (*From* Melmed S, Polonsky K, Larsen PR, et al. Williams textbook of endocrinology. 12th edition. Philadelphia: Saunders; 2011. p. 1136.)

spurt should prompt further evaluation for underlying pathology. Treatment consists primarily of reassurance and observation. Patients experiencing emotional distress related to pubertal delay warrant specialty referral to discuss controversial brief hormonal therapy.[12] Delayed puberty owing to hypothalamic, pituitary, and gonadal disorders can be identified and differentiated by the determination of serum gonadotropin levels. Hypogonadotropic hypogonadism is caused by limited function of the hypothalamus to secrete GnRH or anterior pituitary to secrete LH or FSH. Causes of CNS dysfunction are frequently irreversible and include congenital (midline defect), neoplastic (craniopharyngioma), and infectious (tuberculosis) causes. Chronic illness, malnutrition, and anorexia nervosa are commonly reversible causes of HPG axis suppression. Hypergonadotropic hypogonadism is the result of absence of negative feedback from gonadal sex hormones[39,48] and is indicative of gonadal failure. Karyotyping allows for differentiation between primary and chromosomal causes. The most common chromosomal causes of gonadal failure are Klinefelter syndrome in males and Turner syndrome in females.[40] They are identifiable by the constellation of physical findings, absent to limited development of secondary sexual characteristics, and elevated gonadotropin levels. Adolescents with irreversible causes of hypergonadotropic hypogonadism and gonadal failure require hormonal replacement therapy under the care of specialists to effect puberty.[36] The doses are increased in a step-wise manner to attain sex steroid hormone

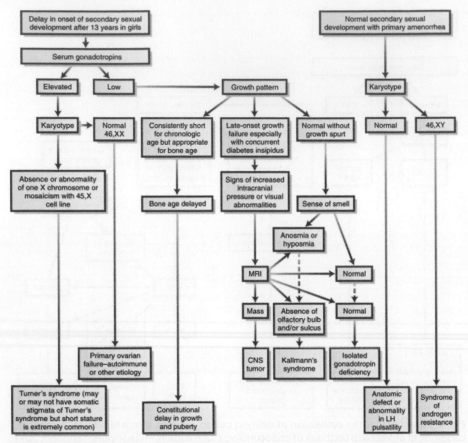

Fig. 10. Flowchart for the evaluation of delayed puberty in girls. (*From* Melmed S, Polonsky K, Larsen PR, et al. Williams textbook of endocrinology. 12th edition. Philadelphia: Saunders; 2011. p. 1137.)

levels appropriate for age and SMR stage. Improvement in health status and nutritional rehabilitation promote recovery of HPG axis activity owing to chronic illness and malnutrition.

Short Stature

Short stature is defined as height below the 3rd percentile or <2 standard deviations below the mean for age and gender.[46] The most common causes of short stature are constitutional delay of growth and puberty and familial short stature.[16] Twenty percent of children identified as having short stature have underlying pathology, with the majority having heights <3 standard deviations below the mean.[46] Careful attention to growth throughout childhood is extremely important as the greatest predictor of adolescent stature is growth trajectory during early childhood.[67] As a result, the evaluation of short stature should begin with a thorough evaluation of family history for instances of short stature as well as establishing the adolescents' natural growth curve by looking at birth anthropometric values and childhood growth curves.[41,67]

A step-wise approach to the adolescent with either short stature or delayed height trajectory is recommended. Physical examination should look for dysmorphic features that may be suspicious for mosaic Down syndrome, Turner syndrome, Noonan syndrome, or skeletal dysplasia.[6,41,44] If the physical examination seems to be normal, screening tests organic etiology should be obtained and include complete blood count, bone morphogenic protein, erythrocyte sedimentation rate, liver function tests, urinalysis, thyroid-stimulating hormone, and bone age.[41,44,47] Abnormal screening test results or delayed bone age by >2 SD warrants referral to endocrinology or the appropriate specialty. If screening test results and bone age studies are normal, the adolescent most likely has familial short stature and can be reassured and observed. Reassurance and observation is also indicated if test results are normal and bone age is slightly delayed, because this is consistent with constitutional delay.[6] If bone age is normal or advanced and puberty is progressing, urgent endocrine referral is indicated to rule out growth hormone deficiency.[44] As puberty progresses, the window to increase height trajectory rapidly closes.

Tall Stature

Tall stature is defined as height >2 standard deviations above the mean for sex, age, and race.[42,47] Based on this definition, 2% to 3% of all adolescents have tall stature.[42] This is most commonly constitutional and owing to genetic predisposition.[6] Tall stature is associated with exogenous obesity and can also be owing to underlying pathology, including hyperthyroidism, precocious puberty, growth hormone excess, and cerebral gigantism. The genetic syndromes leading to tall stature that may not have been diagnosed until adolescence include Marfan syndrome, Klinefelter syndrome, and homocystienuria.

The most important tools in diagnosis of tall stature include historical growth charts for the adolescent, parental heights, the sequence and timing of pubertal progression, and bone age.[47] Adolescents with constitutional tall stature are usually tall from early childhood and have tall parents. They have a normal growth rate and follow the normal progression of puberty, and bone age is compatible with chronologic age. Precocious puberty should be suspected with sudden change in height trajectory (crossing 2 growth curve lines) occurs, signs of virilization or premature sexual development, and advancement in bone age.[47] Pituitary growth hormone excess should be considered if the height trajectory changes without the corresponding development of secondary sexual characteristics.[6,42,47] Tall stature that does not seem to be constitutional warrants referral to an endocrinologist.

Tall stature can be distressing to adolescents, particularly females. Hormonal therapy to blunt height trajectory and achieve a more average adult height can be considered in youth with constitutional stature who find their height distressing.[42] Tall stature owing to organic or hormonal etiology requires treatment of underlying cause.

PSYCHOSOCIAL GROWTH AND DEVELOPMENT

Adolescence is a period of transition through which youth incrementally develop adaptive and functional skills and competencies, and establish self-identities that prepare them to fulfill adult societal roles and expectations. Although commonly conceptualized as a period of storm and stress, data suggest that the transition from childhood to adulthood is relatively smooth for most adolescents.[68] Although this section aims to provide an outline of adolescent psychosocial development, it is important to recognize that this process, which is universal and common to all youth, is also highly variable and individual. Adolescents are a widely heterogeneous group and psychosocial development is a phenomenon that takes place in the modifying milieu of families, peers, communities, and social institutions. The transitions that occur in adolescence do not occur in a linear uniform fashion and youth may progress asynchronously in their achievement of physical and various psychosocial milestones. There are unique developmental considerations for subgroups of adolescents, such as sexual minority and developmentally delayed youth that are discussed elsewhere in this issue.

DEVELOPMENTAL TASKS AND PHASES OF ADOLESCENCE

The developmental tasks of adolescence can be broadly categorized along the domains of cognitive, moral, identity, and relationship development. Progression through the development tasks are incremental and interdependent in nature and can be can be viewed as occurring in the continuum of 3 developmental phases:

- Early adolescence: 11 to 13 years/middle school years
- Middle adolescence: 14 to 18 years/high school years
- Late adolescence, 19 to 21 years/post high school graduation or college years

COGNITIVE DEVELOPMENT

Jean Piaget's Theory of Cognitive Development provides a widely accepted model of cognitive development in adolescence.[69] Early adolescents are in the concrete operational stage and although they demonstrate increased capacity for logical thought, they have difficulty grasping hypothetical concepts. Impulsivity and limitations to understanding cause-and-effect relationships are additional hallmarks of the stage. Youth demonstrate expanding cognitive abilities and intellectual interests and enter the formal operational stage in middle to late adolescence. In this stage, they show the capacity for deductive reasoning, problem solving, and abstract thinking. Along with increased ability for self-regulation and planning, this development of higher-order thinking allows youth to consider future possibilities, assess alternatives, and set and pursue personal goals.

MORAL DEVELOPMENT

Lawrence Kohlberg's Theory of Moral Development[70] describes an evolution in the levels of reasoning that underlie actions and decision making. Unlike other developmental processes, moral development is not linked with chronologic age or stage. Instead, it progresses through 3 levels across the lifespan and reflect an increasingly complex and personal understanding of moral behavior. In the preconventional level, authority is external, and obedience and the avoidance of punishment define ones' moral code. In the conventional level, moral standards of adult role models are internalized and conformity to social roles and expectations are paramount. In post-conventional morality, authority is internal and judgment is based on internalized values and principles such as justice and care, regardless of societal opinion or agreement.

SELF-CONCEPT AND IDENTITY DEVELOPMENT

The establishment self-concept and identity development are defining tasks of adolescence.[71] In establishing a physical self-concept, early adolescents characteristically display preoccupation with pubertal changes and uncertainty about their appearance.[72] Early adolescents also become aware of sexual attractions and feelings in their paths to developing sexual identities. In middle adolescence, pubertal changes are increasingly accepted and personal attractiveness is a primary concern. The acceptance of pubertal changes and being comfortable with one's body are characteristics of late adolescence. Adolescents also consolidate their vocational identities progressively throughout adolescence. Early adolescents engage in fantasy and have idealistic and changing vocational goals. Vocational goals become more realistic later in adolescence as youth acquire the ability to more accurately appraise their attributes and strengths, evaluate alternatives, and plan the pursuit of goals.

RELATIONSHIP DEVELOPMENT

Adolescence is marked by significant shifts in relationships. In the striving for autonomy and independence, the terms of the parent–child relationship are dynamically renegotiated beginning in early adolescence, with increased demands for privacy, decreased interest in parent- and family-based activities, and the reexamination of parental authority. During this stage, relationships with peers provide support and connection and assume increased importance. Middle adolescence marks the peak of distancing from parents and families of origin and immersion in peers and group activities.[34,73] Involvement in romantic relationships is also common and provides adolescents with the context to develop and apply skills in communication, negotiation, and conflict resolution. Although often depicted as the period of greatest vulnerability to negative influences and risk behaviors, middle adolescence is a developmental phase that provides youth the latitude for self-discovery and the opportunity to test adult roles necessary for individuation. Late adolescence marks the integration of adult dynamics in renegotiated parent–child relationships and the consolidation of parent- and family-derived and self-discovered beliefs and value systems.[34,74] Peer groups become less important as youth become more invested in intimate, romantic relationships. Transitions into college or post high school graduation plans entail separation from their families of origin and independent living for a majority of youth.

ADOLESCENCE AS A SOCIAL PHENOMENON: WHEN DOES ADOLESCENCE END?

Although the physical changes of puberty serve to mark the beginning of adolescence, the transition out of adolescence is less well-defined and is subject to sociocultural interpretation. In modern developed societies, the transition from adolescence to adulthood has become increasingly prolonged by shifts in economic, educational, and social factors. The term "emerging adulthood" has been proposed to describe a new life stage extending from the late teens through the mid to late twenties during which many young people do not necessarily settle into committed adult roles, but gradually steer their way toward long-term choices in education, vocation, and relationships.[75] The stage is characterized by continued identity exploration and instability as young people explore possibilities after having achieved independence from their parents and before entering the commitments typical of adult life, such as a long-term employment, marriage, and parenthood.[75-77] In assessing their attainment of developmental tasks, clinicians caring for youth need to consider contemporary sociocultural factors and how such reshape traditionally held developmental expectations of youth.

REFERENCES

1. Colvin CW, Abdullatif H. Anatomy of female puberty: the clinical relevance of developmental changes in the reproductive system. Clin Anat 2013;26(1): 115–29.

2. Fisher MM, Eugster EA. What is in our environment that effects puberty? Reprod Toxicol 2014;44:7–14.

3. Tena-Sempere M. Ghrelin, the gonadal axis and the onset of puberty. Endocr Dev 2013;25:69–82.

4. Lee Y, Styne D. Influences on the onset and tempo of puberty in human beings and implications for adolescent psychological development. Horm Behav 2013; 64(2):250–61.

5. Juul A, Hagen CP, Aksglaede L, et al. Endocrine evaluation of reproductive function in girls during infancy, childhood and adolescence. Endocr Dev 2012;22:24–39.

6. Melmed S, Polonsky KS, Larsen PR, et al. Williams textbook of endocrinology. Philadelphia: Elsevier Health; 2011.

7. Murray PG, Clayton PE. Endocrine control of growth. Am J Med Genet C Semin Med Genet 2013;163C(2):76–85.

8. Apter D. Leptin in puberty. Clin Endocrinol (Oxf) 1997;47(2):175–6.

9. Daftary SS, Gore AC. The hypothalamic insulin-like growth factor-1 receptor and its relationship to gonadotropin-releasing hormones neurones during postnatal development. J Neuroendocrinol 2004;16(2):160–9.

10. Bordini B, Rosenfield RL. Normal pubertal development: part I: the endocrine basis of puberty. Pediatr Rev 2011;32(6):223–9.

11. de Peretti E, Forest MG. Unconjugated dehydroepiandrosterone plasma levels in normal subjects from birth to adolescence in human: the use of a sensitive radioimmunoassay. J Clin Endocrinol Metab 1976;43(5):982–91.

12. Korth-Schutz S, Levine LS, New MI. Serum androgens in normal prepubertal and pubertal children and in children with precocious adrenarche. J Clin Endocrinol Metab 1976;42(1):117–24.

13. de Peretti E, Forest MG. Pattern of plasma dehydroepiandrosterone sulfate levels in humans from birth to adulthood: evidence for testicular production. J Clin Endocrinol Metab 1978;47(3):572–7.

14. Sizonenko PC, Paunier L. Hormonal changes in puberty III: correlation of plasma dehydroepiandrosterone, testosterone, FSH, and LH with stages of puberty and bone age in normal boys and girls and in patients with Addison's disease or hypogonadism or with premature or late adrenarche. J Clin Endocrinol Metab 1975;41(5):894–904.

15. Tanner J. Growth at adolescence. 2nd edition. Oxford (United Kingdom): Blackwell Scientific Publications; 1962.

16. Marshall WA, Tanner JM. Variations in the pattern of pubertal changes in boys. Arch Dis Child 1970;45(239):13–23.

17. Marshall WA, Tanner JM. Variations in pattern of pubertal changes in girls. Arch Dis Child 1969;44(235):291–303.

18. Harlan WR, Harlan EA, Grillo GP. Secondary sex characteristics of girls 12 to 17 years of age: the U.S. Health Examination Survey. J Pediatr 1980;96(6): 1074–8.

19. Sun SS, Schubert CM, Chumlea WC, et al. National estimates of the timing of sexual maturation and racial differences among US children. Pediatrics 2002; 110(5):911–9.

20. Herman-Giddens ME, Slora EJ, Wasserman RC, et al. Secondary sexual characteristics and menses in young girls seen in office practice: a study from the Pediatric Research in Office Settings network. Pediatrics 1997;99(4):505–12.

21. Kaplowitz PB, Oberfield SE. Reexamination of the age limit for defining when puberty is precocious in girls in the United States: implications for evaluation and

treatment. Drug and Therapeutics and Executive Committees of the Lawson Wilkins Pediatric Endocrine Society. Pediatrics 1999;104(4 Pt 1):936–41.

22. Biro FM, Huang B, Daniels SR, et al. Pubarche as well as thelarche may be a marker for the onset of puberty. J Pediatr Adolesc Gynecol 2008;21(6): 323–8.

23. Herman-Giddens ME, Bourdony CJ, Dowshen SA, et al, editors. Assessment of sexual maturity stages in girls and boys. Elk Grove Village (IL): American Academy of Pediatrics; 2010.

24. Biro FM, Huang B, Crawford PB, et al. Pubertal correlates in black and white girls. J Pediatr 2006;148(2):234–40.

25. Roche AF, Wellens R, Attie KM, et al. The timing of sexual maturation in a group of US white youths. J Pediatr Endocrinol Metab 1995;8(1):11–8.

26. Susman EJ, Houts RM, Steinberg L, et al. Longitudinal development of secondary sexual characteristics in girls and boys between ages 91/2 and 151/2 years. Arch Pediatr Adolesc Med 2010;164(2):166–73.

27. Biro FM, Lucky AW, Huster GA, et al. Pubertal staging in boys. J Pediatr 1995; 127(1):100–2.

28. Bordini B, Rosenfield RL. Normal pubertal development: part II: clinical aspects of puberty. Pediatr Rev 2011;32(7):281–92.

29. Tanner J. Fetus into man: physical growth from conception to maturity. Cambridge (MA): Harvard University Press; 1989.

30. Abbassi V. Growth and normal puberty. Pediatrics 1998;102(2 Pt 3):507–11.

31. Tanner JM, Goldstein H, Whitehouse RH. Standards for children's height at ages 2-9 years allowing for heights of parents. Arch Dis Child 1970;45(244):755–62.

32. Bayley N, Pinneau SR. Tables for predicting adult height from skeletal age: revised for use with the Greulich-Pyle hand standards. J Pediatr 1952;40(4):423–41.

33. McKusick V. Heritable disorders of connective tissue. St Louis (MO): Mosby Company; 1066.

34. Neinstein LS, Gordon C, Katzman D, et al, editors. Adolescent health care: a practical guide. 5th edition. Philadelphia: Lippincott, Williams & Wilson; 2007.

35. Frisch RE. Body fat, menarche, fitness and fertility. Humanit Rep 1987;2(6): 521–33.

36. Carel JC, Eugster EA, Rogol A, et al. Consensus statement on the use of gonadotropin-releasing hormone analogs in children. Pediatrics 2009;123(4): e752–62.

37. Brown DB, Loomba-Albrecht LA, Bremer AA. Sexual precocity and its treatment. World J Pediatr 2013;9(2):103–11.

38. Appelbaum H, Malhotra S. A comprehensive approach to the spectrum of abnormal pubertal development. Adolesc Med State Art Rev 2012;23(1):1–14.

39. Blondell RD, Foster MB, Dave KC. Disorders of puberty. Am Fam Physician 1999;60(1):209–18, 223–4.

40. Ducharme JR, Collu R. Pubertal development: normal, precocious and delayed. Clin Endocrinol Metab 1982;11(1):57–87.

41. Hokken-Koelega AC. Diagnostic workup of the short child. Horm Res Paediatr 2011;76(Suppl 3):6–9.

42. Leung AK, Robson WL. Evaluating tall children. Can Fam Physician 1995;41: 457–8, 461–2, 465–8.

43. Wit JM, Clayton PE, Rogol AD, et al. Idiopathic short stature: definition, epidemiology, and diagnostic evaluation. Growth Horm IGF Res 2008;18(2):89–110.

44. Oostdijk W, Grote FK, de Muinck Keizer-Schrama SM, et al. Diagnostic approach in children with short stature. Horm Res 2009;72(4):206–17.

45. De Leonibus C, Marcovecchio ML, Chiavaroli V, et al. Timing of puberty and physical growth in obese children: a longitudinal study in boys and girls. Pediatr Obes 2013. [Epub ahead of print].
46. Mahoney CP. Evaluating the child with short stature. Pediatr Clin North Am 1987; 34(4):825–49.
47. Nwosu BU, Lee MM. Evaluation of short and tall stature in children. Am Fam Physician 2008;78(5):597–604.
48. Loomba-Albrecht LA, Styne DM. The physiology of puberty and its disorders. Pediatr Ann 2012;41(4):e1–9.
49. Faizah M, Zuhanis A, Rahmah R, et al. Precocious puberty in children: a review of imaging findings. Biomed Imaging Interv J 2012;8(1):e6–13.
50. Lazar L, Phillip M. Pubertal disorders and bone maturation. Endocrinol Metab Clin North Am 2012;41(4):805–25.
51. Fuqua JS. Treatment and outcomes of precocious puberty: an update. J Clin Endocrinol Metab 2013;98(6):2198–207.
52. Chaudhary V, Bano S. Imaging of pediatric pituitary endocrinopathies. Indian J Endocrinol Metab 2012;16(5):682–91.
53. Codner E, Roman R. Premature thelarche from phenotype to genotype. Pediatr Endocrinol Rev 2008;5(3):760–5.
54. Ibanez L, Dimartino-Nardi J, Potau N, et al. Premature adrenarche–normal variant or forerunner of adult disease? Endocr Rev 2000;21(6):671–96.
55. Diamantopoulos S, Bao Y. Gynecomastia and premature thelarche: a guide for practitioners. Pediatr Rev 2007;28(9):e57–68.
56. Silverman SH, Migeon C, Rosemberg E, et al. Precocious growth of sexual hair without other secondary sexual development; premature pubarche, a constitutional variation of adolescence. Pediatrics 1952;10(4):426–32.
57. Ucar A, Saka N, Bas F, et al. Precocious adrenarche in children born appropriate for gestational age: is there a difference between genders? Eur J Pediatr 2012;171(11):1661–6.
58. Klein KO, Mericq V, Brown-Dawson JM, et al. Estrogen levels in girls with premature thelarche compared with normal prepubertal girls as determined by an ultrasensitive recombinant cell bioassay. J Pediatr 1999;134(2):190–2.
59. Pasquino AM, Pucarelli I, Passeri F, et al. Progression of premature thelarche to central precocious puberty. J Pediatr 1995;126(1):11–4.
60. Zhu SY, Du ML, Huang TT. An analysis of predictive factors for the conversion from premature thelarche into complete central precocious puberty. J Pediatr Endocrinol Metab 2008;21(6):533–8.
61. Findberg L, Kleinman RE, editors. Saunders manual of pediatric practice. Philadelphia: Saunders; 2002.
62. Kaplowitz P. Clinical characteristics of 104 children referred for evaluation of precocious puberty. J Clin Endocrinol Metab 2004;89(8):3644–50.
63. Midyett LK, Moore WV, Jacobson JD. Are pubertal changes in girls before age 8 benign? Pediatrics 2003;111(1):47–51.
64. de Vries AL. Puberty suppression in adolescents with gender identity disorder: a prospective follow-up study. J Sex Med 2011;8(8):2276–83.
65. Clemons RD, Kappy MS, Stuart TE, et al. Long-term effectiveness of depot gonadotropin-releasing hormone analogue in the treatment of children with central precocious puberty. Am J Dis Child 1993;147(6):653–7.
66. Martinez-Pajares JD, Diaz-Morales O, Ramos-Diaz JC, et al. Peripheral precocious puberty due to inadvertent exposure to testosterone: case report and review of the literature. J Pediatr Endocrinol Metab 2012;25(9–10):1007–12.

67. Sterling R, Miranda JJ, Gilman RH, et al. Early anthropometric indices predict short stature and overweight status in a cohort of Peruvians in early adolescence. Am J Phys Anthropol 2012;148(3):451–61.
68. Arnett JJ. Adolescent storm and stress, reconsidered. Am Psychol 1999;54(5): 317–26.
69. Piaget J. In adolescence: psychological principles. New York: Basic Books; 1969.
70. Kohlberg L. The psychology of moral development: the nature and validity of moral stages. San Francisco (CA): Harper & Row; 1984.
71. Waterman AS. Identity development from adolescence to adulthood: an extension of theory and a review of research. Dev Psychol 1982;18(3):341–58.
72. Susman EJ, Rogel A. Puberty and psychological development. 2nd edition. Hoboken (NJ): John Wiley & Sons, Inc; 2004.
73. Gentry J, Campbell M. Developing adolescents: a reference for professionals. Washington, DC: American Psychological Association; 2002.
74. Simpson AR. Raising teens: a synthesis of research and a foundation for action. Boston: Center for Health Communication, Harvard School of Public Health; 2001.
75. Arnett JJ. Emerging adulthood: the winding road from the late teens through the twenties. New York: Oxford University Press; 2004.
76. Arnett JJ. Emerging adulthood. A theory of development from the late teens through the twenties. Am Psychol 2000;55(5):469–80.
77. Arnett JJ. Conceptions of the transition to adulthood: perspectives from adolescence to midlife. J Adult Dev 2001;8:133–43.

Home

Parents and Family Matter

Strategies for Developing Family-Centered Adolescent Care Within Primary Care Practices

María Verónica Svetaz, MD, MPH[a,b,*],
Diego Garcia-Huidobro, MD[c,d,e], Michele Allen, MD, MS[c]

KEYWORDS

- Positive parenting • Adolescent • Family • Parenting • Positive youth development
- Primary care • Youth

KEY POINTS

- Parental involvement during adolescence is important; however, parents may not recognize that the parenting skills that help teens thrive are different from those they learned for their young children.
- Parenting stress during the teen years can be high, even if there are no other stressors in the family.
- Primary care providers are perfectly positioned to partner with parents, and support them in mastering parenting skills that support healthy youth development.
- Family-centered care does not hinder teens' right and access to confidential care.
- Families need to be supported in the context of their communities and their cultures, considering both their strengths and challenges.

Funding: Aqui Para Ti/ Here For you is partially funded by the Eliminating Health Disparities Initiative (EHDI), from the Minnesota Department of Health.
[a] Department of Family and Community Medicine, Hennepin County Medical Center, 2800 Nicollet Avenue South, Minneapolis, MN 55408, USA; [b] Aqui Para Ti/Here for you clinic for Latino Youth, Hennepin County Medical Center, 2800 Nicollet Avenue South, Minneapolis, MN 55408, USA; [c] Department of Family Medicine and Community Health, University of Minnesota Medical School, 717 Delaware Street Southeast, Suite 166, Minneapolis, MN 55414, USA; [d] Department of Family Social Science, University of Minnesota Medical School, 290 McNeal Hall, 1985 Buford Avenue, St Paul, MN 55108, USA; [e] Department of Family Medicine, School of Medicine, Pontificia Universidad Catolica de Chile, Av Libertador Bernardo O Higgins 340, Santiago, Región Metropolitana, Chile
* Corresponding author. Department of Family and Community Medicine, Hennepin County Medical Center, 2800 Nicollet Avenue South, Minneapolis, MN 55408.
E-mail address: maria.svetaz@hcmed.org

We have an opportunity to revolutionize the way in which we, as a society, think about parenting, in particular the parenting of adolescents.[1] We can raise awareness about the importance of parenting during adolescence, we can shift negative perceptions about parenting and adolescence, and we can provide tools for raising healthy teenagers. The power to do so is well within our grasp, and the effects will reverberate throughout our schools, our courts, our workplaces, our neighborhoods, and our lives.

—Rae Simpson, Raising Teens[2]

INTRODUCTION

The family is the foundational system supporting healthy youth development.[2-7] However, similar to a mobile that includes multiple interdependent pieces, even a well-balanced family can become unsteady when 1 piece shifts. To maintain equilibrium, the system must be flexible and adaptable. Given that a fundamental task of adolescence is renegotiation of the relationship between parents and youth, this developmental stage is particularly challenging for parents seeking to maintain balance within their family system. Despite increased understanding of the importance of parents in the lives of youth, and identification of key strategies and approaches that may help parents to guide their child through adolescence, little support is available to parents during this transition.

Parents receive advice and knowledge about optimal parenting strategies from multiple sources when their children are young, often beginning with prenatal classes and continuing through early childhood education. Yet, although health care, social service, and educational systems provide these messages to parents of young children, similar opportunities are not as widely available during adolescence. For example, when the federal government recently invested in Parenting Home Visiting Programs, only 1 of the 7 funded programs included parents of teenagers.[8,9] Consequently, parents may be left with 2 impressions: First, that they should not need additional parenting support during their children's teenage years, and second, that the strategies they used with their younger children remain appropriate for their teens.

The consequences of the lack of information and support for parents of teens are profound. Results of a recent analysis of parenting skills by the Center on Children and Families indicate that these parenting gaps have consequences for social mobility.[8] This research found that children of parents with strong parenting skills, including high parental warmth and verbal communication skills, are more likely to succeed in life compared with children whose parents have weaker skills. The authors state, "By the end of adolescence, three out of four children with the strongest parents graduate high school with at least a 2.5 GPA, while avoiding being convicted of a crime or becoming a teen parent. By contrast, only 30% of children with the weakest parents manage to meet these benchmarks."[8(p8)] This article presents a clear description of the social benefit of strong parenting skills and identifies the need for interventions focused on building these skills.[8]

Primary care providers are uniquely positioned to provide needed support and education to parents of teens. Although the gap in parenting support is acknowledged within health care preventive guidelines,[10,11] it is not currently being adequately addressed in clinical care or in training for health care providers.[12] Nevertheless, there is evidence to support "best practices" for parenting adolescents and there are strategies primary care providers can use to coach parents in making use of these developmentally appropriate parenting practices. These skills and knowledge support parents in maintaining balance within their family system as their children navigate adolescence to ensure a healthy developmental transition for their teens and themselves. Parents are defined through this article as the significant adult exercising that "role" in a teen's life.

WHY PARENTS AND FAMILY MATTER FOR ADOLESCENTS

Over the last decade, research has reaffirmed that parents play a protective role in the lives of adolescents.[3–7] Developmentally, adolescence is a peer-oriented stage; however, parents are much more influential on the lives of their teens than they believe. Youth self-report that their parents affect the decisions they make.[13,14] For example, 47% of teens say that parents influence their decisions about sex more than friends, and that teens rely on parents more than anyone else when making important decisions.[15] In fact, the positive effects of parents and families on adolescent outcomes are not diminished by the presence of "deviant peers," suggesting that parents can outweigh the influence of negative peer relations on a teenager's life.[16,17]

Given parents' importance, research has identified sets of attributes and skills that characterize parenting associated with optimal youth health outcomes, and importantly has shown that these parenting behaviors can be developed.[18] Four parenting styles have been described based on the levels of control/discipline and emotional nurturance between parents and their children.[7]

- *Authoritative*: This style is notable for an optimal combination of both high nurturance and discipline. It is referred to as "positive parenting" and it will be explored in more detail.[7,18]
- *Authoritarian*: This style is defined by high control, but low emotional support and may sometimes be referred to as "dominating."[7,18]
- *Indulgent*: This style is described by high nurturance but low control, or lack of monitoring, and may be referred to as "permissive."[7,18]
- *Uninvolved*: This style is defined by both low levels of emotional support and low discipline or monitoring and is sometimes referred to as "disengaged."[7,18]

Research indicates that children and teens raised in homes in which parents are characterized as authoritative or "positive" show strong health advantages such as the following:

- Lower engagement in risky sexual behavior,[19]
- Lower smoking and other substance use initiation,[3,20]
- Healthier dietary and physical activity behaviors,[21,22]
- Higher self-esteem, lower incidence of major depression, and fewer suicide attempts,[3,23,24]
- Higher academic performance,[3,25] and
- Lower delinquency and incarceration rates.[26,27]

In 2-parent families, the parenting styles may be the same or different.[28,29] Although having 2 "positive" parents is associated with the best adolescent outcomes, having ≥1 positive parent in the family can protect an adolescent against the negative consequences of the parenting style of the other parent.[28]

Key parenting practices contributing to healthy adolescent behaviors include supervision and monitoring, communication of family values and expectations, and consistent discipline methods.[30,31] Age-appropriate parental monitoring of adolescents' whereabouts also protects against risky health behaviors.[26,32,33] Successful monitoring is an interactive process that depends on youth disclosure and parents' appropriate solicitation of information; it depends on the quality of the parent–youth relationship within the larger family context.[32,33]

Positive qualities of relationships (eg, warmth, support, acceptance, attachment) are not static. They can be bolstered through education and skills building, ultimately protecting adolescents against risky behaviors.[3,20,30] Adolescent development is best supported by a family and home environment that is both flexible and appropriately cohesive.[34] Flexible families are open to new challenges, interpretations, and ideas, and find ways to adjust during the transitions of adolescence; less flexible families find transitions and adapting to change more challenging.[34,35] Healthy levels of family cohesion promote the emotional support that enables individuals or family relationships to remain resilient through challenges. Families at the extremes of cohesiveness may not adequately nurture adolescent transition to adulthood. At 1 extreme, families who are too cohesive may become so enmeshed that it becomes difficult for the adolescent to go through the normal process of individualization.[34–38] At the other extreme, families with low cohesion may be so individualized, there is little emotional involvement and support.[34,35]

Achieving adolescent health-promoting parenting practices and family interactions is challenging, especially in the context with high levels of stress (eg, families with low economic resources facing immigration challenges) and/or low family support (eg, single parents). Parents who are able to utilize positive parenting skills likely have high self-efficacy related to parenting practices. Parenting self-efficacy, defined as a parents' personal belief that he or she can appropriately raise a child, has an important influence on adolescent development.[39] Parenting adolescents per se can generate stress that undermines parenting efficacy for many.[40] Therefore, primary care providers can support and empathize with parents of adolescents to increase parenting efficacy and contribute to positive outcomes in both the teens' and parents' lives.[41]

How Do Community and Neighborhood Factors Affect Parenting Practices and Ultimately Adolescent Health?

There is a growing body of evidence regarding environmental factors that influence healthy adolescent development. These social determinants of health may include poverty, poor housing stock, unsafe neighborhoods, ineffective schools, lack of employment, recent immigration, and language barriers.[42,43] There is clear evidence that neighborhood safety has both direct and indirect effects on adolescent health outcomes[44]; therefore, parenting strategies need be sensitive to these environmental circumstances. Teens in unsafe settings need stricter, more intense monitoring than is necessary in other neighborhoods; parents may be challenged by incorporating these more restrictive guidelines into positive parenting practices.[44] Under these conditions, it is best to encourage youth participation in supervised programming (like after school activities), where teens can develop social connections with peers in a safe way, in addition to have interventions that address multiple areas of family functioning, including emotional support.[45]

Negative social determinants of health contribute to disparities in health outcomes and create significant challenges for primary care providers seeking to optimize health for all adolescent patients.[42,43] Families experiencing negative social determinants of health often have trouble accessing support to address their unmet needs.[46] These environmental stressors may have a direct effect on adolescent outcomes and on parenting efficacy.[45,47,48] Parenting efficacy deterred by these factors can be strengthened by creating supportive relationships with other family members, friends and supportive professionals, and by developing strong cultural and community bonds.[47,48]

Addressing these challenges requires a health care system more attuned to assessing and addressing the ecological contributors to health.[49] A recent Institute of Medicine (IOM)[12] report on gaps in adolescent care delivery called for a focus on the needs of vulnerable adolescents and clearly articulated the need to integrate family-centered approaches into primary care for adolescents. Understanding the impact of these environmental factors on both parents and teens is crucial for providers to support family-centered care.[49]

OPTIMIZING PRIMARY CARE TO MEET THE NEEDS OF ADOLESCENTS AND THEIR FAMILIES
The Current Status

The 2009 IOM report and several national guidelines highlight the need for a new approach within our health system that provides family-centered care to adolescents to optimize health outcomes.[12] Both the American Medical Association through the Guidelines for Adolescent Preventive Services and the American Academy of Pediatrics, through "Bright Futures," state that parents should receive health guidance on parenting behaviors that promote healthy adolescent adjustment at least once during early, middle, and late adolescence.[10,11]

Although delivering education, anticipatory guidance, and support to parents of adolescents is an established standard of care, there are currently several system-level dilemmas to consider regarding translating these recommendations into practice.

Dilemma #1: How Can Health Care Delivery Systems Be Organized to Integrate Families into Adolescent Care?

Although the last IOM report in Adolescent Health Care reflected a general consensus that our primary care delivery system is not currently structured to allow easy integration of families into adolescent care delivery,[12] a number of innovative approaches are emerging that successfully provide high-quality care that supports youth within their family systems. One promising but currently underutilized model is the Patient-Centered Medical Home. The Patient-Centered Medical Home model is well-suited to providing comprehensive adolescent care using an ecological approach[50] by providing the needed time, personnel, and reimbursement to financially compensate for the intensity of this type of care delivery. The newer model, Health Home, allows more comprehensive preventive measures, other services, and a bundle of payment that is well-suited for family-centered interventions.[51]

Dilemma #2: How Can Primary Care Providers Effectively Assess the Health of the Family and Strength of Parenting Practices?

When assessing an adolescent, standard guidelines recommend having separate time both for the teen and the family, and using well-established questionnaires such as those provided in Guidelines for Adolescent Preventive Services and Bright Futures to guide the interaction.[10,11] Links to these questionnaires are presented in **Table 1**. This provide the parent and the teen with confidentiality.

A complete family assessment is indicated when the concerns presented by an adolescent relate to difficult family situations. Examples may include mental or behavioral problems, chronic illness, or situations when the adolescent's actions affect other family members. Important areas to explore during a family assessment of an adolescent and questions targeting these topics are presented in **Box 1**. These questions are designed to assist primary care providers in identifying problems in family relations. Greater issues across the areas indicate need for referral to family therapy.

Table 1
Links to the Guidelines for Adolescent Preventive Services (GAPS) and Bright Futures Parent and Youth Questionnaires

Questionnaire	For Parents	Youth
GAPS	Parent/Guardian Questionnaire http://www.capefearpediatrics.com/var/m_1/14/14e/3376/522775-parent%20english.pdf	Younger Adolescent Questionnaire http://www.capefearpediatrics.com/var/m_1/14/14e/3376/522781-younger%20adolescent%20english.pdf Middle/Older Adolescent Questionaire http://www.drydenfamilymedicine.com/wp-content/uploads/2013/01/Middle-Older-Ado-Q-3818.pdf
Bright Futures	Previsit Questionnaire for Parents of Early Adolescents http://brightfutures.aap.org/pdfs/Other%203/D.Adol.PQ.OC-EA.Parent.pdf Medical Screening Questionnaire http://brightfutures.aap.org/pdfs/Other%203/D.Adol.MSQ.EA.pdf Supplemental Questionnaire for Parents of Early Adolescents https://brightfutures.aap.org/pdfs/Visit%20Forms%20by%20Age%20110/11-14%20Year/D.Adol.SQ.Parent.OC-EA.pdf	Previsit Questionnaire for Early Adolescents http://brightfutures.aap.org/pdfs/Visit%20Forms%20by%20Age%20110/11-14%20Year/D.Adol.PQ.EA.pdf Supplemental Questionnaire for Early Adolescents https://brightfutures.aap.org/pdfs/Other%203/D.Adol.SQ.Patient.EA.pdf Previsit Questionnaire for Middle/Older Adolescents http://brightfutures.aap.org/pdfs/Other%203/D.Adol.PQ.15-17yr.pdf

Data from Elster AB, Kuznets NJ. Guidelines for adolescent preventive services. Baltimore (MD): American Medical Association; 1994; and Hagan JF, Shaw JS, Duncan PM. Bright futures: guidelines for health supervision of infants, children, and adolescents. Elk Grove Village (IL): American Academy of Pediatrics; 2008.

Dilemma #3: What Information Should Providers Share with Parents Regarding Parenting an Adolescent?

Health care providers can be good references for parenting advice beyond the preschool years. Key information for parents to effectively guide their children during adolescence includes the following:

1. Adolescence is a transition toward independence. Some parents are not aware that this process is a normal part of child development, and may feel threatened by their child's new behaviors.[2]
2. You can be an effective parent. Parenting efficacy may be evaluated by asking, "On a scale of 1 to 10, how effective do you think you could be in parenting your teen?" Be prepared for parents coping with high levels of stress in their own lives. By respectfully listening, validating their concerns, and helping them to reflect on their strengths, a clinician can increase parenting self-efficacy. Useful resources to guide parents on how to improve their communication with their child include:
   • Shoulder to Shoulder parents brochure, downloadable at http://www.hcmc.org/services/AquiParaTiHereforYou/APTTeenParentResources/index.htm,
   • A Parent's Guide to Surviving the Teen Years, available at http://kidshealth.org/parent/growth/growing/adolescence.html, and

---

Box 1
Dimensions of a family assessment and associated questions

Family Cohesion and Support

- Do you have a close (or distant) relationship with your parents and siblings? Can you give me examples of a situation where you have felt in close contact with them?
- Do you feel supported by your family? Why or why not? How?

Family Adaptability and Flexibility

- How do you react when something does not result as you had planned?
- How does your family react when something does not result as you had planned?
- Can you give me an example of something that has been challenging for your family? How did they react?
- What have you tried to address this situation?

Family Communication and Conflict Resolution Strategies

- Could you tell me how you solved a recent problem that you had with your family? (Make sure that they provide a detailed description of the situation, including who said what, how the other responded, how the conflict was solved, and how they felt after the situation)

Parental Supervision and Monitoring

- How do you make sure where and with whom your child is when s/he is not at home?
- How do you know what your child is doing when s/he is not at home?

External Resources

- Have you shared your concerns about your child with others? If so, with whom?
- Do you have other family members or friends to ask for advice and support?
- Are you in touch with your child's school teachers?
- Do you attend religious services? If so, do you know people at your place of worship?

- Communicating with Your Teen, available at http://ohioline.osu.edu/hyg-fact/5000/pdf/5158.pdf.

3. Become your teen's "COACH." Parents need to adjust their parenting practices to meet their children at this new phase of development. One model is the COACH system (**Box 2**). Acting as a coach for their teen, parents can focus on guiding their children toward independence and creating opportunities for them in ways that prepares them for the challenges of becoming an adult. At the same time, parents can gain a different perspective. By asking themselves, "How would I react if I were his coach instead of his parent?", parents can focus on their child's behaviors, rather than in their interpretation of what their child is doing.

Box 2
COACH strategies to facilitate changes in parenting styles

C reate confidence

O bserve

A dvise

C almly let them "play"- experience life

H elp them debrief those experiences

4. Be a good communicator. Parents need to master effective parent–youth communication and successful conflict resolution strategies (see links to previous parent–youth communication resources):
   a. Parents should be reminded that an adolescent's willingness to communicate with them is highly influenced by their ability to establish a context where youth feel free to share.[12] Importantly, this does not mean that parents need to agree with their children, but rather that parents should convey that they are willing to listen to them and will treat their opinions with respect.
   b. Clinicians can help to improve parents' communication skills by explaining to them and role modeling what providers know about the basics of motivational interviewing, including skills of active listening, rolling with resistance, and the concept of empathy.[52]
5. Positive parenting works. Parents need to understand that positive parenting works because it creates an emotional context where kids are more open about their opinions and experiences.[53] In the 2001 article "Raising Teens," Simpson identified the 5 key parenting tasks that are crucial in children's teen years (see summary of core content of the report in **Table 2**).[2] The Positive Parenting Pyramid, developed by Rose Allen, former parent educator at the University of Minnesota Extension Service, is an example of a tool that can help to convey how parents can direct teen behavior through establishing foundational relationships and parenting practices (**Fig. 1**).[54]

Dilemma #4: Can a Clinic Be Youth Friendly and Family Oriented? The Challenge of Confidentiality

Confidentiality is a key aspect of adolescent care delivery. A challenge to integrating parents into adolescent care is navigating confidentiality. Evidence suggests that talking or explaining to parents why teens have the right to confidential care can change the predisposition of 30% of the parents.[55] Thus, explaining to parents why confidentiality is important for teenagers is fundamental. It is also important to offer an intimate space for the parent, and to convey that the provider is also available to support and coach them while they adapt their parenting styles to the new needs of their child's adolescence.

PUTTING IT ALL TOGETHER
Lessons Learned from a Case Study of a Family-Oriented, Youth-Friendly Primary Care Clinic: The Aquí Para Ti (APT) Experience

Aquí Para Ti (APT) is a comprehensive, clinic-based, healthy youth development program that provides medical care, coaching, health education, and referrals for Latino youth (all gender) ages 10 to 24 as well as their families in Minneapolis, Minnesota. APT has been at the forefront of health care service delivery innovation for adolescents since it was founded in 2002. Although it was developed for Latino youth, the overarching model is suitable for other ethnic groups. APT addresses positive youth development, health equity, social determinants of health, and family centeredness. The APT model fulfills all the IOM recommendations to improve Adolescent Care (**Table 3**). This multi–award-winning program is currently leading the way in defining best practices for behaviorally appropriate health care homes, has been favorably reviewed by agencies assessing health care improvements, and has been named an innovative program to address health disparities by the Agency for Healthcare Research and Quality's Health Care Innovations Exchange Program and identified as an Innovative approach to Adolescent Health by the Society of Adolescent Health and Medicine (SAHM). Aqui Para Ti is partially funded by the Eliminating Health Disparities Initiatives Grants (EHDI), from Minnesota Department of Health. Aqui Para Ti was officially certified as a Health Care Home in 2010 by the MN State Certification.

Model of care

The main features of APT include the following.

- Parallel family care: This approach protects youth privacy in a family-centered manner. Family members work together to support the healthy youth development of the child. The approach also honors *familism* (a key Latino value that stresses strong family connections and cohesion) and builds family strengths and skills by addressing parents' mental health and parenting needs.
- Culturally inclusive: APT included key Latino values in the design of the program, and created a bilingual, bicultural team that represents, celebrates, and appreciates the community they serve. Cultural concordance, defined by the IOM as a cultural match between those delivering an intervention and the target population,[12] has shown to improve patient outcomes owing to improved communication, patient satisfaction, adherence to recommendations, and increased self-efficacy owing to identification with the team as role models who reinforce a positive sense of ethnic identity.[56]
- Multidisciplinary team: The special developmental needs of adolescents and their families require diverse talents and skill sets. The clinical team is composed of a family physician, 2 care coordinators/health educators, a school/college connector, and a parent educator. The program has an overall Program Coordinator to manage grants and evaluation, staff, and extra clinical activities. This team creates and sustains connections by simultaneously tackling chronic social, mental, and medical conditions and providing holistic care in 1 location (**Fig. 2**).
- Healthy youth development: The team promotes internal assets and external supports using motivational interviewing techniques[52] to record the adolescent's and parent/guardian's goals, perspectives, and readiness to change.[57]
- Dual approach: Prevention–intervention: By fulfilling unmet social, mental, and medical health needs, and building on the existing strengths of the individuals and their families, the team addresses the needs of vulnerable families, and improves health equity.

APT clinical processes

APT functions as a "clinic within a clinic," delivering care during 3 half-day sessions per week and discussing case management as a team during another half-day session per week. Each care session has between 6 and 8 teens, including 2 new teens per session. Teens or parents can come alone or together. Each initial session begins with a pre-planning huddle where the whole team meets to plan the care for the patients to be seen in that specific session (included new patients). Patient visits last 20 to 30 minutes and usually both the teen and his or her parents attend. During the first visit, parents and youth fill out standardized screening questionnaires.[10]

Clinical processes include the following steps.

1. Prepare parents for this process by explaining to them that confidentiality is not meant to contradict or hinder their parenting, rather but to support them. Importantly, this should be done while both the parent and teen are present. The APT team has developed a bilingual English and Spanish document, the "Confidentiality Mantra," that addresses this topic. A copy of the Mantra is available at: http://thenationalcampaign.org/sites/default/files/resource-primary-download/whatresearch_final.pdf.
2. Screen parents and teens. After reading the "Confidentiality Mantra," separate teens and parents and screen them for mood disorders using both the Guidelines for Adolescent Preventive Services questionnaire[10] and the Beck Inventory,[58] for

Table 2
Basic tasks for parents and strategies to promote them

	1. Love and Connect	2. Monitor And Observe	3. Guide and Limit	4. Model and Consult	5. Provide and Advocate
Task for Parents					
Description	Teens need parents to develop and maintain a relationship with them that offers support and acceptance while accommodating the teen's increasing maturity.	Through a process that involves less supervision and more communication, observation, and networking with other adults, teens need parents who are aware of and let teens know they are aware of their activities, including school performance, work experiences, after-school activities, peer relationships, adult relationships.	Teens need parents to uphold a clear but evolving set of boundaries that maintain important family rules and values but also encourage increased competence and maturity.	Teens need parents to provide ongoing information and support about decision making, values, skills, goals, and interpreting and navigating the larger world by teaching through example and ongoing dialogue.	Teens need parents to not only provide adequate nutrition, clothing, shelter and health care but also a supportive home environment and a network of caring adults.
Strategies for Parents					
	Watch for moments to show affection	Keep track of your teen's whereabouts: WHO they hang out with WHAT they are doing WHERE they are WHEN they will be home	Maintain family rules	Set a good example	Network within the community

Acknowledge good times	Keep in touch with other adults	Communicate expectations	Express personal positions	Make informed decisions about school
Expect increased criticism from your teen	Involve yourself in school events	Choose your battles	Model the kind of adult relationships you would like your teens to have	Make similarly informed decisions about extracurricular activities
Spend time simply listening to your teen	Stay informed about your teens' progress	Use discipline as a goal	Answer teens' questions in ways that are truthful.	Arrange or advocate for preventative health care
Treat each teen as a unique individual	Learn and watch for warning signs	Restrict punishment	Maintain or establish traditions	Identify people and programs to support and inform you as a parent
Appreciate and Acknowledge your teen	Seek guidance if you have concerns	Renegotiate responsibilities and privileges	Support your teen's education and vocational training	
Provide meaningful roles for teen in the family	Monitor your teen's experience		Help your teen get information	
Spend time together	Evaluate the level of change		Give teens opportunities to practice reasoning and decision-making.	
Key Messages for Parents				
Most things about their children's world are changing, but don't let your love be one of them.	Monitor your teen's activities because you still can, and it still counts.	Loosen up, but don't let go.	Parents still matter in the teen years and teens still care.	You can't control your teen's world, but you can add to and subtract from it.

Data from Simpson AR. Raising Teens: a synthesis of research and a foundation for action. Boston (MA): Center for Health Communication, Harvard School of Public Health; 2001. Available at: http://www.hsph.harvard.edu/chc/parenting-project/.

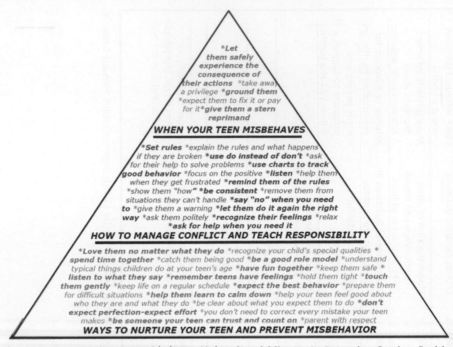

*Let them safely experience the consequence of their actions *take away a privilege *ground them *expect them to fix it or pay for it *give them a stern reprimand

WHEN YOUR TEEN MISBEHAVES

*Set rules *explain the rules and what happens if they are broken *use do instead of don't *ask for their help to solve problems *use charts to track good behavior *focus on the positive *listen *help them when they get frustrated *remind them of the rules *show them "how" *be consistent *remove them from situations they can't handle *say "no" when you need to *give them a warning *let them do it again the right way *ask them politely *recognize their feelings *relax *ask for help when you need it

HOW TO MANAGE CONFLICT AND TEACH RESPONSIBILITY

*Love them no matter what they do *recognize your child's special qualities *spend time together *catch them being good *be a good role model *understand typical things children do at your teen's age *have fun together *keep them safe *listen to what they say *remember teens have feelings *hold them tight *touch them gently *keep life on a regular schedule *expect the best behavior *prepare them for difficult situations *help them learn to calm down *help your teen feel good about who they are and what they do *be clear about what you expect them to do *don't expect perfection-expect effort *you don't need to correct every mistake your teen makes *be someone your teen can trust and count on *parent with respect

WAYS TO NURTURE YOUR TEEN AND PREVENT MISBEHAVIOR

Fig. 1. Teen parenting pyramid. (*From* University of Minnesota Extension Service. Positive parenting of teens: a video-based parent education curriculum. St. Paul (MN): University of Minnesota Extension; 1999.)

screening of depression, on their first visit. Parents are also screened for parenting efficacy and parenting styles on either their second or third visit. Parent and youth complete the questionnaires before the clinical encounter, in separate rooms, to maintain confidentiality.

3. Assess areas of concern for the youth, parents, and provider, which should be organized around the youth's well-being.

4. Counsel youth and parents to help them better understand their health problems by having them work together to prioritize them according to both the teen and family needs.

5. Coach youth and parents by providing them with information, skills, and tools through brief modules based on semistructured scripts and delivered to them by either by one of the team's member.

6. Connect the family with culturally and linguistically appropriate mental health and social services, provide them with referrals to address any unmet needs, and foster personal growth and community connection through different activities.

7. Coordinate the entire plan through weekly case management sessions. In case management, the team designs care plans for new families, taking into consideration the self-identified goals from their visit, determines a risk and need level, and reviews progress for established patients. Care coordination by phone is a crucial element to support the families' success. Families and teens are instructed to call the Program's phone line for troubleshooting problems, make appointments, get transferred to the clinic' nurse if needed, etc. The whole team coordinates 8 AM to 5 PM phone coverage to support their patients' needs during the week. After hours call and weekends are handled by the Clinic ON-Call Physician system.

Table 3
Description of how Aqui para Ti (APT) addresses the Institute of Medicine's (IOM) Adolescent Health Services Delivery Recommendations

IOM Recommendations	APT Innovations & Examples
Focus on the needs of vulnerable adolescents including immigrant populations	Delivers appropriate care for Latino youth and families • Trains providers to use Latino values to guide their approach and interactions • Acknowledge that cultural literacy contributes to trust • Organizes work so that it is family-centered to promote parental skills, well-being, & decision making
Providers must build trust & open communication with adolescents	Provides adolescent-friendly care • Providers are trained in interpersonal skills fostering non-judgmental, respectful communication • They utilize strength-based, youth-guided approach that promotes youth decision-making
Define & train WHAT? to adolescent care competencies	Utilizes an adolescent-focused interdisciplinary team whose members either have skills or experience working with youth or are trained in a defined set of competencies
Prevention, health promotion, and behavioral health should be routine	Utilizes appropriate, standard, screening tools and modularized coaching approaches for health behavior, mental health, and health promoting factors
Protect confidentiality	Assures family-friendly approach to confidentiality
Develop coordinated, linked, & interdisciplinary services for behavioral, reproductive, and mental health	Utilizes case management to coordinate across the health care system and with community resources by: • Referring to vetted behavioral health providers and community agencies • Connecting with schools
Adolescents should have access to care	Screens all youth and families regarding ability to access services & address barriers to care through case management

Data from National Research Council and Institute of Medicine. Adolescent Health Services: Missing Opportunities. Washington, DC: The National Academies Press; 2009.

Using this approach, APT has achieved positive results in teen's overall well-being, mental health, and sexual health. The team tested the model of care with random teen interviews and focus groups with parents. In this evaluation, both parents and youth reported that the APT model was useful to their needs. More information about the APT program and its outcomes is available at http://www.innovations.ahrq.gov/content.aspx?id=2784.

How to Translate the Aquí Para Ti Framework into Your Practice

For providers hoping to move toward a more family-centered approach to adolescent care delivery, the following points are some practical first steps to consider.

Before the clinical visit

1. Identify passionate allies in the clinic that can collaborate with you to build a family-centered adolescent care system. Identify interprofessional staff, including social workers, nurses, and health educators, to work with you to conduct a parallel family visit. If other professionals are not available, make appointments with parents for

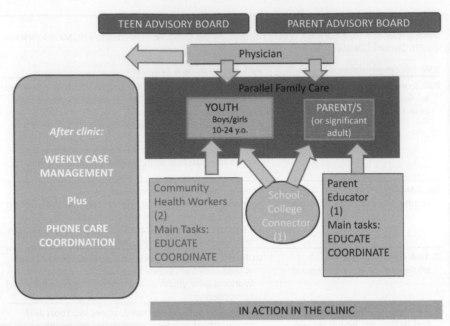

Fig. 2. Aqui Para Ti "Action in clinic" map.

parenting coaching visits. A 30-minute visit can be charged under parenting ICD codes such as "parenting problem" or "parenting stress" on the child's or the parent's insurance. It could be charged under the child's insurance if the teen is present in the clinic, even if the provider spends most of the visit talking only to the parent. The model can be certified as a Patient Centered Medical Home,[50] or as the newer Health Home Model.[51]

2. Find allies outside the clinic: Identify specialists and community agencies that understand the model of care and can complement the approach. Ask internal allies to help identify key individuals at these agencies who can brief your organization about who they are and what they do, and serve as your point person for referrals.

3. Anticipate the practice's needs: It is helpful to have handouts with information that you can give to the parents of teens. Examples of a toolkit can be found on the APT website (see above).

Within the clinical visit

1. Explain confidentiality to parents and youth together as soon as possible during the visit, and establish that this is the way clinicians work with all teens and families. Inform them that this approach allows both teens and parents to receive support from clinicians (or providers).

2. Ideally, assess parents and youth at the same time but in separate rooms using well-established screening questionnaires.[10,11] Providers should review the questionnaire responses and meet with the parent for ≥5 minutes during the initial visit, and then make a plan for follow-up.

3. When providers talk, parents and youth listen. Parents can feel threatened and judged by someone talking to their teens alone. Use motivational interviewing skills when assessing parents.[52] Importantly, parents and families need to be met where they are, and need to feel welcomed and listened to by their health care providers. Keep in mind that, to provide optimal care for youth, both parents

and adolescents need to be the targets of your care and compassion to the same degree.
4. First, do not harm. If clinicians are encouraging parents and their teen to discuss a problem together, help them to set ground rules to ensure that the conversation is safe and useful for everyone:
   a. Constructive comments only
   b. Active listening
   c. No name calling allowed
   d. No embarrassing stories
5. If a teen comes for a visit alone, assess the parent and adolescent relationship and encourage them to tell parents what they talked about during that appointment. For example, say "The fact that I am not going to tell your parents does not mean that you shouldn't." Remember that it is possible to provide family-centered care even when working with only 1 family member.

SUMMARY

There is an increased recognition for the need to create approaches to care delivery for adolescents that are both family centered and youth friendly to improve youth and family outcomes.[10–12]

Primary care providers are in a unique position to strengthen and support parents by delivering evidence-based messages regarding best practices for parenting adolescents. Providers can help parents to successfully maintain balance for themselves and their family by providing empathy, guidance, and support during the sometimes stressful transition of adolescence. Working on parenting is a leverage point in the community; it creates the social capital to raise other children in the household in a positive way and it creates mentors in our neighborhoods who can provide support for other parents and teens in the community.

With intentional planning, providers can become proficient in coaching parents, and foster positive outcomes by working in an integrated, family-centered manner. This article includes guidelines and recommendations that can increase primary care provider's skills and self-efficacy in delivering family-centered adolescent care, while highlighting why adolescent service delivery is a critical priority for primary care.

REFERENCES

1. D'Angelo SL, Omar HA. Parenting adolescents. Int J Adolesc Med Health 2003; 15:11–9.
2. Simpson AR. Raising Teens: a synthesis of research and a foundation for action. Boston (MA): Center for Health Communication, Harvard School of Public Health; 2001. Available at: http://www.hsph.harvard.edu/chc/parenting-project/.
3. Resnick MD, Bearman PS, Blum RW, et al. Protecting adolescents from harm: findings from the National Longitudinal Study on Adolescent Health. JAMA 1997;278:823–32.
4. Resnick MD, Harris LJ, Blum RW. The impact of caring and connectedness on adolescent health and well-being. J Paediatr Child Health 1993;29(Suppl 1): S3–9.
5. Youngblade LM, Theokas C, Schulenberg J, et al. Risk and promotive factors in families, schools, and communities: a contextual model of positive youth development in adolescence. Pediatrics 2007;119(S1):S47–53.
6. Blum RW. Improving the health of youth: a community health perspective. J Adolesc Health 1998;23:254–8.

7. Steinberg L. We know some things: parent–adolescent relationships in retrospect and prospect. J Res Adolesc 2001;11:1–19.
8. Rees RV, Howard K. The parenting gap. Washington, DC: Center on Children and Families at Brookings Institution; 2013.
9. Carnegie Council on Adolescent Development. Great transitions: preparing adolescents for a new century. New York: Carnegie Corporation of New York; 1995.
10. Elster AB, Kuznets NJ. Guidelines for adolescent preventive services. Baltimore (MD): American Medical Association; 1994.
11. Hagan JF, Shaw JS, Duncan PM. Bright futures: guidelines for health supervision of infants, children, and adolescents. Elk Grove Village (IL): American Academy of Pediatrics; 2008.
12. National Research Council and Institute of Medicine. Adolescent health services: missing opportunities. Washington, DC: The National Academies Press; 2009.
13. Collins WA. Parents' cognitions and developmental changes in relationships during adolescence. In: Sigel IE, McGillicuddy-DeLisi A, Goodnow JJ, editors. Parental belief systems: the psychological consequences for children. 2nd edition. Hillsdale (NJ): Lawrence Erlbaum Associates; 2002. p. 175–97.
14. Blum RW. Positive youth development: reducing risk, and improving health. Geneva (Switzerland): World Health Organization; 1999.
15. Albert B. With one voice 2007: America's adults and teens sound off about teen pregnancy. Washington, DC: National Campaign to Prevent Teen and Unplanned Pregnancy; 2007.
16. Van Ryzin MJ, Fosco GM, Dishion TJ. Family and peer predictors of substance use from early adolescence to early adulthood: an 11-year prospective analysis. Addict Behav 2012;37:1314–24.
17. Trudeau L, Mason WA, Randall GK, et al. Effects of parenting and deviant peers on early to mid-adolescent conduct problems. J Abnorm Child Psychol 2012;40: 1249–64.
18. Steinberg L, Lamborn SD, Dornbusch SM, et al. Impact of parenting practices on adolescent achievement: authoritative parenting, school involvement, and encouragement to succeed. Child Dev 1992;63:1266–81.
19. Allen M, Svetaz MV, Hardeman R, et al. What research tells us about Latino parenting practices and their relationship to youth sexual behavior. Washington, DC: The National Campaign to Prevent Teen and Unplanned Pregnancy; 2008.
20. Hill KG, Hawkins JD, Catalano RF, et al. Family influences on the risk of daily smoking initiation. J Adolesc Health 2005;37:202–10.
21. Cislak A, Safron M, Pratt M, et al. Family-related predictors of body weight and weight-related behaviours among children and adolescents: a systematic umbrella review. Child Care Health Dev 2012;38:321–31.
22. Berge JM, Saelens BE. Familial influences on adolescents' eating and physical activity behaviors. Adolesc Med State Art Rev 2012;23:424–39.
23. Clark MS, Jansen KL, Cloy JA. Treatment of childhood and adolescent depression. Am Fam Physician 2012;86:442–8.
24. Bhatia SK, Bhatia SC. Childhood and adolescent depression. Am Fam Physician 2007;75:73–80.
25. Rueger SY, Malecki CK, Demaray MK. Relationship between multiple sources of perceived social support and psychological and academic adjustment in early adolescence: comparisons across gender. J Youth Adolesc 2010;39:47–61.
26. Barnes GM, Hoffman JH, Welte JW, et al. Effects of parental monitoring and peer deviance on substance use and delinquency. J Marriage Fam 2006;68:1084–104.

27. Chung HL, Steinberg L. Relations between neighborhood factors, parenting behaviors, peer deviance, and delinquency among serious juvenile offenders. Dev Psychol 2006;42:319–31.
28. Simons GL, Conger R. Linking mother–father differences in parenting to a typology of family parenting styles and adolescent outcomes. J Fam Issues 2007;28:212–41.
29. McKinney C, Renk K. Differential parenting between mothers and fathers implications for late adolescents. J Fam Issues 2008;29:806–27.
30. Kumpfer KL, Alvarado R. Family-strengthening approaches for the prevention of youth problem behaviors. Am Psychol 2003;56:457–65.
31. Center for Substance Abuse Prevention. The national cross-site evaluation of high risk youth programs: final report. Rockville (MD): Substance Abuse and Mental Health Services Administration; 2000.
32. Kerr M, Stattin H. What parents know, how they know it, and several forms of adolescent adjustment: further support for a reinterpretation of goring. Dev Psychol 2000;36:366–80.
33. Stattin H, Kerr M. Parental monitoring: a reinterpretation. Child Dev 2000;71:1072–85.
34. Olson DH, Russell CS, Sprenkle DH. Circumplex model: systemic assessment and treatment of families. Binghamton (NY): The Haworth Press; 1989.
35. Scabini E, Manzi C. Family processes and identity. In: Schwartz SJ, Luyckx K, Vignoles VL, editors. Handbook of identity theory and research. New York: Springer; 2011. p. 565–84.
36. Cunha AI, Relvas AP, Soares I. Anorexia nervosa and family relationships: perceived family functioning, coping strategies, beliefs, and attachment to parents and peers. Int J Clin Health Psychol 2009;9:229–40.
37. Mayseless O, Scharf M. Too close for comfort: inadequate boundaries with parents and individuation in late adolescent girls. Am J Orthop 2009;79:191–202.
38. Marsiglia FF, Kulis S, Parsai M, et al. Cohesion and conflict: family influences on adolescent alcohol use in immigrant Latino families. J Ethn Subst Abuse 2009;8:400–12.
39. Shumow L, Lomax R. Parental efficacy: predictor of parenting behavior and adolescent outcomes. Parenting: Science Practice 2002;2:127–50.
40. Coleman PK, Karraker KH. Self-efficacy and parenting quality: findings and future applications. Dev Rev 1997;18:47–85.
41. Small SA, Eastman G. Rearing adolescents in contemporary society: a conceptual framework for understanding the responsibilities and needs of parents. Fam Relat 1991;40:455–62.
42. Viner RM, Ozer EM, Denny S, et al. Adolescence and the social determinants of health. Lancet 2012;379:1641–52.
43. Sawyer SM, Afifi RA, Bearinger LH, et al. Adolescence: a foundation for future health. Lancet 2012;379:1630–40.
44. Beyers JM, Bates JE, Pettit GS, et al. Neighborhood structure, parenting processes, and the development of youths' externalizing behaviors: a multilevel analysis. Am J Community Psychol 2003;31:35–53.
45. Gorman-Smith D, Tolan PH, Henry DB, et al. Patterns of family functioning and adolescent outcomes among urban African American and Mexican American families. J Fam Psychol 2000;14:436–57.
46. Marmot M, Wilkinson R. Social determinants of health. 2nd edition. Oxford (England): Oxford University Press; 2005.

47. Clinton M, Lunney P, Edwards H, et al. Perceived social support and community adaptation in schizophrenia. J Adv Nurs 1998;27:955–65.
48. Izzo C, Weiss L, Shanahan T, et al. Parental self-efficacy and social support as predictors of parenting practices and children's socio-emotional adjustment in Mexican immigrant families. Journal of Prevention & Intervention in the Community 2000;20:197–213.
49. Barkley L, Kodjo C, West KJ, et al. Promoting equity and reducing health disparities among racially/ethnically diverse adolescents: a position paper of the Society for Adolescent Health and Medicine. J Adolesc Health 2013;52: e804–7.
50. Walker I, McManus MA, Fox HB. Medical home innovations: where do adolescents fit? The National Alliance to Advance Adolescent Health. Report number (7); December 2011. Available at: http://www.thenationalalliance.org/pdfs/Report7.%20Medical%20Home%20Innovations.pdf.
51. Centers for Medicare & Medicaid Services. 2014. Available at: http://www.medicaid.gov/Medicaid-CHIP-Program-Information/By-Topics/Long-Term-Services-and-Support/Integrating-Care/Health-Homes/Health-Homes.html. Accessed March 28, 2014.
52. Miller WR, Rollnick S. Motivational interviewing: helping people change. New York: Guilford Publications; 2013.
53. Steinberg L. The family at adolescence: transition and transformation. J Adolesc Health 2000;27:170–8.
54. University of Minnesota Extension Service. Positive parenting of teens: a video-based parent education curriculum. St. Paul (MN): University of Minnesota Extension; 1999.
55. Hutchinson JW, Stafford EM. Changing parental opinions about teen privacy through education. Pediatrics 2005;116:966–71.
56. Cooper LA, Powe NR. Disparities in patient experiences, healthcare processes, and outcomes: the role of patient-provider racial, ethnic and language concordance. New York: The Commonwealth Fund (Publication #753); 2004.
57. Rubak S, Sandbæk A, Lauritzen T, et al. Motivational interviewing: a systematic review and meta-analysis. Br J Gen Pract 2005;55:305–12.
58. Beck AT, Steer RA, Carbin MG. Psychometric properties of the Beck Depression Inventory: twenty-five years of evaluation. Clin Psychol Rev 1988;8:77–100.

Education

Primary Care for Adolescents with Developmental Disabilities

Clarissa Calliope Kripke, MD

KEYWORDS

- Developmental disability • Intellectual disability • Interdisciplinary care • Transition
- Youth with special health care needs • Adolescent health • Primary care

KEY POINTS

- Disability is not a trait or characteristic, but a lack of ability to participate fully in society because of the interaction between a persons' functional limitations and the social and physical environment.
- The Americans with Disabilities Act requires health care professionals to ensure access to health care.
- To assist with transition planning, speech, occupational therapy, physical therapy, and neuropsychiatric assessments can help determine strengths and challenges.
- Communication is a basic right that can be enhanced with adaptive technology, support, and appropriate examination room etiquette.

INTRODUCTION
Definition of Developmental Disability

Disability is the inability to exert control and choice over one's life, and to fully participate in and contribute to community. The ability of people to participate fully depends on the interaction between their functional limitations and the social and physical environment in which they live. Environments can be more or less enabling. For example, a student with a learning disability can access the general curriculum if the room has few distractions and the teacher explains instructions verbally. The same student might fail to achieve their potential without those accommodations. Reducing disability can be achieved through improving function or through better adapting the social and physical environment. A developmental disability is a disability that is present during the developmental period when the brain is forming. Because the disability is present during the developmental period, the experience usually shapes part of that person's identity.

Disclosures: None.
Family and Community Medicine, University of California, San Francisco, 500 Parnassus Avenue, MU3E, Box 0900, San Francisco, CA 94143-0900, USA
E-mail address: kripkec@fcm.ucsf.edu

Prim Care Clin Office Pract 41 (2014) 507–518
http://dx.doi.org/10.1016/j.pop.2014.05.005
0095-4543/14/$ – see front matter © 2014 Elsevier Inc. All rights reserved.

There are no specific traits or characteristics that define developmental disability. All people are mixtures of strengths and weaknesses. However, administrative definitions of developmental disability have been developed to define who is eligible for services and supports. Administrative definitions are often based on criteria that describe functional limitations. Other administrative definitions rely on diagnostic labels such as autism, cerebral palsy, and epilepsy. These conditions are not always disabling. People with those diagnoses have a wide range of functional abilities (**Box 1**). More information and resources on care for people with developmental disabilities are available on the Office of Developmental Primary Care websites: http://odpc.ucsf.edu.

Barriers to Accessing Care

Barriers to accessing health care can be physical, financial, or programmatic.[2,3] Physical barriers to medical care include waiting rooms and examination rooms that cannot accommodate wheelchairs and caregivers; bathrooms that are not accessible; or examination tables, scales, or diagnostic equipment that is not fully accessible. Appropriate equipment is needed to ensure physical accessibility, especially when children become too heavy to lift. Many medical practices do not meet the minimum standards for accessibility under the Americans with Disabilities Act. The US Department of Justice has issued guidelines for access to medical care for individuals with mobility disabilities.[4] During adolescence, to facilitate care, people with physical disabilities may also need assessment for home modifications.

Although the Affordable Care Act will reduce financial barriers to care for adolescents with disabilities, many families caring for children with disabilities struggle financially.[5] Families living in states with higher income inequality have higher family financial burdens for funding the health care of children with special health care needs.[6]

Box 1
Federal definition of developmental disability

According to the Developmental Disabilities Assistance and Bill of Rights Act of 2000, a developmental disability is a severe, chronic disability of an individual that:

1. Is attributable to a mental or physical impairment or combination of mental and physical impairments

2. Is manifested before the individual attains the age of 22 years

3. Is likely to continue indefinitely

4. Results in substantial functional limitations in 3 or more of the following areas of major life activity:

5. Self-care

6. Receptive and expressive language

7. Learning

8. Mobility

9. Self-direction

10. Capacity for independent living

11. Economic self-sufficiency

12. Reflects the individual's need for a combination and sequence of special, interdisciplinary, or generic services, individualized supports, or other forms of assistance that are of lifelong or extended duration and are individually planned and coordinated[1]

Programmatic barriers to care include lack of sign language interpreters or print materials available in alternative formats, and inadequate appointment lengths. Programmatic barriers also include lack of training for clinicians and a lack of care coordination. Barriers to care can be reduced through the development of primary care practices that meet the characteristics of patient-centered medical homes.[7] Such practices emphasize coordination with specialty care as well as school-based services, government and community agencies, and adult specialists.[8,9]

Interdisciplinary Team

Health care for people with developmental disabilities requires interdisciplinary, team-based care. Although parents play a central role in their children's care, the role of parents must shift as children reach adolescence. Reaching adolescence should prompt a review of the team membership, roles, and structure. For adolescents who have the capacity to assume more responsibility for managing their own health care needs, a plan should be developed to gradually transfer responsibility from parent to child. Free, online training is available for patients and physicians at http://www.healthytransitionsny.org/.[10] This resource includes videos to model appropriate examination room etiquette and communication about transition topics.

For patients who will continue to require support, parents may intend to continue to be involved in their children's care after their children become adults. However, most children will outlive their parents' capacity to provide support. Therefore it is important for patients to learn to direct and receive some of their support from personal assistants, other family members, friends, and supporters. This approach broadens the circle of support, the number of people with knowledge and expertise about the patient's medical care, and enables the patient to develop healthy independence.

Transition to health care providers who serve adults is best accomplished gradually. Pediatric doctors can ensure a smooth transition by developing a medical summary, calling receiving doctors, and making themselves available for consultation or to comanage care for a period of time.

Examination Room Etiquette

Patients and caregivers are the best sources of information about etiquette. **Box 2** provides some general guidelines. More information can be found on the Office of Developmental Primary Care Web site: http://odpc.ucsf.edu.

Box 2
Examination room etiquette

Assume competence

Ask how your patient communicates best

Speak directly to your patient with a normal adult tone

Wait quietly and expectantly for a response

Do not pretend to understand; check for understanding

Treat assistive devices as personal space

Ask before assisting

Identify yourself to people with visual impairments

Respect privacy

Ensure access to health care

ASSESSMENT
Diagnostic Assessment

In preparation for transition planning, consider repeat diagnostic evaluations and assessments. Knowledge of genetics is rapidly evolving. If the patient has dysmorphic features that suggest a genetic condition, and does not have a diagnosis or a recent evaluation, a referral for genetic consultation is indicated. There is a range in how genetic traits are expressed in individuals. Genetics alone do not determine a person's potential. Likewise diagnostic labels do not describe an individual's strengths, aspirations, or abilities. Genetic and diagnostic information can help connect patients, caregivers, and clinicians to information and support. It can help clinicians identify risks for associated medical problems.

Also, consider repeat physical, speech, and occupational therapy assessments at least every few years. Separate speech assessments may be required for dysphagia and for communication. Neuropsychological, educational, and vocational testing may also be beneficial. Repeating assessments that were done at younger ages is important because some patients improve because of learning adaptive skills, medical interventions, or maturity. This improvement can lead to fewer functional limitations. Others may lose function because of neurodegenerative conditions, injury, arthritis, medical complications, chronic stress, or medication side effects. For patients in the special education system, some of this testing may be requested through the school system. Copies of these assessments should be placed in the medical chart. They are critically important descriptions of the patient's baseline function. Without that information, it can be difficult to make diagnoses in the future, such as for dementia or a slow decline in range of motion or mobility. In addition to school assessments that are focused on helping students access the general curriculum, consider independent assessments that explore a broader range of life and adaptive skills (**Table 1**).

Developing Strengths

By the time people are adolescents, the developmental trajectory is usually clearer than it is in young children. Although the focus of early intervention is often remediating deficits, it is important to recognize that all people also have strengths. Equal emphasis should be on identifying and developing areas of relative strength. All people need opportunities to develop loving relationships, learn new skills, and make a contribution to their families and communities. Adolescents need experiences of success. They also need opportunities to try, fail, and be exposed to the natural consequences.

Adaptive Behavior

Assessments should focus on the conceptual, social, and practical skills that people use in everyday life. Practical skills should include basic and instrumental activities of daily living for work, partnering with health care professionals and personal care staff, decision making, stress management, using transportation, keeping routines and schedules, managing money, and using technology and adaptive equipment.[11]

Communication

The right to communicate is fundamental and it is the foundation of effective patient care. All people communicate and all behavior is communication. Adolescents can be nonverbal, have speech that is hard to understand, or periodically lose speech. They may benefit from adaptive equipment such as voice output devices, letter boards, visual supports, or alternative communication strategies. If this has not

Table 1
Documentation of baseline function

	Domain	Notes
Cognitive	Language, literacy, financial management, sense of time, self-direction, memory, attention, learning style, problem solving, ability to follow rules, abstraction, social skills, and naiveté	Include special education or neuropsychiatric assessments
Neuromuscular	Gait, movement disorder, tone, posture, range of motion, swallow, fine and gross motor control	Patients or physicians can take video footage for documentation. Physical therapists, occupational therapists, speech therapists, neurologists, and orthopedists can do detailed assessments if needed
Seizure	Seizure type, length, and frequency	Any stereotyped behavior or emotion lasting less than 3 min can be seizure
Sensory	Hearing and vision testing; sensory integration and processing; sensitivity to lights, sounds, smells, touch, or foods	Note the patient's typical behaviors when in pain and tips for gaining cooperation with physical examination
Mental health/behavior	Disposition; regulating and triggering stimuli; signs of distress; mental health diagnoses	Note strategies for preventing and managing meltdowns or shutdowns and improving cooperation

been thoroughly explored, it is important to do so while school resources are available for support.

For clinicians who wish to improve their skills, short video clips modeling communication with nonverbal patients are available via iColleague in the MedEd Portal under Mock Clinical Interviews with Nonverbal Standardized Patients. https://www.mededportal.org/icollaborative/resource/904.

ESTABLISHING GOALS OF CARE

Even when healthy, adolescents with developmental disabilities have traits and characteristics that are outside the statistical norm. Everyone has their own balance, even if it is atypical. Strategies to help people be more compliant, behave more normally, or function more independently are not always the best strategies to help patients achieve their own potential. Sometimes people with disabilities thrive when they find alternative ways to function, interdependent relationships, and when they accept help. Accepting help with weaknesses or deficits can allow more energy to develop strengths and special interests. For example, a person may be able to walk, but keep up with their friends better and have less pain when they use a wheelchair. Another may prefer to take an extra class in computer science than to spend elective time in speech therapy to work on producing clearer speech. Adolescents can define for themselves what strategies work best for them, and their own goals and priorities.

TRANSITION PLANNING (PATIENT CENTERED)

The American Academy of Pediatrics, American Academy of Family Physicians, and American College of Physicians have developed protocols and guidance for planning health care transitions.[12] The process starts at age 12 to 13 years and continues until the transition to an adult-focused medical system is complete.[7] Transferring care to adult-oriented clinicians is a process rather than an event, and should involve preparation and communication.

Medical Summary

Transferring key medical and educational records is critical. For people with complex disabilities, by the time they reach adulthood, their records are often too voluminous to be of clinical use. A key component of the transition process is the development of a comprehensive medical summary by the primary care doctor who knows the patient best. In addition to detailed information about baseline function, this summary should include information about the patient's support services, education, and care providers with contact information. It should also include information about all therapeutic trials. It is important to include the ones that were successful and the ones that failed. This information can be critical to diagnosing new symptoms in the future, especially if the patient is unable to give a comprehensive history and family is no longer available to supplement it.

Health Passport

A health passport is a portable record developed and maintained by the patient and caregiver with key clinical and care information. It is important information for caregivers and clinicians. A health passport includes information regarding communication, power of attorney or supporters, diagnoses, medications, allergies, and tips for care (**Box 3**).

Documentation

For adolescents with cognitive or communication disabilities, caregivers play a critical role in recognizing illness, reporting signs and symptoms, and monitoring and implementing health care plans. Parents usually recognize when their children are not

---

Box 3
Tips for care

- How to administer medications
- Feeding plans
- Calming strategies
- Methods to help cope with procedures
- Clues for recognizing pain
- Instructions for transfer or assisting with mobility
- Dressing
- Assisting with hygiene
- Avoiding sensitivities
- Ways to prevent boredom
- Ways to facilitate follow-up

functioning at their baseline. Paid caregivers are less familiar with the patient, and therefore may not always recognize these differences. When the child is diagnosed, parents typically receive training in how to support their children with disabilities. When case workers, professional caregivers, or other relatives assume responsibility, they also need training. Also, as adolescents spend less time with parents, important signs and symptoms can go unrecognized. Documentation systems need to be created to track vital signs, weight, bowel movements, seizures, food intake, menstruation, blood sugars, medication administration, and behaviors. Forms for this purpose as well as other resources are available on the Web site of the Office of Developmental Primary Care (http://odpc.ucsf.edu). Caregivers need clear protocols for when to call a doctor for any change in behavior or function. As adolescents develop more independence from parents, some may assume more responsibility for maintaining documentation.

Maximizing Social Environment

All people thrive in environments in which they are accepted as valued members of the community, and when their communication is acknowledged and supported. It is important to avoid dehumanizing language that suggests that the lives of people with disabilities are less meaningful or that they are less capable of directing their lives or making an important contribution. Words such as unfortunate, suffering, burden, tragic, dependent, and bound suggest that people with disability inherently have a poor quality of life and lack agency.[13] Praising someone for being brave or inspirational merely for being disabled is also a form of low expectations.

Sometimes parents have difficulty accepting their child's disability. Clinicians can help keep the focus on practical problem solving. Physicians can help parents to appreciate their children by celebrating personal accomplishments; helping to interpret behavior positively and developmentally; and modeling comfortable, respectful communication. Any discussion of a child's challenges can start with a review of the child's strengths. It is also helpful to assess the unmet needs of parents and other caregivers. Parents can be encouraged to pursue their own relationships and interests, and can be referred to resources for respite so they can attend to their own well-being. More information on cultural competence when working with people with disabilities can be found on the Office of Developmental Primary Care Web site (http://odpc.ucsf.edu).

Maximizing Physical Environment

Most people are familiar with adaptations to the built environment for people with mobility disorders. These adaptations include things like ramps, automatic doors, and curb cuts. However, other aspects of the physical environment also affect function. For example, helpful environmental supports include signage and other visual supports, lists, instructions, calendars; emergency signals; organization of the physical space, and reduction of visual distractions. The sensory environment can also be more or less enabling. Many people have sensitivities to scents and certain types of lighting and sounds. Reducing high-contrast lighting, strobes, alarms, televisions, and fluorescents can make a medical environment more comfortable.

Improving Function-building Life Skills

Adolescents with developmental disabilities may need to be explicitly taught life skills that other children acquire without specific instruction. Functional life-skill training is often neglected in more academically oriented special education. However, these skills can be as important for successful adulthood as earning an academic degree.

Children enrolled in special education services are entitled to receive services until they receive a diploma or the end of the school year after their 21st birthday. If they are included in an individualized education program, special educators can help prepare adolescents for adult life or can help parents develop a life-skills training program.[14] Components of a comprehensive training plan are listed in **Box 4**.

Self-determination

Adolescents with disabilities should be supported to participate in meetings in which issues that concern them are addressed. They should also be educated about citizenship and their right to vote. A transition plan can include voter registration. Because people with disabilities are disproportionately affected by government policy decisions, it is important to exercise their right to participate in the political process. Self Advocates Becoming Empowered has a tool kit for providing this education for people with cognitive disabilities.[15] Participation in youth leadership and self-advocacy activities can help build these critical skills.[16]

Also, adolescents should participate in informed consent decisions. Capacity to make an informed consent decision should be assessed for each decision. Capacity can fluctuate. Not all decisions require the same cognitive ability. Informed consent requires a person to understand the options, the risks, and benefits of each, weigh them against each other and communicate a choice. Patients should receive support such as plain language explanations, pictures, videos, or demonstrations. Many people who do not have the capacity to make a specific decision can still contribute information about values and priorities, and these should be considered. Some people who do not have the capacity to make an informed consent decision do have the capacity to select someone to serve as power of attorney.

Prevention of Abuse and Neglect

People with disabilities need skills to resist and protest, lest they become easy targets for abuse. This requirement is important regardless of the adolescent's support needs or functional limitations. For people with cognitive and communication challenges, it is important to teach students a method for communicating when they are being mistreated. Adolescents with disabilities should be encouraged to set boundaries; make choices; and spend time alone with peers and away from parents, teachers, and other authority figures. Clinicians should inquire about abuse and neglect during

---

Box 4
Developing skills

Academic skills

Activities of daily living

Assistive and adaptive devices

Communication

Functional life skills

Healthy lifestyle

Self-advocacy

Self-care

Social skills

Vocational skills

appointments, and be alert to the possibility when a patient is having difficulty. For any suspected or reported abuse, the accused should be separated from the patient during the investigation. All complaints should be followed up.

Bullying

Bullying of people with disabilities is more common than in the general population.[17] The US Department of Education finds that bullying of a student with a disability that results in the student not receiving meaningful education benefits constitutes a denial of their rights to free, appropriate public education. Schools are directed to take a variety of actions to address and prevent bullying.[18] If students use communication aids, vocabulary about bullying should be included. It is also important to teach and support students to set personal boundaries, including retaining control of assistive devices, maintaining personal space, and limiting touch.

Isolation/Seclusion

Peers can bully, but so can parents, teachers, caregivers, and professionals. Bullying from authority figures can include isolation and seclusion, exclusion, aversive therapies, physical or chemical restraint, and derogatory language.

NAVIGATING PUBERTY
Changing Roles

At the age of majority, adolescents assume legal responsibility for making their own health care decisions and control release of information protected by the Health Insurance Portability and Accountability Act. An Advanced directive and health care power of attorney should be discussed. To ensure continuity, it is helpful to have these conversations before the age of majority. Guardianship and conservatorship are legal proceedings available in most states for people who have cognitive disabilities. They are often unnecessary if supports are in place for decision making and/or if the patient has a valid power of attorney for health care and representative payee or financial trustee to assist with finances. Clinicians can provide paperwork for a health care power of attorney. For more complete planning, referrals can be made to case workers and estate lawyers with expertise in disability.

Family Adjustment: Acceptance

When children are young, their developmental trajectories are often unclear. Some parents go through a process of grieving for a child they hoped for and did not have. Others pursue treatments they hope will lead to a cure. Parents are often unaware of how expressing their disappointment about missed expectations can affect the self-esteem of their children. Even nonverbal children are sensitive to these messages from their parents. Focusing on deficits and weaknesses can distract from appreciating the positive qualities of their children, and their unique perspective and experience. Clinicians can help by pointing out growth, progress, accomplishments, and positive characteristics and by taking the time to genuinely enjoy their interactions with their patients. Clinicians can refer parents to their local parent training and information center for support (http://www.parentcenterhub.org/find-your-center/). Like all adolescents, youth with disabilities benefit from opportunities to make a contribution to family and community through chores, volunteer work, or employment.

Sexuality

People with disabilities can and often do have sex. Individual education programs can include goals for health and sexuality education. Many adolescents with cognitive disabilities benefit from explicit education about the unwritten social rules of negotiating sexual relationships.[19] Youth also need explicit explanations of the laws and social rules of sexual activity. Adolescents with disabilities who require support to access medical care still need confidential care. Like all adolescents, privacy and confidentiality are critical for discussions of gender and sexual identity, sexuality, prevention of sexually transmitted infection, and pregnancy.

Rates of sexual abuse are high in the population. People with disabilities are often taught to comply with authority. However, youth also need skills to protest and resist authority when appropriate. This skill is important for preventing and identifying abuse.

Accessing Service Systems

Some patients' needs have been met primarily by the school district or other programs accessible to children, but not to adults. If the patient is or will become eligible for public benefits or programs, it is helpful to start the process of applying for these programs early, because this helps to avoid disruption in needed services. Families are often unprepared for the decrease in the level of support they receive that usually accompanies graduation from school.

Person-centered Planning

Person-centered planning is an ongoing process of helping people with disabilities plan for their future. Person-centered planning is a team process in which people come together to support a person with a disability to develop relationships, participate in community, and increase their control over their lives. It is a structured planning process that starts with a personal profile; shares visions for the future; and develops plans, services, and supports to achieve the goals. Many tools to structure this process are available online.[20] Person-centered planning teams benefit from a case coordinator or social worker with expertise in public health insurance programs, Department of Rehabilitation, Department of Developmental Services, Department of Housing and Urban Development, and Social Security programs.

MONITORING HEALTH AND SAFETY
Care Management

Many adolescents with disabilities benefit from care management services. These services are sometimes available through the state Department of Developmental Services, patient-centered medical homes, or health plans. Parents and guardians typically do a lot to coordinate care for their children, but still benefit from working with people with expertise in transition planning.

Circles of Support

Circles of support are informal support networks such as family, friends, and community members who share responsibility for access, inclusion, and support of a disabled person. Adolescence is a good time to discuss expanding and engaging circles of support. Siblings sometimes take on a greater role in providing support.

Crisis Intervention

Families can become overwhelmed with the needs of adolescents in crisis. For adolescents with challenging behavior, parents may need access to respite or crisis homes, training in behavior modification techniques, or assistance with diagnosing the cause of the patient's distress. Unrecognized medical problems and pain are a common cause of challenging behavior. Physicians should maintain lists of local resources. To find local resources, every state has federally funded parent centers that offer training information and assistance to families of children with disabilities.[21]

Estate Planning

Parents may want to consult an estate attorney with expertise in disability. Giving or leaving money to support a child with a disability can inadvertently make them ineligible for government programs that their children need. With careful financial planning, even small amounts of financial support can improve the lives of people with disabilities. Organizations such as the Special Needs Alliance and the Arc of the United States can provide guidance to families developing plans for long-term care.[22,23]

SUMMARY

Helping adolescents with disabilities to develop the skills and supports to direct their own lives ensures better quality of life in adulthood. Wellness is more than being free of illness; it is being in balance, participating, and being included in all aspects of life. Health professionals have a lot of influence over the lives of people with developmental disabilities. They have a key role in helping people get access to medical care and adaptive technology. They also have a role in determining access to education, employment, transportation, housing, services, supports, assistive equipment, adaptive technology, and public benefits. In many situations they have a key role in ensuring the opportunity for their patients to make decisions and form and maintain relationships. Systematic assessment and planning processes can improve quality of life as adolescents transition from child-oriented to adult-oriented services.

ACKNOWLEDGMENTS

I thank Special Hope Foundation for supporting this work.

REFERENCES

1. Title I, Subtitle A. Sec. 102. Definitions. [42 USC 15002] 8. Available at: http://www.acl.gov/Programs/AIDD/DDA_BOR_ACT_2000/p2_tl_subtitleA.aspx. Accessed November 6, 2013.
2. The National Council on Disability. The current state of health care for people with disabilities. Washington, DC: 2009. Available at: http://www.ncd.gov/publications/2009/Sept302009. Accessed November 6, 2013.
3. Reis J, Breslin M, Iezzoni L, et al. It takes more than ramps to solve the crisis of healthcare for people with disabilities. Chicago: Rehabilitation Institute of Chicago; 2004. Available at: www.tvworldwide.com/events/hhs/041206/PPT/RIC_whitepaperfinal82704.pdf. Accessed November 6, 2013.
4. US Department of Justice. Access to medical care for individuals with mobility disabilities. Washington, DC: 2010. Available at: http://www.ada.gov/medcare_mobility_ta/medcare_ta.htm. Accessed November 6, 2013.
5. Ne'eman A. The Affordable Care Act and the I/DD community: an overview of the law and advocacy priorities going forward. Washington, DC: Autistic Self Advocacy Network; 2013. Available at: http://autisticadvocacy.org/wp-content/uploads/2013/09/ACA-ASAN-policy-brief.pdf. Accessed November 6, 2013.
6. Parish S, Rose R, Dababnah S, et al. State-level income inequality and family burden of U.S. families raising children with special health care needs. Soc Sci Med 2012;74:399–407.

7. National Center for Medical Home Implementation. [homepage on the Internet]. Elk Grove Village (IL). Available at: http://www.medicalhomeinfo.org/. Accessed December 27, 2013.

8. American Academy of Pediatrics, American Academy of Family Physicians, American College of Physicians, Transitions Clinical Report Authoring Group. Supporting the health care transition from adolescence to adulthood in the medical home. Pediatrics 2011;128:182–200. Available at: http://pediatrics.aappublications.org/content/early/2011/06/23/peds.2011-0969. Accessed December 20, 2013.

9. Institute of Medicine. The future of disability in America. Washington, DC: The National Academies Press; 2007. Available at: http://www.iom.edu/Reports/2007/The-Future-of-Disability-in-America.aspx. Accessed June 21, 2014.

10. Healthy Transitions. Moving from pediatric to adult health care. [homepage on the Internet]. Available at: http://www.healthytransitionsny.org/. Accessed November 6, 2013.

11. Schalock R, Borthwick-Duffy S, Bradley V, et al. Intellectual disability: definition, classification, and systems supports. 11th edition. Washington, DC: American Academy of Intellectual and Developmental Disabilities; 2009.

12. American Academy of Pediatrics, American Academy of Family Physicians, American College of Physicians-American Society of Internal Medicine. A consensus statement on health care transitions for young adults with special health care needs. Pediatrics 2002;110:1304–6. Available at: http://pediatrics.aappublications.org/content/110/Supplement_3/1304.full.pdf.

13. Rousseau MC. Evaluation of quality of life in complete locked-in syndrome patients. J Palliat Med 2013;16:1455–8.

14. Wrightslaw. [Homepage on the internet]. Available at: http://www.wrightslaw.com/. Accessed November 19, 2013.

15. Self advocates becoming empowered. Project Vote toolkit. Available at: http://www.sabeusa.org/govoter/. Accessed June 21, 2014.

16. Welcome to the autistic community. AutismNow. Available at: http://autismnow.org/2013/11/26/new-resource-available-welcome-to-the-autistic-community/. Accessed February 7, 2014.

17. Twyman KA, Saylor CF, Saia D, et al. Bullying and ostracism experiences in children with special health care needs. J Dev Behav Pediatr 2010;31:1–8.

18. United States Department of Education Dear Colleague letter. Available at: http://www2.ed.gov/policy/speced/guid/idea/memosdcltrs/bullyingdcl-8-20-13.pdf. Accessed November 19, 2013.

19. Baladerian N. The rules of sex: social and legal guidelines for those who have never been told. Disability and Abuse Project 2006. Available at: http://www.disabilityandabuse.org/. Accessed June 21, 2014.

20. Person centered planning. 2013. Pacer Center. Available at: http://www.pacer.org/tatra/resources/personal.asp. Accessed November 19, 2013.

21. Parent Technical Assistance Center Network. [Homepage on the internet]. Available at: http://www.parentcenternetwork.org/. Accessed November 19, 2013.

22. Special Needs Alliance [Homepage on the Internet]. Available at: http://www.specialneedsalliance.org/home. Accessed November 19, 2013

23. The Arc [Homepage on the Internet]. Available at: http://www.thearc.org/. Accessed November 19, 2013.

Eating

Body Image and Health
Eating Disorders and Obesity

Carolyn Bradner Jasik, MD

KEYWORDS

- Obesity • Eating disorders • Binge eating • Anorexia nervosa • Bulimia nervosa
- Hyperlipidemia • Diabetes • Disordered eating

KEY POINTS

- Eating behavior in adolescents can be as high risk a behavior for future health as other risk-taking behaviors and is related to developmental changes during puberty.
- Disordered eating can present as a wide range of behaviors and can result in being either underweight or overweight.
- It is essential for primary care providers to recognize the signs and symptoms of abnormal eating patterns early, screen for fluctuations in weight, and be familiar with the basics of management and referrals.
- In particular, using a multidisciplinary approach strongly predicts clinical response. The early involvement of mental health (as needed), nutrition, and social work colleagues can have an important impact on behavior change.

INTRODUCTION

Adolescence is a time of rapid changes in development, including body shape, behavior, and cognition. Although teen pregnancy, substance use, and mental health are the most significant risks to adolescent health, the 2 health behaviors that may have the largest overall impact on adult morbidity are changes in diet and physical activity that occur during adolescence. This impact can manifest as a spectrum of behaviors that range from extreme dieting, to unhealthy habits, to overeating. In extreme cases this can result in obesity and eating disorders such as anorexia nervosa and bulimia nervosa. Both ends of the weight spectrum can have serious health consequences such as heart disease, diabetes, bone loss, and infertility.

Changes in diet and activity that occur during adolescence can become some of the riskiest of adolescent behaviors and merit close monitoring by health professionals because of the impact on adult health. Prior work from Irwin and colleagues[1] indicates

Disclosures: None.
University of California, San Francisco, 3333 California Street, Suite 245, Box 0503, San Francisco, CA 94143, USA
E-mail address: jasikc@peds.ucsf.edu

Prim Care Clin Office Pract 41 (2014) 519–537
http://dx.doi.org/10.1016/j.pop.2014.05.003
0095-4543/14/$ – see front matter © 2014 Elsevier Inc. All rights reserved.

that high-risk behaviors tend to occur together and are influenced by biological, social, and psychological factors. Screening and intervening on adolescent eating behavior must take an approach that not only considers the behavior but the context in which it occurs, much like other high-risk behaviors such as unprotected sex and substance use. The psychosocial context of the behavior and the mental health sequelae that result can strongly influence the impact of the eating behavior on the adolescent.

This article presents a framework for screening and intervention in abnormal eating and activity patterns across the adolescent weight spectrum. Eating behavior and its associated psychological impact are at the core of adolescent malnutrition and obesity. Interventions that are designed to increase weight in undernourished teens, or reduce weight in obese teens, must address the behavior to facilitate change.

The care related to obese and malnourished adolescents is highlighted, but the concepts are also applicable to healthy-weight teens in primary care. How to take a nutrition and activity history and highlight the early warning signs of overeating and undereating is covered first, followed by the specifics of early identification, diagnosis, and treatment of obesity and eating disorders in teens.

Case Example

MS is a 12-year-old boy who presents to the clinic for a yearly physical and vaccines. He has no complaints. His mother stops his clinician in the hall and explains that she is concerned because he used to play sports in elementary school, but since he started middle school all he does is play video games and use the computer. His mother recently had a gastric bypass and is concerned about MS's weight. The family history is notable for obesity (mother and father), obstructive sleep apnea (maternal grandfather), and hypertension (father). His weight is 60 kg (132 lbs) and his height is 143 cm (56.2 inches).

ASSESSING EATING BEHAVIOR AND ACTIVITY IN ADOLESCENTS

An adolescent preventive health visit begins with measurement of the patient's height and weight and calculation of the body mass index (BMI).[2] The calculated BMI should be plotted on the growth chart and the percentile determined. Any BMI measurement should be interpreted in the context of prior measurements, in particular looking for large increases, or decreases, in a short period of time. Such changes can be a sign of the onset of unhealthy eating behavior. A preventive visit should also include a brief nutrition and physical activity assessment. **Box 1** summarizes the steps for how to approach the initial assessment for abnormal eating patterns, activity, and BMI in primary care.

Formal quantitative nutrition assessments, preferably by a registered dietician, may be the gold standard, but are not always realistic in primary care. These assessments typically include a food frequency questionnaire, food record, or detailed interview.[3] Instead, primary care providers (PCPs) can do a brief nutrition and activity screen that includes nutrition content, eating behavior, and activity.[4,5] This assessment can be done via interview or questionnaire. One example of a validated activity and nutrition assessment is the Block food frequency questionnaire.[6]

Providers often limit themselves to asking about dietary intake and do not screen for eating behavior. What an adolescent eats is inextricably linked to why, when, how, and with whom they eat. Eating behavior refers to a patient's routine for eating and can be grouped with activity as healthy, unhealthy, disordered, and extreme.[7–9] **Table 1** summarizes this framework with a modified list of the different types of adolescent eating behaviors proposed by Neumark-Sztainer and colleagues[7–9] at the University of Minnesota.

Box 1
Key steps for an adolescent nutrition and BMI assessment in primary care

Step 1. Eating behavior and activity assessment

• Brief eating behavior and activity assessment (see **Tables 2** and **3**)

• Categorize behaviors as extreme, disordered, unhealthy, or healthy (see **Table 1**)

Step 2. Mental health assessment

• Brief mental health screen for depression, anxiety, family history and so forth (see **Table 4**)

Step 3. Psychosocial assessment

• Brief psychosocial screen for housing problems, school issues, substance abuse, child abuse, or partner violence (see **Table 4**)

Step 4. BMI calculation

• Calculate BMI and plot on the growth curve

• Classify as underweight (BMI $\leq$ 5th), healthy weight (BMI = 5th–84th), overweight (BMI = 85th–94th), or obese (BMI $\geq$ 95th)

Step 5. Medical assessment

• Thorough medical evaluation for current health status, family risk, current/suspected comorbidities, medications, symptoms, and physical findings (see **Table 6**)

• Laboratory and screening tests to aid medical work-up

Step 6. Weight management and referrals (see **Table 7**)

Data from Katzman DK, Peebles R, Sawyer SM, et al. The role of the pediatrician in family-based treatment for adolescent eating disorders: opportunities and challenges. J Adolesc Health 2013;53(4):433–40; and Barlow SE, Expert C. Expert committee recommendations regarding the prevention, assessment, and treatment of child and adolescent overweight and obesity: summary report. Pediatrics 2007;120(Suppl 4):S164–92.

Table 1
Eating and activity behavior spectrum

	Healthy	Unhealthy	Disordered	Extreme
Description	Eating intuitively and making healthy food choices	Making poor choices, excessive snacking, excessive sedentary time, and not eating mindfully	Unhealthy emotional eating and activity associated with mild psychological dysfunction	Dangerous eating and activity associated with medical complications and major psychological dysfunction
Examples	Family meals Packing a lunch Intuitive eating (eating when hungry) Participation in sports Regular exercise	Fast food School lunch Eating in front of TV, computer Unbalanced choices Calorie counting Prolonged sedentary time	Eating alone Lying about intake Hiding food Night eating Skipping meals Bingeing without loss of control Hyperexercising for weight loss	Restricting Bingeing with loss of control Purging/vomiting Compensatory exercise Diet pills or laxatives

Healthy eating includes meals that are prepared at home and are eaten with other people at regular times. Family meals are associated with lower rates of obesity and eating disorders.[10,11] Another sign of healthy eating is when teens report only eating when they are hungry. Patients with long-standing overeating or restriction lose physiologic hunger and satiety cues.[12]

Unhealthy eating refers to eating habits that are not health promoting and may be disordered. However, the adolescent eating behavior is not so extreme that it leads to large changes in weight. This behavior can be an early sign of obesity and/or eating disorder risk and is associated with a risk for gaining weight.[13–15] New-onset calorie counting can also be an early warning sign of an emerging eating disorder. However, this is typically only once there is evidence of psychological dysfunction such as depression or anxiety. Once unhealthy eating behavior is also accompanied by feelings of loss of control, guilt, anxiety, or depression, it has evolved into disordered eating. Examples are listed in **Table 1**.[7]

At the extreme end of the spectrum are behaviors that can have serious health consequences. When teens have lost control over their eating there are significant psychological impacts on both the child and the family. Behaviors include major dietary restriction, bingeing with loss of control, purging with exercise or vomiting, diet pills, and laxatives.[16] It is essential to know when extreme or disordered eating is present because it significantly changes the treatment plan from standard lifestyle counseling to a referral for eating-disorder treatment.

Unlike the assessment of other high-risk behaviors, the nutrition and activity screen should be done with the parent present. Family participation in interventions for both obesity and eating disorders is key, so having the parent present facilitates this. However, it is also important to confirm key components with adolescents during the confidential interview in case they are concealing certain behaviors, especially if the patient is already significantly underweight or overweight. **Table 2** summarizes the key components of the nutrition interview, emphasizing the importance of assessing eating behavior in addition to food content. The method summarized in **Table 2** offers an

Table 2
Components of the brief nutrition and eating behavior assessment

Concept	Sample Interview Questions
Who	Do you eat together as a family or alone in your room?
What	What did you eat over the past 24 h for breakfast, lunch, and dinner? Did you have any snacks? What do you usually have to drink: water, milk, juice, or soda?
Where	Do you eat fast food? Do you eat school lunch? Do you eat in front of the TV, video games, or computer?
When	Do you skip any meals like breakfast or lunch? Do you ever skip meals on purpose or to make up for an earlier meal?[a]
Why	How do you know when it is time to eat? Do you get hungry? Do you overeat or skip meals when you are stressed or anxious?[a] Do you have a hard time limiting your intake of favorite foods?[a]
How	Do you eat your food from a plate? Do you eat quickly? Do you ever lie about what you ate?[a] Do you ever hide food from your parents or others?[a] Do you ever feel as though you have lost control over your eating?[a] Do you ever exercise, take pills, or vomit to make up for food you ate?[a]

[a] Ask only for obese or underweight adolescents, or those with existing mental health problems.

easily remembered format that can be adapted to any clinical situation. Screening questions for extreme behaviors should be reserved for patients who have evidence of a rapid increase or decrease in weight or existing mental health problems.

A typical method for assessing food content (the what) is the 24-hour recall, in which the interviewer asks the family for a full account of what they ate and drank in the past day.[4] Families often need multiple prompts to report all the details. It is helpful to ask whether the day before was typical and, if not, ask for a more typical intake. A written 24-hour food record form can be administered, but an in-person assessment is better. Particular attention should be paid to whether the teen reports imbalance in content or portions, such as excessive carbohydrates or lack of fruits or vegetables. It is also important to determine whether food is typically prepared at home or purchased through school lunch or as fast food. These factors are known to be associated with obesity.[17] Standardized tool kits that can aid in a brief food content assessment such as 5-2-1-0 Let's Go! have been developed by public health departments.[18,19]

Beverages are a key component of the dietary history given the strong association between sugar-sweetened beverages (SSB) and weight gain.[20] Intervention studies have shown that a reduction in SSB consumption can have a positive impact on weight status and ameliorate the negative health effects of obesity.[21,22] Using the model of the 24-hour recall mentioned earlier, the provider should ask about all beverages consumed, specifically asking individually about water, soda, juice, and sports drinks. The provider should get a sense of the quantity of SSBs consumed at each time.

An adolescent's level of physical activity can be healthy or unhealthy depending on the context. Teens ideally engage in 60 minutes a day of moderate activity and maintain their weight in a healthy range.[2] When asking teens about their level of physical activity, the provider should determine the level of sedentary activity, current level of activity, and existing barriers to either limiting or increasing activity. Similar to the nutrition assessment, if the patient recently experienced a large change in weight or has preexisting mental health issues, the provider should screen for excessive or compensatory exercise. **Table 3** provides sample interview questions when talking to adolescents about their levels of activity.

Excessive sedentary time (more than 2 hours per day) can be both a risk factor for weight gain and a potential sign of social isolation or depression.[17] A full eating and activity assessment must include questions about current screen time and access to electronic and mobile devices in their room and home.

The success of recommended changes in nutrition and activity are linked to participation of the family. Therefore, providers should consider including the diet of all other family members living in the home, which sends a message that their choices affect their teen's choices.[17,23] This also offers the opportunity for the provider to reinforce key concepts in parenting. Being able to provide structure, set limits, and follow through on recommendations is essential to achieving a healthier lifestyle.[23]

Case Example (Continued)

MS's mother reports that he often eats alone in his room and she sometimes finds candy wrappers under his bed. When she confronts him about this, he denies it and blames his younger brother. MS has had a tough time adjusting to middle school because his best friends from elementary school went to a different school. His mother worries that he might be depressed or at least anxious because he does not seem to want to leave the house. MS is quiet throughout the interview, but does admit to feeling out of control with his eating.

Table 3
Components of the brief activity assessment

Concept	Sample Interview Questions
Screen time	How many hours a day do you watch TV/movies or sit and play video/computer games? Do you have a TV in the room where you sleep? Do you have a computer in the room where you sleep?
Current activity	How much time a day do you spend in active play (faster breathing/heart rate or sweating)? Do you currently play any sports regularly?
Barriers to activity	Do you have access to a gym or park near your home? Do you have any physical limitations to exercise? If you are not currently in sports, have you ever played a sport? If you are not currently active, are there any kinds of activity you enjoy?
Extreme activity behavior	Do you ever exercise alone or in private? Do you ever exercise after eating to make up for what you ate? Do you ever lie about how much you exercise?

Ask only for obese or underweight adolescents or those with existing mental health problems.

Data from Rogers VW, Motyka E. 5-2-1-0 goes to school: a pilot project testing the feasibility of schools adopting and delivering healthy messages during the school day. Pediatrics 2009;123(Suppl 5):S272–6; and 5-2-1-0 Let's Go! Available at: http://www.letsgo.org/. Accessed July 14, 2014.

THE PSYCHOSOCIAL CONTEXT OF EATING BEHAVIOR

The presence of disordered eating as MS is describing may merit a referral to an eating disorder program and a mental health evaluation, regardless of his BMI status, especially if he is already showing signs of psychological dysfunction associated with the behavior. The standard psychosocial assessment of an adolescent, the HEADSSS assessment, is a key component of the primary care nutrition and eating evaluation, specifically screening for mental health risk and psychosocial context. The presence of risk factors in either of these domains requires referral to either mental health treatment and/or a higher level of weight management than can be provided in primary care. When a teen has preexisting mental health struggles, or new anxiety or depression associated with rapid weight loss or gain, standard primary care messages for nutrition and activity change are not effective. Adolescents with significant depression are more likely to engage in unhealthy dieting practices and less likely to be able to adopt improved diet and exercise.[24]

The mental health aspects of adolescent obesity in particular have received little attention despite evidence documenting the co-occurrence of depression and stigma.[25] Furthermore, disordered eating behaviors, extreme dieting, and depression lead to increased weight gain over time.[26,27] Prior studies report that 11% to 15% of adolescents entering treatment of obesity have significant depressive symptoms,[28] and 10% to 30% report disordered eating behavior.[29–32] Therefore, before a referral to weight management, PCPs should screen for mental health risk in adolescents to maximize their responses to lifestyle change.

The patient's social and developmental context can also strongly affect both their eating behaviors and also their ability to respond to lifestyle change recommendations. **Table 4** summarizes the key psychosocial and developmental areas to screen for when evaluating eating behavior. If any of these areas are positive, early involvement of a social worker and/or mental health provider are key in addition to considering referring to a higher level of weight management such as an eating disorder program or multidisciplinary weight management program.

Table 4
Mental health and psychosocial associated findings that may complicate lifestyle change in adolescents

Concept	Psychosocial/Mental Findings
Mental health	Depression, anxiety Bipolar, schizophrenia Posttraumatic stress disorder Parental mental health diagnosis
Social risk: home	Divorce, split households Single parent Unstable housing, financial problems Food insecurity
Social risk: education	Learning disability, developmental delay Bullying, school avoidance
Social risk: substance use	Active substance abuse in patient Parental substance abuse
Social risk: safety	History of sexual or physical abuse Exposure to or witnessing violence
Social risk: sexual activity	LGBTQ youth with low family acceptance Intimate partner violence

The presence of significant psychosocial risk complicates response to standard treatment of being underweight or obese in primary care. Patients with significant psychosocial stressors are better served by a multidisciplinary care environment such as an eating disorder program or weight management clinic.

Case Example (Continued)

MS screens positive for depression in the clinic. The clinician probes further and does not think his reported eating habits are highly disordered. The clinician initiates a referral to therapy, but elects to further manage his weight status in primary care. MS's BMI is 29.3 kg/m², which is greater than the 95th percentile for his age and gender. The clinician informs the mother that he is in the obese range. The patient reports that he drinks 2 to 3 regular sodas a day, recently began to stop on the way home from school to buy snacks, and usually eats in front of the TV/computer. The review of systems is otherwise negative. The rest of the examination is unremarkable. He is Tanner stage I for pubic hair and II for genitalia.

ADOLESCENT OBESITY SCREENING, TREATMENT, AND REFERRALS

Although 18% of adolescents are obese, there are few evidence-based solutions for prevention or treatment.[33] The American Academy of Pediatrics (AAP) Expert Committee Recommendations and US Preventive Services Task Force suggest that PCPs should screen all adolescents for obesity with BMI and a brief nutrition/activity assessment as described earlier at their annual visits.[17,34] The visit usually starts with BMI measurement and classification and then a thorough medical evaluation to screen for causes of the obesity and potential medical complications, as indicated in **Box 1**.

Medical risk includes family history, past medical history, current symptoms, and medical comorbidities. Most patients who are overweight or obese receive lifestyle counseling in primary care that consists of setting brief, achievable goals, with monthly follow-up. Referrals for multidisciplinary weight management and/or subspecialty care depend on the initial assessment and associated medical findings.

Screening

BMI should be calculated as weight (kg)/height (m^2) annually for adolescents and plotted on the growth curve. In adults, weight status is determined using BMI alone but in adolescents the healthy BMI is linked to the percentile on the US Centers for Disease Control and Prevention (CDC) growth chart (**Table 5**).[17]

BMI interpretation should be based not just on the current measurement, but on how it compares with past measurements. Dramatic increases, or decreases, even if they are not greater than the cutoff for obesity or less than the cutoff for underweight, should be monitored. If a patient has gained a lot of weight over a short period of time, or currently has a BMI greater than the 85th percentile, the patient should receive extra screening and follow-up beyond the general screening mentioned earlier.

Blood pressure is also measured in triage and should be considered carefully when evaluating how to proceed with obesity management. Obese adolescents are more likely than other teens to have hypertension.[35] In addition to interpreting the BMI and blood pressure, the PCP then conducts a thorough history to assess for comorbidities and possible causes of the obesity. This interview and the physical examination facilitate treatment and referrals beyond primary care. The key concepts and associated medical findings are summarized in **Table 6** as recommended by the AAP Expert Committee Recommendations.[17] The presence of these medical risk factors may make it harder to respond to standard lifestyle counseling and are a reason to refer to multidisciplinary care.

The goal of the medical risk assessment is to (1) diagnosis an organic cause of the obesity; (2) diagnose and treat comorbidities; and (3) determine whether the patient can safely initiate lifestyle change and treatment of comorbidities within primary care, or whether they need a referral to either a medical subspecialist and/or multidisciplinary weight management. Obesity is usually caused by modifiable diet and activity factors. However, it is important to rule out genetic syndromes (eg, Prader-Willi, Bardet-Biedl), endocrinopathies (eg, hypothyroid, Cushing), and iatrogenic (eg, medications, hypothalamic obesity). Suggestive signs of genetic syndromes include obesity since childhood, persistent hyperphagia, and poor linear growth. In addition, screening for certain medications that cause obesity is important, such as psychotropic medications.

Treatment

As noted earlier, there are few evidence-based solutions for prevention or treatment of obesity; many of the treatment recommendations are based on expert opinion. The AAP Expert Committee Recommendations describe 2 phases of primary care management of obesity: stage 1, prevention plus; and stage 2, structured weight management.[17] Stage 1 refers to monthly visits with a PCP to reinforce lifestyle change and monitor for comorbidities. Stage 2 refers to a structured weight management clinic that is located within primary care with dietician/social work support and specific content and monitoring. Most primary care practices do not have access to stage 2

Table 5
Determining BMI weight status in adolescents

	Adolescents (Age 12–17 y)	Adults (18+ y)
Underweight	BMI <5th percentile	BMI <18.5
Normal weight	Fifth ≤ BMI <85th percentile	18.5 ≤ BMI<25
Overweight	85th ≤ BMI <95th percentile	25 ≤ BMI<30
Obese	95th ≤ BMI percentile	30 ≤ BMI

Table 6
Associated medical findings that complicate lifestyle change in overweight/obese adolescents

Concept	Associated Findings
BMI status	Poor linear growth (endocrinopathy such as hypothyroidism, Cushing, Prader-Willi[a])
Vital signs	Increased blood pressure/hypertension[b]
Family history	Type 2 DM, hypertension Stroke, hypercholesterolemia Mental health (eating disorder, depression, anxiety)
Past medical history	Type 2 DM[b] Hypertension[b] Hypercholesterolemia[b] Mental health (eating disorders, depression, anxiety)[a,b]
Medications	Corticosteroids[a] Antiseizure (valproic acid, carbamazepine)[a] Psychotropics (lithium, SSRIs, amitriptyline)[a] Antipsychotics (risperidone)[a] Depo-Provera[a]
Review of systems	Anxiety, irritability, behavior problems, poor concentration, sleep problems (depression[a,b]) Psychosis, mania (bipolar[a,b]) Polyuria, polydipsia, weight loss (type 2 DM[b]) Headache (pseudotumor cerebri[b]) Snoring/waking up at night (sleep apnea[b]) Abdominal pain (constipation[b], GERD[b], gallbladder disease[b]) Hip or knee pain (slipped capital femoral epiphysis[b]) Irregular menses or amenorrhea (polycystic ovarian syndrome[b])
Physical examination	Acanthosis nigricans (insulin resistance[b]) Hirsutism ± acne (polycystic ovarian syndrome[b]) Striae, buffalo hump (Cushing[a]) Papilledema (pseudotumor cerebri[b]) Enlarged tonsils (sleep apnea[b]) Undescended testes (Prader-Willi[a])
Diagnostic testing: laboratory tests	Increased glucose, Hemoglobin A1C (Type 2 DM[b]) Increased liver enzymes (nonalcoholic fatty liver disease[b]) Increased LDL, total cholesterol (hyperlipidemia[b]) Increased TSH, low T4 (hypothyroidism[a]) Increased testosterone, androgens (polycystic ovarian syndrome[b])
Diagnostic testing: other	ECG: left ventricular hypertrophy (hypertension[b]) Brain MRI: increased intracranial pressure/dilated ventricles (pseudotumor cerebri) Abdominal ultrasonography: gallstones (gallbladder disease[b]) Sleep study: sleep apnea[b] Ambulatory blood pressure monitoring: hypertension[b]

Abbreviations: DM, diabetes mellitus; ECG, electrocardiogram; GERD, gastroesophageal reflux disease; LDL, low-density lipoprotein; MRI, magnetic resonance imaging; SSRI, selective serotonin reuptake inhibitor; TSH, thyroid-stimulating hormone.
[a] Causes for obesity.
[b] Comorbidities.

programs. Weight management referral could be either a stage 2 or stage 3, a tertiary care center program. In the absence of major medical, social, or mental health risk, it is reasonable to begin a lifestyle modification plan with adolescents with a BMI between the 85th and 94th percentiles and those greater than the 95th percentile while waiting for a referral to a structured program. The initial approach to treatment of an overweight or obese patient is summarized in **Table 7** and the key messages are summarized in **Table 8**. Management of the underweight patient is discussed later.

The goal is a safe amount of weight loss; about 1 kg (2 lbs)/wk for an obese adolescent.[17] At the first visit, it is best to assess readiness to change. If the patient is at the precontemplative stage, clinicians can use motivational interviewing techniques to try to motivate the patient and family.[36] The strongest predictor of success is when the parents are also ready to make a change. Patients should return monthly to monitor progress and screen for rapid fluctuations in weight.

Referrals

The presence of any comorbidity, or cause for the obesity, may merit a referral to a subspecialist for management. However, as obesity becomes more common, providers will need to become more comfortable managing conditions such as hypertension, hyperlipidemia, polycystic ovarian syndrome, and type 2 diabetes mellitus (DM). The diagnosis and treatment of comorbidities is beyond the scope of this article. **Table 9** summarizes the screening, initial treatment, and indications for referral for common comorbidities of obesity in adolescents.

Case Example (Continued)

The clinician recommends to MS that he return in 1 month to review his fasting test results and reinforce the lifestyle counseling. Two goals are set: to eliminate sugar beverages and to walk with his mother 3 times a week. However, he does not obtain the tests and does not return to clinic again for 5 months. Before the clinician enters the room, the nurse informs the clinician of MS's "amazing" progress because his weight is now 41 kg (90 lbs) and his height is 145 cm (57 inches). His BMI is now 19.5 kg/m², which is at the 70th percentile for age and gender. The clinician notes the 19-kg weight loss and plots MS's BMI on the growth curve. MS's vital signs are also notable for a heart rate of 46 beats per minute and temperature of 35.1°C. The clinician is concerned that MS may have lost weight too quickly and the vital signs are confusing given that the BMI is between the 5th and 85th percentile, which is considered in the normal range.

ADOLESCENT EATING DISORDERS SCREENING AND REFERRALS

Extreme disordered eating behavior such as loss of control, binge eating, restricting, and purging warrants a referral to a multidisciplinary eating disorder program regardless of the patient's BMI status. Early identification of disordered eating behaviors can prevent the medical complications and complex treatment required for a patient once they begin to show medical complications of extreme dieting practices. **Table 1** summarizes disordered and extreme eating behaviors that can be elicited during a preventive health visit. If the behavior is mild and not associated with significant malnutrition or obesity, it is reasonable to undertake initial screening and work-up from within primary care. If the behavior is associated with a BMI less than the 5th percentile and/or rapid fluctuations up or down in weight, an eating disorder should be suspected.

Once the extreme eating behavior has become entrenched and is associated with rapid changes in weight, the patient may meet diagnostic criteria for an eating

Table 7
Key steps for primary care treatment and referrals by BMI status

	BMI ≤ 5th Underweight	BMI = 5th–84th Healthy Weight	BMI = 85th–94th Overweight	BMI ≥ 95th Obese
Initial Treatment				
Goals/approach	Weight gain using a family-based treatment model (Katzman et al[38])	Healthy eating and activity behavior	Stabilize BMI and/or weight loss; AAP stage 1 or 2 primary care weight management	Weight loss; AAP stage 1 or 2 primary care weight management
Lifestyle change counseling	Boasted calories, 3 meals/3 snacks family meals, ±minimize exercise	Reinforce healthy eating/activity behavior (see **Table 8**)		
Referrals/consults depending on initial assessment and availability	Social word if psychosocial risk present; Mental health if suspected diagnosis; Nutritionist for detailed assessment or specialized counseling (except diabetes); Medical subspecialists depending on comorbidities (see **Tables 9** and **11**)			
Follow-up	Weekly or monthly depending on severity	Routine care	Monthly for 3–6 mo	
Referral for Multidisciplinary Weight Management				
Eating disorder clinic referral indications	Refer immediately: extreme eating/activity behavior present, BMI extremely low, vital signs unstable, significant mental health or psychosocial risk, medical comorbidities/complications present; Refer early: lack of primary care expertise, time, services to manage patient; Refer later: patient fails 3–6 mo treatment trial, disordered eating/activity behavior still present, and medical work-up negative			
Stage 3 or 4 weight management program (per AAP guidelines) Referral Indications	Not applicable			Refer immediately: BMI extremely high, significant mental health or psychosocial risk, medical comorbidities/complications present; Refer early: lack of primary care expertise, time, services to manage patient; Refer later: patient fails 3–6 mo treatment trial

Data from Katzman DK, Peebles R, Sawyer SM, et al. The role of the pediatrician in family-based treatment for adolescent eating disorders: opportunities and challenges. J Adolesc Health 2013;53(4):433–40; and Barlow SE, Expert C. Expert committee recommendations regarding the prevention, assessment, and treatment of child and adolescent overweight and obesity: summary report. Pediatrics 2007;120(Suppl 4):S164–92.

Table 8
Key lifestyle modification messages for overweight and obese adolescents

Concept	Key Messages
Food content	No SSB
	5 fruits and vegetables per day
	Choose whole grains that are high in fiber
	Choose lean protein; plant based is best
Eating behavior	Do not skip meals, especially breakfast
	Eat together as a family
	Pack lunch for school
	Limit meals outside the home
	Involve the whole family in the changes
Activity	Be physically active for 1 h/d
Sedentary time	Limit screen time to 2 h/d

disorder. The overall lifetime prevalence of eating disorders among adolescents aged 13 to 18 years in the United States is 0.3% for anorexia nervosa, 1.6% for binge-eating disorder, and 0.9% for bulimia nervosa. The female/male ratio was higher for binge-eating disorder and bulimia nervosa, but not for anorexia nervosa.[37] Patients with eating disorders are usually defined as underweight, with a BMI less than the 5th percentile. However, adolescents with eating disorders can be of normal weight, underweight, or overweight.[38] As discussed earlier, the disordered eating behavior provides the earliest sign of a problem.

Screening and Diagnosis

As with obesity, the BMI should be calculated and plotted on the growth chart. Rapid changes up or down in weight or a BMI that is significantly lower than is expected for the patient's age, sex, and gender can be a sign of a malnourished state. A patient at significant risk (eg, MS) can present with a BMI that is appropriate for age; however, compared with prior BMI values, rapid change is noted. Patients' ideal body weights are determined based on their BMI percentiles before initiation of extreme eating behavior and, for girls, the weight at which they last menstruated.[39] However, for patients like MS, it can be confusing if they have a prior history of obesity and it is unclear what a healthy BMI is for them.

Once an eating disorder is suspected based on BMI calculation and/or nutrition interview, the next diagnostic steps for the PCP are the following:

1. Gather enough history to generate a preliminary diagnosis
2. Screen for comorbidities and other causes of malnutrition, and
3. Determine the medical severity of the situation

Most patients with extreme dieting practices are eventually referred to a multidisciplinary eating disorder clinic or mental health provider, but the PCP has an important role in supporting these providers. Katzman and colleagues[38] recommended that the PCP can provide medical monitoring while the adolescent is undergoing family-based treatment of eating disorders to support the mental health team. The acuity of a referral to a subspecialty clinic depends on the severity of the medical and mental health presentation in primary care.

Table 10 summarizes the elements of the history that would suggest an eating disorder diagnosis based on the Diagnostic and Statistical Manual of Mental Disorders, Fifth Edition, diagnostic criteria for the 3 most common eating disorders: anorexia nervosa, bulimia nervosa, and binge-eating disorder.[40] As with a confidential

Table 9
Initial management of obesity comorbidities and causes in primary care and indications for referral

| Comorbidities | Primary Care Management | | | | | | Subspecialty Referral | |
| | Screening/ Diagnosis | | | | Initial Treatment | Indications for Referral | Discipline |
	VS	HX	PE	DT			
Hypertension	●	—	—	●	Lifestyle modification[a] Antihypertensive[b]	Noncompliance, abnormal ECG, symptomatic, failed multiple medications	Nephrology, cardiology
Dyslipidemia	—	●	—	●	Lifestyle modification[a] Statin[b]	Noncompliance, failed multiple medications, liver toxicity	Lipid clinic
Impaired glucose tolerance/diabetes	—	●	●	●	Lifestyle modification[a] Metformin[b]	Noncompliance, failed multiple medications, requires insulin injections	Endocrinology
Hypothyroidism	—	●	●	●	Thyroid replacement	Diagnosis unclear, noncompliance, unresponsive to treatment	Endocrinology
Nonalcoholic fatty liver disease	—	●	●	●	Lifestyle modification[a]	Suspected cirrhosis, suspected infectious/autoimmune hepatitis, biopsy needed	Hepatology
Depression, anxiety	—	●	—	—	Therapy referral, psychotropic medications[b]	Failed initial medication, unable to find therapist, diagnosis unclear, multiple diagnoses, requires multiple medications	Psychiatry
Eating disorder	—	●	●	●	Triage for medical stability	Refer all patients	Multidisciplinary eating disorder clinic
Polycystic ovarian syndrome	—	●	●	●	Combined hormonal contraceptives, metformin	Excessive hirsutism, suspect androgen-secreting tumor, late-onset congenital adrenal hyperplasia, or other hyperandrogen state	Reproductive endocrinology
Obstructive sleep apnea	—	●	●	●	Lifestyle modification[a]	Refer all patients	Sleep laboratory/pulmonology/otolaryngology
Slipped capital femoral epiphysis	—	●	●	●	Hip radiograph	Refer all patients	Orthopedics
Cholelithiasis	—	●	—	●	Abdominal ultrasonography	Refer all patients	Surgery
Pseudotumor cerebri	—	●	—	●	Brain CT/MRI	Refer all patients	Neurology/ophthalmology

Abbreviations: CT, computed tomography; DT, diagnostic testing; HX, history; PE, physical examination; VS, vital signs.

[a] The specific dietary recommendations differ by comorbidity and depend on whether the condition presents in isolation or along with other comorbidities.

[b] Indications for medical therapy and choice of individual agent depends on multiple factors.

Table 10	
Eating disorder history elements	
Suspected Diagnosis	**History Elements**

Anorexia nervosa
  Subtypes: restricting type,
    binge-eating/purging type
	Significant restriction in intake to a low body weight
	Intense fear of gaining weight or being fat
	Distorted body image
	Unable to recognize or acknowledge the severity of low
	  body weight

Bulimia nervosa	Binge eating: eating a lot of food with loss of control Compensatory behavior: self-induced vomiting, laxatives, diuretics, fasting, exercise Self-worth linked to weight

Binge-eating disorder	Binge eating: eating a lot of food with loss of control
	Disordered eating pattern: eating rapidly, eating until
	  uncomfortable, eating when not hungry, eating
	  alone, feeling guilty afterward
	No compensatory behavior

Adapted from American Psychiatric Association. Diagnostic and statistical manual of mental disorders. Fifth edition (DSM-5) ed. Arlington (VA): American Psychiatric Association; 2013; and *Data from* Call C, Walsh BT, Attia E. From DSM-IV to DSM-5: changes to eating disorder diagnoses. Curr Opin Psychiatry 2013;26(6):532–6.

psychosocial history, it is important to interview adolescents privately to gauge the extent of their dieting behaviors. Extreme dieting behavior can be a secretive, private, and emotionally charged topic. Adolescents may be more likely to reveal the details without a parent present. In addition to the screening questions presented in **Tables 2** and **3**, there are more dedicated screening instruments for primary care, such as the SCOFF and Eating Disorder Screen for Primary Care.[41,42] The AAP has also developed guidelines for assessing eating disorders.[43] Typical questions include:

- Weight: what is the most and least you have ever weighed? Do you think your current weight is healthy? What is a healthy weight for you?
- Exercise: how much, how often, and at what intensity do you exercise? How do you feel if you miss a workout?
- Nutrition: 24-hour diet recall with attention paid to portion sizes, variety (are certain foods off-limits?), recent veganism/vegetarianism
- Beverages: caffeinated drinks, water
- Eating habits: food rituals, eating alone, calorie counting, fat/carbohydrate counting, surfing the Web for diet tips
- Extreme dieting behaviors (see **Tables 2** and **3**): binge eating, purging (vomiting, exercise, pills)
- Mental health history: prior diagnoses, therapy history, medication history

Treatment

Based on the initial history, the provider can begin to generate a hypothesis for an eating disorder diagnosis. The next step is to screen for comorbidities and possible other explanations for the rapid weight loss (or gain). When a patient has malnutrition and may or may not endorse disordered eating behavior, providers should review associated medical findings that could explain the malnutrition. In addition, the provider needs to determine the level of medical severity. **Table 7** reviews the initial primary care management for adolescents with suspected extreme or disordered eating/activity behavior in primary care. **Table 11** summarizes the medical risk factors that

Table 11
Associated medical findings that complicate lifestyle change in malnourished adolescents

Concept	Associated Findings
BMI status	Poor linear growth (renal disease, liver disease, hypothyroid, growth hormone deficiency, cystic fibrosis[a])
Vital signs	Bradycardia (sinus bradycardia[b], heart block[a]) Orthostatic hypotension: orthostatic changes (+20 beats per min, −10 mm Hg decrease in blood pressure)[b] Hypothermia (malnutrition[b], hypothyroid[a])
Family history	Obesity, eating disorders Depression, other mental illness (especially anxiety disorders and obsessive-compulsive disorder) Substance abuse by parents or other family members
Past medical history	Type 2 DM[a] Inflammatory bowel disease[a] Celiac disease[a]
Mental health history	Prior eating disorder[a] Depression[b] Anxiety[a,b] Substance use (cigarettes, drugs, alcohol)[a,b] History of abuse[a]
Medications	Stimulants (attention-deficit/hyperactivity disorder[a]) Anabolic steroids[a]
Review of systems	Irregular menses[b] Dizziness, presyncope, syncope, fatigue (dehydration[b]) Pallor, easy bruising or bleeding[b] Cold intolerance, hair loss, dry skin (hyperthyroid[a]) Palpitations, chest pain, shortness of breath? Exercise intolerance? Abdominal pain, bloating, reflux, constipation[b] (inflammatory bowel disease[a]) Vomiting/regurgitation (GERD)[b] Fevers, night sweats, weight loss (malignancy, human immunodeficiency virus[a]) Headache, vomiting (brain tumor[a]) Frequent hand washing, rituals (obsessive-compulsive disorder[b]) Muscle cramps (hypokalemia[b])
Physical examination	Flat or anxious affect Slow cognition Cachexia; facial wasting Cardiac murmur (one-third with mitral valve prolapse) Lanugo Sialoadenitis (parotitis most frequently reported) Angular stomatitis, palatal scratches, oral ulcerations, dental enamel erosions Bruising/abrasions over the spine related to excessive exercise Delayed or interrupted pubertal development Atrophic breasts; atrophic vaginitis (postpubertal) Russell sign (callous on knuckles from self-induced emesis) Cold extremities; acrocyanosis; poor perfusion Peripheral edema
Diagnostic testing: laboratory tests	Hypokalemia, hypomagnesemia, hyponatremia (purging[b]) Anemia, leukopenia (malnutrition[b]) Hypercholesterolemia Increased liver enzymes Sick euthyroid
Diagnostic testing: other	ECG: sinus bradycardia (malnutrition[b]) Low bone mineral density: osteoporosis[b] Gastric emptying scan: delayed[b]

Malnourished refers to a patient with a BMI <5th percentile, or a history of rapid decrease in weight.
[a] Causes for malnourished state.
[b] Comorbidities.

can complicate primary care weight management of the malnourished patient, could explain the malnutrition entirely, and require a referral to an eating disorder clinic or medical subspecialty.

It is also important during the initial evaluation to rule out comorbid conditions and/or other causes for the malnutrition such as hyperthyroidism, inflammatory bowel disease, collagen vascular disease, or malignancy. Although the patient may also have extreme dieting behavior, these diagnoses also require a referral to a medical subspecialist. Most of the comorbidities associated with the malnutrition, such as hypothermia, bradycardia, and orthostasis, improve with refeeding the patient or resumption of a more normalized eating pattern.

The principal treatment of eating disorders is to resume a normalized eating pattern that includes regular meal times, variety, and eating with family. For patients who are underweight or have abnormal vital signs related to rapid weight loss, regaining some of the lost weight until they reach their ideal body weights, resume menses, or stabilize vital signs is also a principal goal. This goal is primarily accomplished through multidisciplinary support at an eating disorder program. These programs usually consist of a physician/nurse practitioner, social worker, dietician, psychiatrist, and therapist. For anorexia nervosa, the primary treatment is family based and requires the parents' active participation with a therapist in refeeding their child.[38] After an initial assessment, it is important for PCP to evaluate an adolescent with extreme dieting behavior to screen for severe malnutrition and bradycardia, which put the patient at risk for refeeding syndrome.[38] These patients need to be hospitalized emergently and should be referred directly to an eating disorder center or local emergency department for transport.

The AAP guidelines specify the criteria for hospitalization as[43]:

- Seventy-five percent of ideal body weight or ongoing weight loss despite intensive management
- Acute refusal to eat
- Body fat less than 10%
- Heart rate less than 50 beats per minute during the day and less than 45 beats per minute at night
- Systolic blood pressure less than 90 mm Hg
- Orthostatic changes in heart rate (+20 beats per minute) or blood pressure (−10 mm Hg)
- Temperature less than 35.6°C (96°F)
- Arrhythmia: prolonged QTc
- Syncope
- Hypokalemia less than 3.2 mmol/L, chloride less than 88 mmol/L
- Suicide risk
- Intractable vomiting
- Failure of outpatient management

SUMMARY

Disordered and extreme eating behavior In adolescents can be as high risk as many of the other behaviors that traditionally are screened for in primary care. Being skilled in assessing and categorizing eating behavior in terms of healthy, unhealthy, disordered, and extreme potentially allows the PCP to identify concerning behavior early, before it leads to rapid increases or decreases in weight. The PCP has an opportunity for early intervention by recognizing abnormal eating and activity behavior before it starts to adversely affect health.

Once a dramatic change in BMI status has occurred, the provider needs to know the key medical comorbidities and alternate causes for which to screen and treat. Having access to a network of obesity, eating disorder, and medical subspecialists who can serve as a resource is important to providing all the care that the teen needs. The PCP has an essential role not only in early recognition but also in care coordination as the adolescent and family navigate the care team.

REFERENCES

1. Irwin CE Jr, Igra V, Eyre S, et al. Risk-taking behavior in adolescents: the paradigm. Ann N Y Acad Sci 1997;817:1–35.
2. Hagan JE, Shaw JS, Duncan PM, editors. Bright futures: guidelines for health supervision of infants, children, and adolescents. 3rd edition. Elk Grove Village (IL): American Academy of Pediatrics; 2008.
3. Livingstone MB, Robson PJ, Wallace JM. Issues in dietary intake assessment of children and adolescents. Br J Nutr 2004;92(Suppl 2):S213–22.
4. Ross MM, Kolbash S, Cohen GM, et al. Multidisciplinary treatment of pediatric obesity: nutrition evaluation and management. Nutr Clin Pract 2010;25(4):327–34.
5. Krebs NF, Himes JH, Jacobson D, et al. Assessment of child and adolescent overweight and obesity. Pediatrics 2007;120(Suppl 4):S193–228.
6. Block G, Gillespie C, Rosenbaum EH, et al. A rapid food screener to assess fat and fruit and vegetable intake. Am J Prev Med 2000;18(4):284–8.
7. Neumark-Sztainer D, Wall M, Story M, et al. Dieting and unhealthy weight control behaviors during adolescence: associations with 10-year changes in body mass index. J Adolesc Health 2012;50(1):80–6.
8. Neumark-Sztainer D, Hannan PJ. Weight-related behaviors among adolescent girls and boys: results from a national survey. Arch Pediatr Adolesc Med 2000; 154(6):569–77.
9. Neumark-Sztainer D, Story M, Hannan PJ, et al. Weight-related concerns and behaviors among overweight and nonoverweight adolescents: implications for preventing weight-related disorders. Arch Pediatr Adolesc Med 2002;156(2):171–8.
10. Haines J, Kleinman KP, Rifas-Shiman SL, et al. Examination of shared risk and protective factors for overweight and disordered eating among adolescents. Arch Pediatr Adolesc Med 2010;164(4):336–43.
11. Neumark-Sztainer D, Larson NI, Fulkerson JA, et al. Family meals and adolescents: what have we learned from Project EAT (Eating Among Teens)? Public Health Nutr 2010;13(7):1113–21.
12. Denny KN, Loth K, Eisenberg ME, et al. Intuitive eating in young adults. Who is doing it, and how is it related to disordered eating behaviors? Appetite 2013; 60(1):13–9.
13. Lachat C, Nago E, Verstraeten R, et al. Eating out of home and its association with dietary intake: a systematic review of the evidence. Obes Rev 2012;13(4): 329–46.
14. Robinson TN, Matheson DM, Kraemer HC, et al. A randomized controlled trial of culturally tailored dance and reducing screen time to prevent weight gain in low-income African American girls: Stanford GEMS. Arch Pediatr Adolesc Med 2010; 164(11):995–1004.
15. Nestle M. School meals: a starting point for countering childhood obesity. JAMA Pediatr 2013;167(6):584–5.
16. Marcus MD, Kalarchian MA. Binge eating in children and adolescents. Int J Eat Disord 2003;34(Suppl):S47–57.

17. Barlow SE, Expert C. Expert committee recommendations regarding the prevention, assessment, and treatment of child and adolescent overweight and obesity: summary report. Pediatrics 2007;120(Suppl 4):S164–92.
18. Rogers VW, Motyka E. 5-2-1-0 goes to school: a pilot project testing the feasibility of schools adopting and delivering healthy messages during the school day. Pediatrics 2009;123(Suppl 5):S272–6.
19. 5 -2-1-0 Let's Go! Available at: http://www.letsgo.org/. Accessed July 14, 2014.
20. Grimes CA, Riddell LJ, Campbell KJ, et al. Dietary salt intake, sugar-sweetened beverage consumption, and obesity risk. Pediatrics 2013;131(1):14–21.
21. Ebbeling CB, Feldman HA, Osganian SK, et al. Effects of decreasing sugar-sweetened beverage consumption on body weight in adolescents: a randomized, controlled pilot study. Pediatrics 2006;117(3):673–80.
22. Hu FB. Resolved: there is sufficient scientific evidence that decreasing sugar-sweetened beverage consumption will reduce the prevalence of obesity and obesity-related diseases. Obes Rev 2013;14(8):606–19.
23. van der Kruk JJ, Kortekaas F, Lucas C, et al. Obesity: a systematic review on parental involvement in long-term European childhood weight control interventions with a nutritional focus. Obes Rev 2013;14(9):745–60.
24. Fulkerson JA, Sherwood NE, Perry CL, et al. Depressive symptoms and adolescent eating and health behaviors: a multifaceted view in a population-based sample. Prev Med 2004;38(6):865–75.
25. Neumark-Sztainer D, Falkner N, Story M, et al. Weight teasing among adolescents: correlations with weight status and disordered eating behaviors. Int J Obes Relat Metab Disord 2002;26(1):123–31.
26. Neumark-Sztainer D, Wall M, Guo J, et al. Obesity, disordered eating, and eating disorders in a longitudinal study of adolescents: how do dieters fare 5 years later? J Am Diet Assoc 2006;106(4):559–68.
27. Field AE, Austin SB, Taylor CB, et al. Relation between dieting and weight change among preadolescents and adolescents. Pediatrics 2003;112(4):900–6.
28. Zeller MH, Modi AC. Predictors of health-related quality of life in obese youth. Obesity (Silver Spring) 2006;14(1):122–30.
29. Decaluwe V, Braet C. Prevalence of binge-eating disorder in obese children and adolescents seeking weight-loss treatment. Int J Obes Relat Metab Disord 2003; 27(3):404–9.
30. Berkowitz R, Stunkard AJ, Stallings VA. Binge-eating disorder in obese adolescent girls. Ann N Y Acad Sci 1993;699:200–6.
31. Isnard P, Michel G, Frelut ML, et al. Binge eating and psychopathology in severely obese adolescents. Int J Eat Disord 2003;34(2):235–43.
32. Glasofer DR, Tanofsky-Kraff M, Eddy KT, et al. Binge eating in overweight treatment-seeking adolescents. J Pediatr Psychol 2007;32(1):95–105.
33. Ogden CL, Carroll MD, Kit BK, et al. Prevalence of obesity and trends in body mass index among US children and adolescents, 1999-2010. JAMA 2012;307(5):483–90.
34. US Preventive Services Task Force, Barton M. Screening for obesity in children and adolescents: US Preventive Services Task Force recommendation statement. Pediatrics 2010;125(2):361–7.
35. Sorof J, Daniels S. Obesity hypertension in children: a problem of epidemic proportions. Hypertension 2002;40(4):441–7.
36. Gourlan M, Sarrazin P, Trouilloud D. Motivational interviewing as a way to promote physical activity in obese adolescents: a randomised-controlled trial using self-determination theory as an explanatory framework. Psychol Health 2013;28(11): 1265–86.

37. Swanson SA, Crow SJ, Le Grange D, et al. Prevalence and correlates of eating disorders in adolescents. Results from the national comorbidity survey replication adolescent supplement. Arch Gen Psychiatry 2011;68(7):714–23.
38. Katzman DK, Peebles R, Sawyer SM, et al. The role of the pediatrician in family-based treatment for adolescent eating disorders: opportunities and challenges. J Adolesc Health 2013;53(4):433–40.
39. Golden NH, Katzman DK, Kreipe RE, et al. Eating disorders in adolescents: position paper of the Society for Adolescent Medicine. J Adolesc Health 2003;33(6): 496–503.
40. American Psychiatric Association. Diagnostic and statistical manual of mental disorders. Fifth edition (DSM-5). Arlington (VA): American Psychiatric Association; 2013.
41. Morgan JF, Reid F, Lacey JH. The SCOFF questionnaire: assessment of a new screening tool for eating disorders. BMJ 1999;319(7223):1467–8.
42. Cotton MA, Ball C, Robinson P. Four simple questions can help screen for eating disorders. J Gen Intern Med 2003;18(1):53–6.
43. Rosen DS, American Academy of Pediatrics Committee on Adolescence. Identification and management of eating disorders in children and adolescents. Pediatrics 2010;126(6):1240–53.

Activity

Common Issues Encountered in Adolescent Sports Medicine
Guide to Completing the Preparticipation Physical Evaluation

Blair Heinke, MD[a],*, Justin Mullner, MD[b]

KEYWORDS

- Preparticipation physical evaluation • Sudden cardiac death • Concussion
- Musculoskeletal • Sports medicine • Adolescents

KEY POINTS

- The preparticipation physical evaluation is an essential tool used to screen adolescents for potential health risks associated with physical exertion.
- Cardiac screening with history and physical examination is often sufficient but diagnostic tests, such as ECG, can add additional, useful information if there are risk factors associated with sudden cardiac death (SCD).
- Concussion is an increasingly common injury in adolescents, so effective diagnosis and management are essential for primary care providers (PCPs).
- Musculoskeletal injuries are common among adolescents, specifically injuries of the shoulder, knee, and spine.

INTRODUCTION

Participation in athletic activities among children and adolescents is on the rise in the United States. Approximately 35 million US children ages 5 to 18 play organized sports each year.[1] The Centers for Disease Control and Prevention estimates that high school athletes suffer approximately 2 million injuries per year, resulting in 500,000 doctor visits and 30,000 hospitalizations annually.[2] In addition to traumatic injuries, early specialization in sports has led to increased incidence of overuse injury in adolescents. Head injuries among adolescents are also on the rise. Emergency department

Disclosure: None.
[a] Medstar Georgetown University Hospital, Georgetown University, 3800 Reservoir Road, North West, Washington, DC 20007, USA; [b] Atlantic Health Sports Medicine, 111 Madison Avenue, Suite 400, Morristown, NJ 07960, USA
* Corresponding author.
E-mail address: blair.e.heinke@gunet.georgetown.edu

Prim Care Clin Office Pract 41 (2014) 539–558
http://dx.doi.org/10.1016/j.pop.2014.06.001
0095-4543/14/$ – see front matter © 2014 Elsevier Inc. All rights reserved.

visits for sports-related concussions in adolescents nearly doubled between 1997 and 2007,[3] likely secondary to increased participation in organized athletics as well as improved awareness surrounding concussion. Additionally, SCD is the leading cause of mortality in athletic young people, with an incidence in athletes ages 13 to 19 in the United States reported to be 0.35 per 100,000.[4]

Due to the quickly escalating patient volume, PCPs, regardless of training or interest in sports medicine, are called on to complete preparticipation evaluations (PPEs) and to see adolescents with acute injuries. PCP familiarity with concussion management, basic musculoskeletal injury care, and identification of dangerous cardiac conditions are essential to providing this service.

A majority of secondary schools in the United States require a PPE before allowing any child to participate in athletics. PPEs serve as the primary way to identify underlying medical conditions that may become dangerous during intense physical activity. PCPs should be aware that regardless of expertise level, they likely will be called on to clear athletes for participation and identify dangerous risk factors. Additionally, a PPE is often the initial gateway for adolescents to access the health care system without parental supervision. PCPs can use these physicals to discuss healthy lifestyle choices; review immunizations; screen for depression, anxiety, and drug use; or use other psychosocial screening tools.[5]

A complete PPE starts with a thorough history to screen for medical problems, medication use, past and familial cardiac conditions, history of concussions, and previous and current injuries. Physical examination components are included in **Table 1**.

Preparticipation Cardiac Screening

A thorough history and physical examination can identify an athlete at risk for SCD. The most important aspects of a patient's history are personal and family cardiac history. Personal cardiac history includes previously identified heart murmur, hypertension, syncope, exertional chest pain or dyspnea, and previous cardiac testing. Significant family history includes unexplained or sudden death in individuals under 50 years of age. Unfortunately, this is often complicated by nonspecific complaints, incomplete or inaccurate history, and insidious onset of disease. Therefore, PCPs must pay special attention to history and physical examination findings, especially surrounding cardiac disease, and be prepared to look deeper into these issues if questions arise.

An American Heart Association consensus panel developed recommendations regarding history and physical examination findings that are most meaningful in identifying risk factors for SCD (**Box 1**).

Although athletes are encouraged to complete history forms prior to the PPE visit, this information is especially vital, so providers should take time to review these historical questions with patients and family members during a visit. Providers can quickly repeat questions involving previous symptoms (chest pain, shortness of breath, and so forth), previous cardiac testing or diagnosis, and family history of heart disease or any sudden death. Further screening questions include[6]

1. Have you ever passed out or nearly passed out during or after exercise?
2. Have you ever had pain, tightness, or pressure in your chest during exercise?
3. Does your heart ever race or skip beats during exercise?
4. Has a doctor ever told you that you have any heart problems?
5. Has a doctor ever ordered a test for your heart?
6. Do you get more tired or short of breath more quickly than your friends?

Table 1
Preparticipation evaluation physical examination components

System	Key Examination Components	Notes
General	Height Weight	Calculate body mass index to screen for obesity, anorexia, and drastic weight changes
Eyes	Visual acuity Pupil symmetry	Functionally 1-eyed athletes defined as best corrected vision <20/40 require eye protection Anisocoria or unequal pupils should be noted at baseline
Lungs	Breath sounds	Asthmatics need medical optimization of breathing and education
Heart	Blood pressure Radial and femoral pulses Heart rate/rhythm Murmurs Marfan syndrome stigmata	Hypertension should be identified, worked up, and controlled Screening for coarctation of aorta Identify cardiac arrhythmia Initial finding for structural heart disease
Abdomen	Tenderness Masses Organomegaly	Athletes with hepatosplenomegaly should be excluded from certain high-impact sports
Skin	Rashes, lesions	Identify and isolate contagious conditions (ie, boils, herpes simplex, impetigo, scabies, molluscum)
Genitalia (male only)	Testicle masses	Identify absent or undescended testicles unitescle athletes should wear protective gear Added benefit of early identification of testicle masses
Musculoskeletal	Neck, back Shoulder Elbow, wrist, hand Hip Knee Ankle Foot Gait	Range of motion, scoliosis Joint appearance, range of motion, strength, and stability of all joints Duck walk and 1-foot hop can be used to identify pain and range of motion in lower extremities

Data from Neinstein LS. Adolescent health care: a practical guide. 4th edition. Philadelphia: Lippincott, Williams and Wilkins; 2005.

7. Has any family member died of heart problems or experienced unexpected or unexplained sudden death before age 50?
8. Does anyone in your family have a heart problem, pacemaker, or defibrillator?
9. Has anyone in your family ever had unexplained fainting, unexpected seizures, or near drowning?

Cardiac Physical Examination

The cardiac examination portion of the PPE can be daunting and requires great attention to identify murmurs and arrhythmias. The most common pathologic causes of systolic murmurs in athletes include atrial and ventricular septal defects, patent ductus arteriosus, and pulmonary or aortic outflow tract abnormalities, including hypertrophic cardiomyopathy (HCM). PCPs are in good position to discuss risks with athletes and their families if referral to a cardiologist is necessary for clearance to play. PCPs should

---

Box 1
American Heart Association consensus panel recommendations for preparticipation examination screening

Family history

1. Premature SCD

2. Heart disease in surviving relatives less than 50 years old

Personal history

3. Heart murmur

4. Systemic hypertension

5. Fatigue

6. Syncope/near-syncope

7. Excessive/unexplained exertional dyspnea

8. Exertional chest pain

Physical examination

9. Heart murmur (supine/standing)

10. Femoral arterial pulses (to exclude coarctation of aorta)

11. Stigmata of Marfan syndrome

12. Brachial blood pressure measurement (sitting)

Data from Maron BJ, Thompson PD, Puffer JC, et al. Cardiovascular preparticipation screening of competitive athletes: a statement for health professionals from the Sudden Death Committee (Clinical Cardiology) and Congenital Cardiac Defects Committee (Cardiovascular Disease in the Young), American Heart Association. Circulation 1996;94:850–6.

---

not clear any patient with an abnormal cardiac examination without consultation with a cardiologist; however, it is important to know the features of a pathologic murmur to explain reasoning for a referral to patients, families, coaches, and specialists. The most common characteristics of a pathologic murmur are intensity of grade 3 or higher, diastolic murmurs, and an increase in intensity as a patient goes from supine to standing. A commonly missed murmur, characteristic of atrial septal defects, is a fixed splitting of the S2 heart sound, heard best at the left upper sternal border.[7] Any of these characteristics should prompt referral to a cardiologist. The murmur associated with HCM (the most common cause of SCD in the United States) is a crescendo-decrescendo systolic murmur, best heard along the left sternal border. The HCM murmur can be identified by an increase in intensity when the athlete stands. The increased intensity of the murmur occurs as a result of the decreased venous return associated with standing or Valsalva maneuver. As venous return decreases, left ventricular (LV) end-diastolic volume decreases, and the already narrowed outflow tract becomes more obstructed, increasing the intensity of the murmur.[7]

Electrocardiogram

In addition to history and physical examination, some experts recommend universal ECG screening for dangerous cardiac abnormalities that otherwise may be missed by PPE. These screening ECGs are the topic of much debate. ECG findings suggestive of pathologic cardiac abnormalities may be difficult to identify. Newly developed criteria for ECG interpretation in athletes, the Seattle Criteria, allow for more effective differentiation between cardiac hypertrophy associated with fitness from that associated with pathologic structural changes.[8] The financial burden of ECG screening is another obstacle, due to not only the great costs associated with performing and interpreting such a large number of ECGs but also costs associated with the follow-up needed for abnormal results. Finally, it is not clear how often these screening tests must be performed, because the pathologic changes evolve as young athletes mature.[7]

The American Medical Society for Sports Medicine (AMSSM), in collaboration with several other cardiology societies and sporting bodies, released guidelines to aid in ECG interpretation for athletes. These guidelines, called the Seattle Criteria, identify ECG abnormalities that can be normal in highly trained athletes.[8] The *British Journal of Sports Medicine*, in partnership with the AMSSM, released a training module that is freely accessible to help providers learn more about ECG interpretation in athletes.[9]

SUDDEN CARDIAC DEATH

SCD is a tragic event that has generated considerable media attention due to the impact on the community and concerned parents. SCD in athletes is caused predominantly by underlying cardiac abnormalities that remain undiagnosed despite PPEs.[8] Cardiovascular abnormalities can be difficult to detect in young and otherwise healthy adolescents; thus, the first presentation of a cardiac condition is often fatal.

The causes of SCD can be broken down into categories, including structural, electrical, and other. Structural causes of SCD include HCM, anomalous coronary artery, arrhythmogenic right ventricular cardiomyopathy (ARVC), Marfan syndrome, mitral valve prolapse, dilated cardiomyopathy, myocarditis, and coronary artery disease. Electrical causes of SCD include ion channelopathies, such as Brugada syndrome, Wolff-Parkinson-White syndrome, long QT syndrome, and catecholaminergic polymorphic ventricular tachycardia. Other causes include commotio cordis (a direct blow to the chest), stimulant medications, illicit drugs, and primary pulmonary hypertension. The leading causes of SCD are listed in **Box 2**.[10]

Hypertrophic Cardiomyopathy

HCM is the most common cause of SCD in young athletes in the United States. It is inherited as an autosomal dominant trait from 1 of 11 different genes coding for proteins affecting the development of cardiac sarcomeres.[11] HCM has a prevalence of 1 in 500 in the general population[12] and often higher in select populations, such as male basketball players. HCM is primarily a disease of the myocardium characterized by idiopathic hypertrophy involving the interventricular septum. The hypertrophy is often asymmetric leading to outflow obstruction. In addition to structural abnormalities, there is associated disruption in the alignment of the sarcomeres leading to altered electrical function. The most common finding in HCM on echocardiogram is asymmetric hypertrophy of the LV wall, particularly involving the basal septum.[13] A septal wall thickness greater then 15 mm is considered diagnostic for HCM.[13] HCM can be difficult to differentiate from the normal physiologic hypertrophy of a young athlete's heart. There is a gray zone of LV wall thickness, between 13 and 15 mm, that could be caused by either HCM or by high-level cardiovascular training. Specialists must often make difficult choices when diagnosing HCM and additional factors may be considered when disqualifying an athlete, including family history of HCM, unusual patterns of LV hypertrophy, LV cavity size less than 45 mm, marked left atrial enlargement, distinctly abnormal ECG patterns, abnormal LV filling, and female gender.[13] A short period of deconditioning (approximately 3 months' restriction from exercise) may decrease LV wall thickness by 2 to 5 mm. Repeat echocardiogram distinguishes

Box 2
Leading causes of sudden cardiac death (descending order of prevalence)

HCM

Coronary artery anomalies

Commotio cordis (blunt chest trauma)

LV hypertrophy

Myocarditis

Marfan syndrome

ARVC

Tunneled coronary artery

Aortic stenosis

Dilated cardiomyopathy

Myxomatous mitral valve degeneration

Mitral valve prolapse

Drug abuse

Long QT syndrome

Cardiac sarcoidosis

Brugada syndrome

Wolf-Parkinson-White

Data from Giese EA, O'Connor FG, Depenbrock PJ, et al. The athletic preparticipation evaluation: cardiovascular assessment. Am Fam Physician 2007;75:1008–14.

training-induced hypertrophy from the pathologic hypertrophy of HCM by demonstrating return of LV wall thickness to normal levels.[13] Any athlete with suspected HCM or other cardiac condition should be held out of any physical activity. Return to play guidelines can be found in the 36th Bethesda Conference,[14] but clearance decisions should not be made until after consultation with a cardiologist.

PREPARTICIPATION CONCUSSION SCREENING

A structured concussion history is an important part of a PPE and can help identify athletes with previous or persistent concussions, some of which may have been unrecognized or unreported. Clinicians should be comfortable with assessment of current symptoms, counseling about risks associated with recurrent concussions, and monitoring for any long-term cognitive issues. Concussion screening also provides an opportunity for providers to educate athletes and families about concussions and potentially provide referral to a specialist for management of persistent concussion symptoms.[15]

Screening questions include

1. Have you ever had a head injury or concussion?
2. Have you ever had a hit or blow that caused confusion, prolonged headaches, or memory issues?[6]

Interest in concussion management has risen recently as many former professional athletes came forward reporting long-term neurologic complications secondary to concussion, including 58,000 former National Football League (NFL) players involved in a lawsuit against the NFL.[16] Although the actual incidence of concussion is unknown, more than 248,000 children visited an emergency department in 2009 for traumatic head injuries related to recreational sports.[3] Concussions are becoming an important public health problem as the long-term complications of concussion are recognized. Cognitive changes affecting thought, sensation, language, and emotion are linked to concussion. Current management and research of concussions is driven both by concern surrounding chronic impairment and by fear of allowing athletes to return to play prematurely with resultant, potentially fatal, second impact syndrome.[17]

Acute Concussion Diagnosis and Management

Adolescents often present to PCPs with a history of head injury or mention being "dinged" or "dazed" after a rough game. It is important to investigate these injuries further because surveys have indicated that approximately 43% of adolescent athletes admit that they have knowingly hidden concussion symptoms to stay in a game.[18] The American Academy of Neurology (AAN) recently released a position statement that is a major departure from the previous AAN guidelines released in 1997. These clinical management recommendations are focused on long-term cognitive impairment and concern for second impact syndrome. Additionally the 4th International Consensus Conference of Concussion in Sports, most recently held in Zurich in 2012,[15] offers a similar and widely accepted consensus statement regarding concussion diagnosis and management. Current research has yet to define a standardized method of assessing concussion severity and resolution, so guidelines are driven by expert opinion.

The Zurich consensus statement offers the definition: "concussion is a brain injury and is defined as a complex pathophysiologic process affecting the brain, induced by biomechanical forces." These biomechanical forces may occur as a direct blow to the head, face, or neck or as impulsive or rotational force is transmitted from a blow to the body.[15]

In the past, concussions were graded as mild, moderate, and severe based on duration of symptoms and loss of consciousness. All current guidelines have discarded the use of any grading scale, however, because these have failed to predict clinical course or long-term outcome.[19] History of the initial injury is important, but grading of concussions or predicting severity for patients based on the history is not possible and can create unreasonable expectations. Athletes, parents, and coaches may remain focused on the presence or absence of loss of consciousness, but it should be emphasized that loss of consciousness has not been shown to be predictive of severity or duration of symptoms.

The AAN and Zurich guidelines emphasize that no athlete with suspected concussion should return to play on the same day regardless of how mild or short-lived the symptoms may seem.[15,19] It is also important to note that there are no provocative tests that can be used to clear to athletes to return to play on the same day if a diagnosis of concussion is made.[17] A provider who performs a PPE for an adolescent with or without a history of concussion has a unique opportunity to emphasize these important recommendations.

Health care professionals may be called on to see patients to provide individualized management because the AAN places greater emphasis on clinical judgment and less on rigid algorithms previously followed.[19] Guidelines recommend that younger athletes be managed more conservatively than adults because they seem to be more susceptible to concussion from the same amount of force and require longer to recover. Unfortunately, guidelines fail to define specific ages below which athletes should be considered "younger" and do not define "more conservative management."[15,19]

Many currently practicing sports medicine physicians consider this threshold to be 13 years of age and younger. The Zurich conference recommendations also encourage these younger athletes to complete the return to play protocol after only 1 to 2 weeks of complete resolution of symptoms instead of immediately after they become symptom-free. The protocol should then be completed over an extended course, longer than the 5- to 7-day period suggested for older athletes (**Box 3**, **Tables 2** and **3**).[15,19]

For health care providers with limited training and experience in concussion management, the use of a standardized assessment tool is helpful for evaluating a concussed athlete. The third edition of the Sideline Concussion Assessment Tool (SCAT3) can be used for athletes over the age of 12 years and there is now a pediatric version that has been validated for individuals 5 to 12 years of age.[15] The SCAT3 is available in multiple platforms; it can be downloaded freely from the Internet.[20] The SCAT assessment is also available in smartphone application format. None of these tools is meant to rule out concussion or be a substitute for thorough evaluation by a health care provider. **Tables 2** and **3** highlight many of the key points used to evaluate an athlete with potential concussion; all of this information is available and described in detail in the SCAT3 test forms.

The Post Concussion Symptom Scale, a portion of the SCAT3, can be easily administered to patients in the office, and evidence indicates that these tools accurately identify concussions in athletes after significant biomechanical force is transmitted to the head, with sensitivity 64% to 89% and specificity 91% to 100%.[21] The Standardized Assessment of Concussion (SAC), another part of the SCAT3, assesses orientation, immediate memory, concentration, and delayed recall. The SAC is thought to have a sensitivity of 80% to 94% and specificity of 76% to 91% for concussion.[15,21] The SCAT3 is often done on the sideline at the point of injury and can be repeated in the office to provide a means to track changes in objective and subjective symptoms. Computer-based assessments, such as Immediate Post-Concussion Assessment and Cognitive Testing (ImPACT) and Headstart, may also be useful in identifying concussions, but constraints, such as the need for a baseline testing, additional training required for providers, and cost, currently limit usefulness.

Box 3
Key consensus guidelines for concussion management

1. Concussions should not be graded and no concussion "severity" can be determined by presence or absence of loss of consciousness.

2. No same-day return to play for any athlete with suspected concussion, regardless of duration of symptoms.

3. Concussion management should be managed based on individual needs of every athlete.

4. Clinical management of concussion is driven as much by concerns for long-term consequences as by fear of second impact syndrome.

5. Graded return to play should occur in a stepwise progression, with each step taking approximately 24 hours, only after an athlete becomes asymptomatic.

Data from McCrory P, Meeuwisse WH, Aubry M, et al. Consensus statement on concussion in sport: the 4th International Conference on Concussion in Sport Held in Zurich, November 2012. Br J Sports Med 2013;47:250–8; and Giza CC, Kutcher JS, Ashwal S, et al. Summary of evidence-based guideline update: evalution and management of concussion in sports. Report of the Guideline Development Subcommittee of the American Academy of Neurology. Neurology 2013;80(24):2250–7.

Table 2
Signs and symptoms of acute concussion

Clinical Doman	Explanation	Best Test to Identify This
Symptoms	Somatic symptoms: Headache, "pressure in head," neck pain, nausea or vomiting, dizziness, blurred vision, sensitivity to light, sensitivity to sound Cognitive symptoms: Feeling "in a fog," feeling "slowed down," difficulty concentrating, difficulty remembering, fatigue or low energy, confusion, drowsiness Emotional symptoms: Lability, more emotional, irritability, increased sadness, feeling nervous or anxious	Symptom evaluation portion of SCAT
Physical signs	Loss of consciousness, amnesia, poor balance	Balance examination—modified Balance Error Scoring System Upper limb coordination—finger-to-nose task
Behavioral changes	Irritability	Per teammates, parents, coaches
Cognitive impairment	Slow reaction time	SAC
Sleep disturbance	Insomnia	Per patient history

Data from McCrory P, Meeuwisse WH, Aubry M, et al. Consensus statement on concussion in sport: the 4th International Conference on Concussion in Sport Held in Zurich, November 2012. Br J Sports Med 2013;47:250–8.

After diagnosis of an acute concussion, clinicians should understand the clinical course to provide management and return to play recommendations. Concussions may result in the rapid onset of short-lived impairment of neurologic function that resolves spontaneously. These symptoms may occur immediately after the trauma or develop in several minutes to hours after the inciting incident.[15,19] Physicians should recognize that concussed athletes may experience an impaired sense of the severity of the injury, resulting in refusal to seek appropriate medical attention.[22] These symptoms largely reflect a functional neurologic disturbance rather than a structural injury. Therefore, there is often no abnormality seen on standard neuroimaging studies, such as CT or MRI.[19] For this reason, neuroimaging should not be used to diagnose concussion but may be warranted to rule out other traumatic brain injuries, such as intracranial hemorrhage, in the event of neurologic symptoms, including loss of consciousness, posttraumatic amnesia, Glasgow Coma Scale score less than 15, focal neurologic deficits (unequal pupils and cranial nerve deficits), and evidence of a skull fracture, or in athletes with unexplained clinical deterioration.[17]

Recovery

After the immediate diagnosis and management of a concussed athlete (ie, decision to order imaging, SCAT testing, and removal from play), PCPs must be prepared to manage recovery. Although referral to a concussion expert may be warranted, it is often not available or practical. Most adolescents recover in less than 1 month but 10% to 20% of adolescent concussions take longer to fully improve.[6,23] During the initial stages of recovery, the Zurich guidelines recommend physical and cognitive

Table 3
Components of the SCAT3

Component	Description	Purpose
Post Concussion Symptom Scale	Rate the following symptoms on a scale of none = 0 to severe = 6: Headache "Pressure in head" Neck pain Nausea and vomiting Dizziness Blurred vision Balance problems Sensitivity to light Sensitivity to noise Feeling slowed down Feeling in a "fog" "Don't feel right" Difficulty concentrating Difficulty remembering Fatigue or low energy Confusion Drowsiness Trouble falling asleep More emotional Irritability Sadness Nervous or anxious	Subjective scale to follow symptoms through the course of the concussion from onset to resolution
SAC	Immediate memory: read patient a list of 5 words, ask patient to repeat words back in any order. Concentration: read patient a list of numbers and ask to repeat them in reverse order (ie, "if I say 8-9-6 you say 6-9-8"). Months in reverse order	Cognitive assessment including orientation, concentration, immediate and delayed memory
Balance Error Scoring System test	Double-leg stance: stand without shoes, feet together, and hands on hips. Close eyes and try to maintain stability for 20 s. Single-leg stance: stand on nondominant without shoes and place hands on hips. Close eyes and try to maintain stability for 20 s. Tandem stance: stand heel to toe and place hands on hips. Close eyes and try to maintain stability for 20 s.	Assess balance
Maddocks score	At what venue are we at today? Which half is it now? Who scored last in this match? What team did you play last week/game? Did your team win the last game?	Sideline diagnosis of concussion
Glasgow Coma Scale	Best eye response Best motor response Best verbal response	Recorded in case of subsequent deterioration

Data from McCrory P, Meeuwisse WH, Aubry M, et al. Consensus statement on concussion in sport: the 4th International Conference on Concussion in Sport Held in Zurich, November 2012. Br J Sports Med 2013;47:250–8.

rest until acute symptoms resolve. The current published data regarding the nature, duration, and efficacy of this rest period are meager. Some experts agree, however, that rest is a cornerstone of initial concussion management[15] and a 24- to 48-hour period of cognitive rest involving removal from social activities, school, and stimuli, such as cell phones, television, and computers, can be considered a sensible approach. The use of acetaminophen for headache management has not been shown detrimental, whereas NSAIDs are often avoided until structural damage is completely ruled out.[23] See **Box 3** for main points of concussion management.

After symptom resolution, a stepwise return to sport is recommended. The approach prescribed by the Zurich conference is seen in **Table 4**.[15] This graded return to activity includes completion of 1 step, followed by a 24-hour period before progression to the next step. If concussion symptoms return during any stage of the return to play protocol, patients should be transitioned back to previous step after an additional 24 hours of rest. There is evidence that adolescents take longer to recover from concussion and the AAN recommends that conservative concussion management may include a more gradual return to play protocol spanning a 2-week period in this population.[19] The Zurich consensus statement suggests that in cases when recovery extends past 10 days, management should include a multidisciplinary team experienced in sports-related concussion.[15]

Increased public awareness in regard to concussion has led to legislation in 43 out of 50 states, with 4 additional states pending legislation, designed to protect young athletes from improper concussion management.[19] These laws include components to educate parents, coaches, and administrators about concussion diagnosis and complications. There are also laws that immediately remove athletes with suspected concussion from further athletic participation. Legislation also dictates that athletes must have return to activity assessed exclusively by a licensed health care professional.[19] These laws will likely bring more student athletes into providers' offices for consultation after concussion. Legislation is also meant to raise awareness regarding concussion consequences among parents and coaches. This may lead to increased

Table 4
Graduated return to play protocol

Return to Play Stage	Activities Permitted
Rest	Limit physical and cognitive rest as much as possible (avoid TV, video games, sporting activity of any kind; some athletes may be permitted to miss classes).
Light aerobic exercise	Walking, swimming, stationary biking at <70% intensity for short intervals (20–30 min/d); avoid resistance training.
Sport-specific exercise	Simple drills, such as skating drills in hockey, running drills in soccer; continue to avoid any contact activities; continue to avoid resistance training.
Noncontact practice	Progress to more complex drills, such as passing drills in soccer, running routes, and receiving in football. Patient can restart resistance training.
Full-contact practice	After progressing through all steps without issue, athlete should be cleared for normal play without restriction
Full participation	Game day

Data from McCrory P, Meeuwisse WH, Aubry M, et al. Consensus statement on concussion in sport: the 4th International Conference on Concussion in Sport Held in Zurich, November 2012. Br J Sports Med 2013;47:250–8.

acceptance of decisions to hold athletes out of activity when concussion is suspected, lessening the burden of this decision for the provider.

Preparticipation Evaluation of Musculoskeletal Injuries

Musculoskeletal injuries are often an area of concern for adolescents and should be addressed during routine PPE. Providers caring for adolescent athletes should be able to diagnosis and provide treatment plans for common musculoskeletal injuries. These injuries may require additional evaluation prior to clearance. The musculoskeletal history associated with a PPE should include the following questions:

1. Have you ever had an injury to a bone, muscle, ligament, or tendon that caused you to miss practice or a game?
2. Have you ever had a broken bone or dislocated joint?
3. Have you had an injury that required radiographs, MRI, CT scan, injection, therapy, a brace, a cast, or crutches?
4. Have you ever had a stress fracture?
5. Have you ever been told that you have or have you had a radiograph for neck instability or atlantoaxial instability?
6. Do you regularly use a brace, orthotics, or other assistive device?
7. Do you have a bone, muscle, or joint injury that bothers you?
8. Do your joints become painful or swollen, feel warm, or look red?
9. Do you have any history of juvenile arthritis or connective tissue disease?[23]

By addressing all positive answers to these questions during a PPE, providers can offer guidance for current injuries, acute and chronic, and prevent additional musculoskeletal injuries. Common musculoskeletal injuries among adolescent athletes are discussed. Although many of these issues are not specific to adolescents, there are some predisposing factors that put adolescents at increased risk for these injuries.

Traumatic Shoulder Injury

Traumatic shoulder instability can occur in athletes playing high-impact sports, but low-impact shoulder injury also occurs, mostly in adolescents with inherent joint laxity. Shoulder stability is maintained via static stability from ligaments and dynamic stability from muscular control. Shoulder dislocation is defined as complete dissociation of the humeral head from the glenoid and occurs as an anterior dislocation in 95% of cases.[24] A shoulder subluxation is characterized as a partial dislocation that spontaneously reduces. A shoulder dislocation or subluxation typically occurs due to a direct blow to the shoulder or due to indirect blow to an abducted and externally rotated arm.[25] There is an 80% chance of recurrence with shoulder dislocations in patients under 30 years of age[24] secondary to instability from ligamentous injury, capsular damage, and compensatory weakness that occurs with muscular disuse after the injury (**Fig. 1**).[26]

Dislocations typically require manual reduction by a physician. This is ideally done on the sideline before the muscles tighten up but may require sedation to accomplish in a clinic or emergency department setting. It is beyond the scope of this article to discuss reduction techniques, but they should not be attempted unless the provider is experienced in one or more of these maneuvers. Reduction improves pain and allows for a more thorough examination. A basic shoulder examination, including range of motion, strength, provocative tests (labral tests, apprehension, and relocation test), and a neurologic evaluation for injury to the axillary and musculocutaneous nerves should be performed. Video examples of the shoulder examination are available online at https://www.youtube.com/watch?v=g8xtOqZFTwo.[27] Radiologic

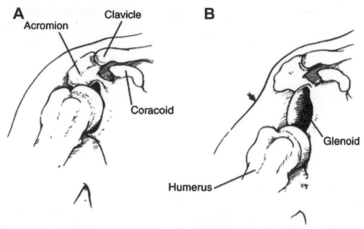

Fig. 1. Shoulder dislocation. (*Courtesy of* P. Auerbach MD, Stanford, CA; with permission. *From* Auerbach PS. Medicine for the outdoors: the essential guide to first aid and medical emergencies. 5th edition. Philadelphia: Elsevier; 2009.)

imaging is indicated for all dislocations to rule out bony injury and confirm proper realignment. Radiographs in AP and lateral planes are sufficient to identify fractures; however, the axillary view is often necessary to confirm proper reduction of the joint. Common fractures identified include Bankart lesions, Hill-Sachs lesion, and more rarely humeral head and distal clavicle fractures. Bankart lesions result from trauma as the humeral head translates anteriorly and damages the glenoid labrum or the glenoid itself (bony Bankart). A Hill-Sachs lesion is a depression in the posterior humeral head resultant from a dislocation (**Fig. 2**).[24]

MRI with or without arthrogram can be used to better define soft tissue damage but is typically not indicated in immediate injury management. An initial period of immobilization in shoulder sling for approximately 2 weeks is indicated to manage pain. As pain begins to improve, early rehabilitation to improve range of motion and strengthen the rotator cuff is important. In some cases, patients require only home range-of-motion exercise and isometric strengthening; however, patients with persistent pain or recurrent dislocations should be referred for formal physical therapy evaluation and treatment. Referral to orthopedics is indicated if the shoulder cannot be reduced, dislocation is recurrent, or neurovascular injury or fracture is identified.[24] Many young athletes return to play with nonoperative management, but complete resolution of pain and normal range of motion and adequate strength are indicated prior to allowing an athlete to return to play. Adolescents may attempt to minimize symptoms to return to play quickly and providers must be prepared to hold out athletes to avoid recurrent dislocations.[28]

Nontraumatic Shoulder Injury

Nontraumatic overuse injuries are also a common problem for developing overhead athletes (ie, throwing athletes, volleyball players, and swimmers). Sports specialization and year-round seasons can contribute to these overuse injuries because athletes do not get an opportunity to rest the shoulder. Studies of pediatric and adolescent baseball players indicate that players may develop biomechanical problems, including glenohumeral internal rotation deficit, glenohumeral hyperangulation, and scapular dyskinesis, due to epiphyseal changes from traction and rotational stresses.[26] Overuse injuries, if identified early, may be treated with relative rest and rehabilitation,

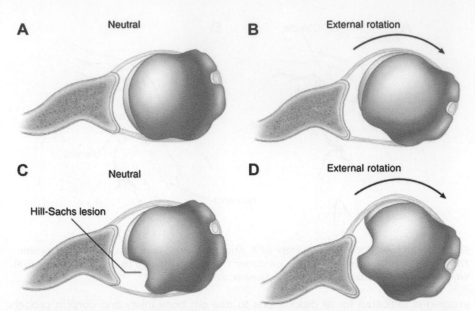

Fig. 2. Hill-Sachs lesion. (*Modified from* Burkhart SS, Danaceau SM. Articular arc length mismatch as a cause of failed Bankart repair. Arthroscopy 2000;16(7):740–4; with permission.)

but delayed diagnosis can lead to labral tears and rotator cuff injuries that may require surgical intervention. Physicians caring for young overhead athletes should determine repetitiveness of overhead motions (eg, pitch counts in baseball), location in the overhead motion at which pain occurs, and performance issues related to onset of pain (such as decreased velocity, control, or stamina that may indicate injury).[25]

A shoulder examination should include range of motion, strength, and tests to determine labral and rotator cuff integrity.[27] Radiographs should be obtained to evaluate growth plates. The rotator cuff can be adequately visualized with MRI but if labral tear is suspected, magnetic resonance arthrogram (with intra-articular contrast) may be indicated to further evaluate. PPEs are vital for early recognition of overuse injuries that may initially be treated conservatively with rest and physical therapy. They also provide an opportunity to explore and discuss pitch count limits and the amount of off-season rest, lack of which may be contributing to stress injuries. Identification of these injury patterns can protect developing athletes from sustaining further damage that may set them back significantly or even cause them to quit a sport altogether.

Anterior Knee Pain

Anterior knee pain is one of the most common musculoskeletal complaints among adolescents. The most common causes of anterior knee pain are patellofemoral pain syndrome (PFPS), patellar tendonitis, Osgood-Schlatter disease, and articular cartilage injuries.[29] Anterior knee pain is more common in young women compared with men because of an increased Q angle, which is the angle created by the intersection of a line between the anterior superior iliac spine to the midpatella with a line from midpatella to tibial tuberosity. A Q angle greater than 13° to 18° for female patients and greater than 10° to 15° for male patients is considered elevated (**Fig. 3**).

There are videos online detailing how to properly measure the Q angle, for example, https://www.youtube.com/watch?v=Murq9XJSKig.[30] Muscle imbalance may occur

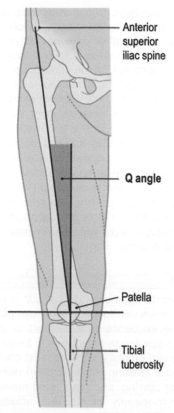

Fig. 3. Q angle. (*From* Porter S. Dictionary of physiotherapy. Philadelphia: Elsevier Butterworth-Heinemann; 2005; with permission.)

as a result of vastus medialis muscle weakness or iliotibial band tightness. A high Q angle and muscle imbalances lead to increased force across the patellofemoral joint, which can cause inflammation and cartilage damage.[28] Patients with PFPS often describe increased pain going up and down stairs and may report a sensation of insta-bility during running and cutting activities. Swelling is rarely noted.[28] Physical exami-nation may reveal crepitus with knee extension, abnormal patellar tracking, pain with grind test (downward force placed on the patella as the quad is activated), and tender-ness with palpation of the medial or lateral retinaculum. The quadriceps muscles, in particular the vastus medialis, are often weakened on the affected leg.[28,29]

Imaging is not indicated in the absence of severe swelling or trauma. Treatment is a combination of rehabilitation to improve quadriceps strength. Rest, ice, and nonste-roidal antiinflammatory drugs (NSAIDs) aim to reduce swelling, and bracing can be helpful to aid patellar tracking.[29]

Patellar tendonitis is another cause of anterior knee pain and is also called jumper's knee. In older adolescents with closed growth plates, the patellar tendon itself may become inflamed with overuse and poor flexibility. As the long bones grow rapidly dur-ing adolescence, muscle and tendons often lengthen at a slower rate putting excess force on the apophysis. In younger athletes (10–14 years of age), growth plates are not fused and tibial tubercle apophysitis, also known as Osgood-Schlatter disease, can occur due to chronic tensile stress of the patellar tendon on the tibial tubercle apophysis. This causes the apophysis to pull away from tibia, producing an increasingly prominent tibial tubercle and associated pain.[29] Individuals with patellar apophysitis or tendonitis are often basketball or volleyball players. There is rarely an acute injury that precedes the onset of symptoms. Pain is located either directly over the patellar tendon or at the attachment of the tendon on the anterior tibial tubercle. Patients also report a positive theater sign, pain increased with long episode of sitting with bent knees, as in a movie theater. Physical examination reveals tenderness over the patellar tendon or anterior tibial tubercle, tight quadriceps musculature, and absence of joint instability or swelling.[29] The treatment of both conditions is aimed at reduction of inflammation, with NSAIDs, ice, and rest from any activities that cause pain. Physical therapy can be used to correct muscle imbalance and improve flexibility. A strap placed across the patellar tendon (cross strap or Cho-Pat strap) also reduces stress across the tendon and relieves pain. Patients may return to activity as symptoms allow. A short rest period from vigorous activities for 2 to 3 weeks is often long enough to provide relief and allow gradual return to sport.[29] Patellar tendonitis may require referral to an orthopedic specialist in cases refractory to rest and conservative therapy for several months.

Anterior Cruciate Ligament

Injuries to the anterior cruciate ligament (ACL) occur in both adolescent and adult patients, but management varies depending on age, symptom severity, and functional status. Women have a higher incidence of ACL injury than men, with the highest prevalence in the 15- to 20-year age range for women.[31] Evaluation for ACL injury begins by establishing the mechanism of injury, with the most common mechanism noncontact sudden deceleration and twisting. Athletes often describe hearing a "pop," are typically unable to continue playing, and have rapid onset of swelling. The physical examination findings used to identify an ACL tear include a positive Lachman test (sensitivity = 77.7%, specificity >95%) and positive anterior draw (sensitivity = 22.5%, specificity >95%).[32] Radiographs are often normal in patients with ACL tears, but a small fleck of bone noted near the lateral joint line, called the Segond fracture, is indicative of a torn ACL. All patients with suspected ACL tear require orthopedic referral, but urgent referral is only necessary if imaging reveals tibial tubercle avulsion fracture.

Nonoperative management of complete ACL tears in young athletes have shown poor outcomes, so definitive treatment requires surgical management.[33] At time of referral, providers should recommend modalities to decrease swelling and pain, including ice, compression, and protected weight bearing. Improved surgical outcome occurs with restoration of a patient's range of motion and optimization of strength prior to surgery. No prophylactic bracing has been shown to prevent ACL injuries, but there are studies that indicate certain exercises can prevent ACL tears.[33]

The Adolescent Spine

Young athletes have higher rates of low back pain than their nonathlete counterparts and etiology of back pain is unlike that of adults.[34] Spondylolysis occurs at a rate of approximately 2% to 3% in the general population but is as high as 11% in young female gymnasts.[35] Spondylolysis is defined as a defect of the pars interarticularis portion of the vertebrae and is related to repetitive hyperextension motions seen in sports like gymnastics, volleyball, and diving and in football linemen. It occurs most commonly at that L5 level. Spondylolisthesis, or vertebral slippage, can occur if pars fractures occur bilaterally. The risk for progression to fracture is increased during

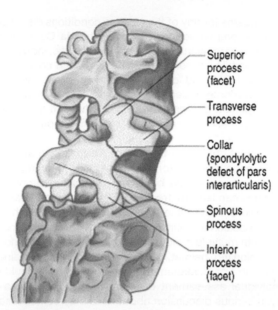

Superior process (facet)

Transverse process

Collar (spondylolytic defect of pars interarticularis)

Spinous process

Inferior process (facet)

Fig. 4. Spondylolysis. (*From* Lagatutta F. Spondylolysis. In: Slipman CW, Derby R, Simeone FA, et al, editors. Interventional spine: an algorithmic approach. 1st edition. Philadelphia: Elsevier; 2008; with permission.)

puberty when growth is accelerated or if an athlete continues sports activities that aggravate the pain (**Fig. 4**).[28,36]

Pain associated with spondylolysis may be acute or insidious in onset. The pain typically worsens with activity and improves with rest. Symptoms are usually present for several months prior to presentation. Although the stork sign is thought to indicate pars interarticularis irritation, there are no pathognomonic physical examination findings to confirm diagnosis of spondylolysis. Diagnosis can be made with standing anteroposterior (AP) and lateral radiographs of the lumbar spine. Oblique views likely do not improve diagnostic accuracy. If no fractures are seen on radiograph and clinical suspicion is high, single-photon emission CT scan or MRI is highly sensitive for occult fractures. Treatment consists of rest and physical therapy for a period of 3 to 6 months until symptom-free followed by gradual return to physical activity. Bracing is controversial, but recent studies indicate that it is likely no better than recovery without a brace. Surgery, including laminectomy or posterior fusion, is rarely indicated. As symptoms improve, there is often no radiographic evidence of bony healing, so repeat films are not necessary. Orthopedic referral is often helpful for management but referral is not required in the absence of spondylolisthesis.[28,36]

CLEARANCE TO PLAY

If an athlete passes the initial screening history questions and physical examination without any red flags, this should be documented and the athlete may be cleared to play sports. Clearance may be given for participation in specific activities, for example, noncontact sports, if injury or illness precludes participation in contact sports. Clearance can also be held until referral and further testing are completed by a specialist. PCPs should take the time during the PPE to discuss red flag symptoms with athletes, families, and coaching staff and encourage immediate follow-up if any of these symptoms occurs.[6]

If the PPE raises concerns for any of the cardiac conditions discussed previously, a cardiology referral is recommended. The 36th Bethesda Conference (available for review online http://www.cardiosource.org) outlined specific, individual recommendations for determining eligibility in competitive athletes with congenital heart defects, valvular heart disease, HCM and other cardiomyopathies, mitral valve prolapse, myocarditis, Marfan syndrome, Ehlers-Danlos syndrome, pericarditis, and systemic hypertension.[14] Management of these conditions is beyond the scope of this article and PCPs encountering these conditions are strongly encouraged to refer patients to specialists for clearance.[14]

There are no such strict guidelines to clear or disqualify an athlete with history of concussion; however, concussion history is part of the PPE for important reasons discussed previously. Clearance should be based on the fundamental principles that (1) multiple concussions can lead to irreparable brain damage in an additive manner and (2) an athlete is more susceptible to a concussion after each successive head injury.[17] PCPs are in a position to counsel athletes and their families or coaches about the risks associated with multiple concussions and to discuss that no effective means for preventing concussion (eg, helmet, neck strengthening, or padding) exists beyond cessation of contact sport participation. Clearance decisions should be made based on a clinician's individual assessment of each athlete. In athletes with significant concussion history, a serious discussion about risks may be necessary to determine if continued participation is prudent and a referral to a multidisciplinary concussion management team may be helpful.[15]

Clearance for athletes with abnormal findings in the musculoskeletal history and physical evaluation may also warrant further investigation prior to clearance. PCPs detecting musculoskeletal injuries must determine if the injury can be made worse by continued participation in sport, such as a shoulder injury in a baseball pitcher, or if an injury may result in athletes' inability to protect themselves during a contact sport. Athletes with limited strength or range of motion may not be able to block or move sufficiently to avoid further injury. An example of this is a quarterback in football who cannot move quickly due to knee pain; this quarterback may be repeatedly sacked due to his limited mobility, thus sustaining a concussion or traumatic injury (fracture, ACL tear, and so forth). Early diagnosis and treatment often prevent more serious injuries, and clearance should be denied until an athlete receives treatment of musculoskeletal limitation. PCPs are in a good position to address these issues before the season begins and recommend treatments or referral to an orthopedic specialist. It is also suggested that athletes or parents keep track of the documentation surrounding their condition and clearance because these likely are required for clearance at future PPEs.

SUMMARY

The PPE is essential in the safe participation of young athletes in sporting activities. The PPE not only allows for assessment of potentially fatal cardiac conditions but also helps address and prevent long-term impairment secondary to concussion or musculoskeletal injury. A complete PPE includes documentation of medical history, personal and family cardiac history, and past concussions and a thorough physical examination, including screening functional musculoskeletal examination. ECG can be useful in detection of cardiac abnormalities but universal screening is not yet recommended. Although some aspects of clearance for athletic participation go beyond the scope of PCPs, PCPs have a unique opportunity to interact with and educate a young, healthy population at this important developmental life stage. Ongoing research in concussion and cardiac issues in sports continues to improve the accuracy and usefulness of the PPE.

REFERENCES

1. Minnesota Amateur Sports Commission, USA Today Survey, Michigan state youth statistics. September 9, 1990.
2. Centers for Disease Control and Prevention (CDC). Sports-Related Injuries Among High School Athletes, United States, 2005-06. MMWR Morb Mortal Wkly Rep 2006;55(38):1037–40.
3. Centers for Disease Control and Prevention. Nonfatal traumatic brain injuries related to sports and recreation activities among persons aged ≤19 years, United States, 2001-2009. MMWR Morb Mortal Wkly Rep 2011;60(39):1337–42.
4. Maron BJ, Gohman TE, Aeppli D. Prevalence of sudden cardiac death during competitive sports activities in Minnesota High School Athletes. J Am Coll Cardiol 1998;32:1881–4.
5. Goldenring JM, Rosen DS. Getting into adolescent heads: an essential update. Contemp Pediatr 2004;21(1):64–80.
6. Bernhardt DT, Roberts WO. Preparticipation physical evaluation. 4th edition. Elk Grove Village (IL): American Academy of Pediatrics; 2010. p. 39–66, 107–19.
7. Mcconnell ME, Adkins SB, Hannon DW. Heart murmurs in pediatric patients: when do you refer? Am Fam Physician 1999;60(2):558–64.
8. Drezner JA, Ackerman MJ, Anderson J, et al. Electrocardiographic interpretation in athletes: the 'Seattle Criteria'. Br J Sports Med 2013;47:122–4.
9. Available at: http://learning.bmj.com/learning/module-intro/.html?moduleId=10042584. Accessed January 3, 2014.
10. Giese EA, O'Connor FG, Depenbrock PJ, et al. The Athletic preparticipation evaluation: cardiovascular assessment. Am Fam Physician 2007;75:1008–14.
11. Basavarajaiah S, Wilson M, White G, et al. Prevalence of hypertrophic cardiomyopathy in highly trained athletes. J Am Coll Cardiol 2008;51:1033–9.
12. Maron B. Contemporary insights and strategies for risk stratification and prevention of sudden death in hypertrophic cardiomyopathy. Circulation 2010;121:445–56.
13. Ramaraj R. Hypertrophic cardiomyopathy. Etiology, diagnosis and treatment. Cardiol Rev 2008;16:172–80.
14. Maron BJ, Zipes DP. 36th Bethesda Conference: eligibility recommendations for competitive athletes with cardiovascular abnormalities. J Am Coll Cardiol 2005; 45(8):1318–21.
15. McCrory P, Meeuwisse WH, Aubry M, et al. Consensus statement on concussion in sport: the 4th International Conference on Concussion in Sport Held in Zurich, November 2012. Br J Sports Med 2013;47:250–8.
16. Belson K. NFL agrees to settle concussion suit for $765 million. NY Times 2013;A1.
17. Giza CC, Kutcher JS, Ashwal S, et al. Summary of evidence-based guideline update: evaluation and management of concussion in sports. Report of the Guideline Development Subcommittee of the American Academy of Neurology. Neurology 2013;80(24):2250–7.
18. Torres DM, Galetta KM, Phillips HW, et al. Sports-related concussion: Anonymous Survey of a Collegiate Cohort. Neurol Clin Pract 2013;3(4):279–87.
19. Gomez JE, Hergenroeder AC. New guidelines for Management of Concussion in Sport: Special Concern for Youth. J Adolesc Health 2013;53:311–3.
20. Available at: http://bjsm.bmj.com/content/47/5/259.full.pdf. Accessed January 3, 2014.

21. McCrea M, Barr WB, Guskiewicz KM, et al. Standard regression-based methods for measuring recovery after sport-related concussion. J Int Neuropsychol Soc 2005;290:2556–63.
22. Buzzin SM, Guskiewicz KM. Sports-related concussion in the young athlete. Curr Opin Pediatr 2006;18:376–82.
23. Vidal PG, Goodman AM, Colin A, et al. Rehabilitation strategies for prolonged recovery in pediatric and adolescent concussion. Pediatr Ann 2012;41(9):1–7.
24. Howard TM, Butcher JD. The Little Black Book of Sports Medicine. 2nd edition. Sudbury (MA): Jones and Barlett Publishers; 2006. p. 72–4.
25. Lyman S, Fleisig GS, Waterbor JW, et al. Longitudinal study of elbow and shoulder pain in youth baseball pitchers. Med Sci Sports Exerc 2001;33(11):1803–10.
26. Olson SJ, Flesig GS, Dun S, et al. Risk factors of shoulder and elbow injuries in adolescent baseball pitchers. Am J Sports Med 2006;34(6):905–12.
27. Oxford Medical Education. Available at: http://www.oxfordmedicaleducation.com/; https://www.youtube.com/watch?v=g8xtOqZFTwo. Accessed January 3, 2014.
28. Madden CC, Putukian M, Young CC, et al. Netter's Sports Medicine. 1st edition. Philadelphia: Saunders Elsevier; 2010. p. 60–1.
29. Fulkerson JP. Diagnosis and treatment of patients with patellofemoral pain. Am J Sports Med 2002;30(3):447–56.
30. Available at: https://www.youtube.com/watch?v=Murq9XJSKig. Accessed January 3, 2014.
31. Ireland ML. Anterior cruciate ligament injury in female athletes: epidemiology. J Athl Train 1999;34(2):150–4.
32. Katz JW, Fingeroth RJ. The diagnostic accuracy of ruptures of the ACL comparing the lachman test, the anterior drawer sign, and the pivot shift test in acute and chronic knee injuries. Am J Sports Med 1986;14(1):88–91.
33. Postma WF, West RV. Anterior cruciate ligament injury-prevention programs. J Bone Joint Surg Am 2013;95:661–9.
34. Bono CM. Low-back pain in athletes. J Bone Joint Surg Am 2004;86(2):382–96.
35. Standaert CJ, Herring SA. Spondylolysis: a critical review. Br J Sports Med 2000; 34:415–22.
36. Standaert CJ, Herring SA. Expert opinion and controversies in sports and musculoskeletal medicine: the diagnosis and treatment of spondylolysis in adolescent athletes. Arch Phys Med Rehabil 2007;88:537–40.

Teens, Technology, and Health Care

Francesco Leanza, MD[a,b,*], Diane Hauser, MPA[a,b]

KEYWORDS

- Teens • Technology • Text messaging
- Computer-based or Web-based interventions • Chronic disease management
- Social media • Teen sexual health

KEY POINTS

- Teens prefer to receive text messages rather than e-mails as a form of communication.
- Computer-based screenings are acceptable to teens and helpful to providers for identifying and preventing high-risk behaviors.
- Web sites that address specific domains of teen health care should be easy to use, youth centered, connected to an organization that is recommended by the provider, and trustworthy.
- Social media can play a role in teen health, but should be connected to the teen's personal experience with a group or organization that focuses on the teen's specific condition (ie, other teens with the same condition).

INTRODUCTION

The use of technology and social media is ubiquitous among teens. Ninety-five percent of American teens are online at least sometimes, and this connectivity increasingly moves with them on a rapidly developing array of mobile devices.[1] It has been noted that trends in mobile connectivity among teens are a harbinger of future behaviors among adults, expanding the relevance of teen-focused technology initiatives. Smartphones, social media sites, and online videos and gaming have much potential to promote health and healthy behaviors in teens.

There is a growing body of research on teens and the use of technology with regard to their health care. To date, studies are small and imperfect. As a result it is difficult to extrapolate to the general population given that most studies are not considered high

[a] Department of Family Medicine and Community Health, Icahn School of Medicine at Mount Sinai, One Gustave L. Levy Place, New York, NY 10029, USA; [b] Institute for Family Health, 16 East 16th Street, New York, NY 10003, USA
* Corresponding author. Department of Family Medicine and Community Health, Icahn School of Medicine at Mount Sinai, One Gustave L. Levy Place, New York, NY 10029, USA
E-mail address: fleanza@institute2000.org

Prim Care Clin Office Pract 41 (2014) 559–566
http://dx.doi.org/10.1016/j.pop.2014.05.006
0095-4543/14/$ – see front matter © 2014 Elsevier Inc. All rights reserved.

quality from an evidence-based perspective. However, trends are emerging that are helpful when designing interventions for further study.

Health Information Seeking Among Teens

In the general population of online teens, 31% obtain health, dieting, or physical fitness information from the Internet according to a 2010 survey of adolescents and young adults by the Pew Internet & American Life project.[2] This survey also found that 17% of online teens report using the Internet to learn about health topics that are difficult to discuss with others, such as drug use and sexual health. Research on how teens search for and use health information is limited, with most studies using qualitative methods and small samples. One study found that adolescents do not search for health information with a critical eye.[3] This small study showed that participants used a "trial-and-error approach to formulate search strings, scanned pages randomly instead of systematically, and did not consider the source of the content when searching for health information."[3] Another study that tracked use of suggested health Web sites for adolescents with asthma and diabetes found that 60% of participants accessed at least one site over a 6-month period. Perceived usefulness and content, particularly stories, targeted toward teens were predictors of continued use of a Web site. Teens were more likely to use sites for information than for self-management purposes.[4] One study of sources of information about suicide found that teens often use online sources for information about suicide, with 59% citing online sources.[5] A survey of more than 700 young people who had previously reported knowledge of others who had attempted or committed suicide and had associated experiences of hopelessness and suicidal ideation found that the Internet and social networking sites were important sources of suicide stories for this group. However, only discussion forums were associated with increased suicidal ideation. The investigators suggest that social networking sites may provide increased exposure to suicide, and also greater social support.

Some Web sites contain low-quality and/or erroneous information. A study of sexual health information Web sites visited by teens found that 17% of sites reviewed contain at least one inaccuracy, and these were most likely to be related to complex (eg, contraception) or controversial (eg, abortion) topics.[6] In another study, specifically of sexually transmitted infection (STI) sites available to teens, key information, such as primary prevention and partner testing, was often missing.[7] To address concerns about the accuracy of online information, the organization Common Sense Media (commonsensemedia.org) draws on a national advisory board to rate media sites targeting children and teens, with specific reviews of health-related sites. Although teens are increasingly seeking health information online, the impact of the information on teen's health behavior is unclear and may not always be accurate. Health care professionals and organizations that work with teens should identify online health information that is both accurate and teen friendly.

Use of Technology for Health Care Engagement and Promotion Among Teens

A variety of technologies have been used to engage teens in their health both outside and inside the health care system. Because cell phone texting is currently the preferred form of communication among teens, a variety of adolescent health education initiatives involve texting.[8] In San Francisco, Internet Sexuality Information, Inc partnered with the city's Department of Public Health to publicize a text messaging program, SEXINFO, through traditional media, which enables adolescents to find services related to sexual health. Teens use their phones to choose from a menu of concerns (eg, D4 to find out about human immunodeficiency virus [HIV]), and receive information about services via text. Surveys found high awareness and use of services among the targeted youth.[9] Through a program known as Hook-up, supported by the California Family Health Council, teens can sign up to receive weekly texts on "sex info and life advice."[10] A recent review of studies assessing the impact of digital media designed to prevent STIs and HIV found that study design issues, such as lack of biological outcomes and comparison groups, makes it difficult to determine whether the digital interventions were effective.[11]

Although use of texting has been studied to reach teens outside the clinic, the use of personal digital devices (PDAs) for health screening has been studied for use within the clinical setting. A study that used PDAs to conduct health screenings using a modified Guidelines for Adolescent Preventive Services (GAPS)[12] indicated that teens were more likely to think that their visit was confidential, that they were listened to more carefully, and to be satisfied with the visit. The use of PDAs increased discussions of certain behaviors, such as fruit/vegetable intake, tobacco use, and alcohol use.[13] A review article by Hassan and Fleegler[14] highlighted several important studies regarding the use of technology to screen adolescents in clinics:

- A randomized study substantiated that teens self-disclose as accurately on computer surveys as they do on paper.[15]
- Several studies have concluded that computer-based surveys are perceived as confidential and nonjudgmental, resulting in accurate answers to sensitive questions.[13,16,17]
- Screening teens for psychosocial concerns just before a provider visit increases the number of concerns identified and addressed during the visit.[18]

These studies substantiate that computerized versions of the traditional paper screen are acceptable, valid, and increase concerns identified by teens and addressed by providers. Although the best technology for screening teens has not been established, PDAs show promise.

Interventions to prevent risky behaviors or increase healthy behaviors have also been studied to some extent. In Hassan and Fleegler's[14] review article, several computerized interventions to decrease risky behavior were highlighted:

- In an efficacy study at the University of California, Los Angeles, of computerized HIV prevention for adolescents, Lightfoot and colleagues,[19] found that teens in the computerized group were less likely to engage in sexual activity and reported fewer partners.
- In a screening and brief online intervention for college freshman at Boston University, unhealthy alcohol use was decreased.[20]

A systematic review of technology-based interventions (Web and computer) designed to increase preadolescent and adolescent physical activity found that increases in activity occurred. Location of interventions varied from school to camp to activities at home. The interventions included physical activity, improving diet, counseling, and group sessions. Half the studies were by self-report and the other half measured body mass index, body weight, percent body fat, and/or activity as measured by accelerometer. These findings were small and not sustained and require further study. The number of studies addressing physical activity did not adequately address the effectiveness of technology-based interventions.[21]

Technology is quickly becoming pervasive in the interaction between teens and their health. Texting is being used to reach out to teens, computer-based screens are being used to assess for high-risk behaviors, and studies show that teens respond to online or computer-based interventions.

Tools to Manage Chronic Illness

Research on the use of technology to manage chronic illness in teens has mostly been limited to qualitative feasibility studies. Most studies show how technology improves knowledge about disease; a smaller number evaluate improvement of adherence or disease-based outcomes associated with a particular condition. Applebaum and colleagues,[22] at the University of Chicago, performed surveys and focus groups with a small group of chronically ill teens and their parents in a pediatric university-based rheumatology practice and general pediatric practice. Several of the following themes emerged from the focus groups:

- Teens prefer appointment reminders by text, not e-mail, because they rarely check their inboxes.
- Online portals are acceptable as a means to store personal medical information and provide a forum for communication between patients and providers.
- Online portals should be presented in a fun, interactive, and customizable way.

Teens in the study also wanted an easy way to retrieve medication lists, test results, and personal information with minimal data entry required. The patients in the study had chronic illness and felt uncomfortable searching the Internet on their own for information regarding their illnesses. They preferred to have their provider recommend reputable online sources; ideally sources that were interactive and provided easy-to-understand information about their conditions and medications. Portable memory devices, such as thumb drives, for teens were discouraged because they are easily lost. Social media were acceptable as means to connect with other teens with similar conditions, but not as means to access information and communicate with providers, because this could affect the teens' privacy. In addition, teens in the focus groups thought that they would not connect with other teens unless they had met them previously. Teens wanted peer-based support groups. Support groups are seen as a venue to share information and socialize with peers who understand what it means to have the same illness. The teens with chronic illness in the study did not want to engage with peers at their schools, because "They ask dumb questions and they do not understand."[22]

Feasibility studies substantiate that texting to improve management and knowledge of chronic disease, such as type 1 diabetes and cystic fibrosis (CF), is acceptable. A small study using the Computerized Automated Reminder Diabetes System (CARDS) showed that teens are more likely to check their blood sugar if they are reminded by text rather than e-mail. However, response to texts waned after 3 months.[23] In another study with young type 1 diabetic patients, Sweet Talk, a text messaging support system, sent text messages tailored to the individual. Messages from Sweet Talk included reminders to take medications and check blood sugars, provided lifestyle advice such as to eat healthily and exercise, and offered general newsletters and tips from other youth with diabetes. The Sweet Talk systems also allowed teens to text data and questions to their diabetes care teams. Patient messages were in several categories: blood glucose readings, diabetes questions, diabetes information, personal health administration, and social messages. The study did not find any associations with frequency of messaging and clinical or psychosocial outcomes.[24] Although it is unclear whether texting improves clinical measures in diabetes, there is some indication that texting is a preferred method for reminders.

Studies that addressed disease self-management, adherence to medication, and treatment in teens had mixed results. Many of the studies have small samples and few show improvement with adherence. A small, randomized controlled trial using Your Way, an Internet-based program to improve self-management in adolescents with type 1 diabetes, found that Web-based interventions may improve self-management through enhancing problem-solving skills. Glycemic control as measured by hemoglobin A1c remained stable in the intervention group and worsened in the control group. The sample size was small and the data were analyzed as treated rather than as intent to treat.[25] In a small feasibility, usability, and utility pilot study at Columbia University in New York, the use of CFFONE, a cell phone technology that is Web enabled, provides education about CF, and connects teens with CF through social networking, showed that it was considered somewhat helpful by teens and helpful by parents and adults. Future studies will examine whether the program improves adherence and health outcomes of teens with CF.[26] In a systematic review of Internet and cell phone–based smoking cessation programs among adolescents, the Internet was found to be more effective when used as an adjunct to multiple approaches (counseling, group counseling, acupressure, medications) to cessation versus using the Internet alone. Most interventions had specific Web sites about smoking cessation (chat rooms, Web-based curricula and interventions).[27]

Research is showing that teens with chronic health conditions are knowledgeable consumers of health care technology. There are clear themes that are consistent across the studies. Teens want reliable and trustworthy sources of information regarding their illnesses, and to interact with their providers through online portals. Reminders regarding specific disease treatment plans are acceptable. Social media are acceptable, but must be used in a controlled setting and with peers who have the same condition.

SEXUAL AND REPRODUCTIVE HEALTH

Use of technology by teens with regard to sexual and reproductive health has been studied more than other domains of teen health. Texting is an acceptable mode of communication regarding sexual health if it is anonymous, confidential, and the information is reliable and from a trusted source.[28] There are several innovative ways in which text messaging is being used to promote adolescent sexual health, including:

- Providing health education.
- Offering medication reminders (eg, birth control pill reminders).
- Providing information about available health care services.[28] Although studies have looked at many ways to provide this information, there are limited effectiveness studies that measure whether there is an improvement in sexual health outcomes as a result of the text messaging.

With sensitive topics such as sexual health, youth have increased concern about privacy, especially when they are potentially accessing the Internet on a public versus private computer. Data from a few qualitative studies assessing the use of the Internet among HIV-positive youth supported the use of the Internet for social support and education. A qualitative study of HIV-positive youth in Ontario, Canada, used semi-structured interviews to understand their perspectives on the use of the Internet as a tool to learn about living with HIV. Although these teenagers primarily used the Internet for social networking and entertainment, they acknowledged that a youth-centered, interactive Web site with confidential chat rooms and message boards would be acceptable to them for health information. Privacy was very important.[29] Another qualitative study focusing on HIV-positive African American youth showed that using remote videoconferencing, when privacy was maintained in a secure location, was convenient, efficient, and had a positive impact on their knowledge. The effect of this program on CD4 count and viral load was not studied.[30]

Another promising use of technology with teens is to improve treatment of STIs. Two studies assessed the use of text messaging to decrease time to treatment of chlamydia. Although 1 study found that texting decreased the time to treatment compared with phone or clinic follow-up and that fewer staff hours were needed to do follow-up as a result,[31] the other study found no difference between texting and regular follow-up.[32] Both studies were small and neither was a randomized controlled trial, but these studies indicate that texting is at least as useful as traditional methods for follow-up on abnormal tests, and it has the potential to be better. As software becomes more sophisticated and electronic health records use patient portals it may be more cost-effective and efficient to use technology to notify patients of results and to schedule follow-up.[31]

SUMMARY

Although in its nascency, research in teens and technology has come far in a short period of time. There are already emerging patterns in the literature. Teens prefer text messaging for communication. Computer-based screenings are acceptable to teens and helpful to providers to increase identification and interventions based on high-risk behaviors. Web sites that address specific domains of teen health care should be easy to use, youth centered, connected to an organization that is recommended by the provider, and trustworthy. Social media can play a role in teens and health, but should be connected to the teen's personal experience with a group or organization that focuses on the teen's specific condition (ie, other teens with the same condition). Technology and its role in chronic disease management, including improvement of disease parameters and adherence to medications, shows promise as an intervention.

In a recent article in the *Journal of Adolescent Health* summarizing a conference that set a research agenda for the intersection of youth, technology, and new media with regard to sexual health, scientists and technology experts made key recommendations that included:

- Partner with established community-based organizations skilled in the use of technology to do research
- Petition local institutional review boards to include members with expertise in technology research
- Use theoretic models to understand why technology and social media interventions work
- Use technology in research from the onset
- Use technology and incentives to recruit large, diverse sample sizes
- Conduct research projects that focus on health outcomes with large sample sizes[33]

Experts agree that further research on teens and technology is critical. To date, studies have been small and imperfect. As a result it is difficult to extrapolate to the general population given that most studies are not considered high quality from an evidence-based perspective. The body of research on patient-oriented outcomes that matter to teens is limited, but it is the area that needs the most development along with studies with larger sample sizes and vigorous research protocols. Teens use technology more than any other demographic and future study using interventions that intersect with teens, technology, and their health is important.

REFERENCES

1. Madden M, Lenhart A, Duggan M, et al. Teens and technology 2013. Washington, DC: Pew Internet & American Life Project; 2013. Available at: http://www.pewinternet.org/~/media//Files/Reports/2013/PIP_TeensandTechnology2013.pdf. Accessed January 27, 2014.
2. Lenhart A, Purcell K, Smith A, et al. Social media & mobile internet use among teens and young adults. Washington, DC: Pew Internet & American Life Project; 2010. Available at: http://www.pewinternet.org/~/media//Files/Reports/2010/PIP_Social_Media_and_Young_Adults_Report_Final_with_toplines.pdf. Accessed January 27, 2014.
3. Hansen DL, Derry HA, Resnick PJ, et al. Adolescents searching for health information on the Internet: an observational study. J Med Internet Res 2003;5(4):e25.
4. Chisolm DJ, Johnson LD, McAlearney AS. What makes teens start using and keep using health information web sites? A mixed model analysis of teens with chronic illnesses. Telemed J E Health 2011;17(5):324–8.
5. Dunlop SM, More E, Romer D. Where do youth learn about suicides on the internet, and what influence does this have on suicidal ideation? J Child Psychol Psychiatry 2011;52(10):1073–80.
6. Buhi ER, Daley EM, Oberne A, et al. Quality and accuracy of sexual health information web sites visited by young people. J Adolesc Health 2010;47(2):206–8.
7. Meyer KL, Ahlers-Schmidt CR, Harris KR, et al. STI testing information available to teens on the internet: what's missing? J Pediatr Adolesc Gynecol 2011;24(2):e17–9.
8. Lenhart A, Ling R, Campbell S, et al. Teens and mobile phones. Washington, DC: Pew Internet & American Life Project; 2010. Available at: http://pewinternet.org/~/media//Files/Reports/2010/PIP-Teens and Mobile-2010-with-topline.pdf. Accessed January 27, 2014.
9. Levine D, McCright J, Dobkin L, et al. SEXINFO: a sexual health text messaging service for San Francisco youth. Am J Public Health 2008;98(3):393–5.
10. Carroll JA, Kirkpatrick RL. Impact of social media on adolescent behavioral health. Oakland (CA): California Adolescent Health Collaborative; 2001. Available at: http://www.californiateenhealth.org/wp-content/uploads/2011/09/SocialMediaAug2011.pdf. Accessed March 26, 2014.
11. Chávez NR, Shearer LS, Rosenthal SL. Use of digital media technology for primary prevention of STIs/HIV in youth. J Pediatr Adolesc Gynecol 2013. pii:S1083-3188(13):00239-8.
12. Elster A, Kuznets N, editors. AMA guidelines for adolescent preventive services (GAPS): recommendations and rationale. Baltimore (MD): Williams & Wilkins; 1994.
13. Olson AL, Gaffney CA, Hedberg VA, et al. Use of inexpensive technology to enhance adolescent health screening and counseling. Arch Pediatr Adolesc Med 2009;163(2):172–7.
14. Hassan A, Fleegler EW. Using technology to improve adolescent healthcare. Curr Opin Pediatr 2010;22(4):412–7.
15. Mangunkusumo RT, Moorman PW, Van Den Berg-de Ruiter AE, et al. Internet-administered adolescent health questionnaires compared with a paper version in a randomized study. J Adolesc Health 2005;36(1):70.e1–6.
16. Mackenzie SL, Kurth AE, Spielberg F, et al. Patient and staff perspectives on the use of a computer counseling tool for HIV and sexually transmitted Infection risk reduction. J Adolesc Health 2007;40(6):572.e9–16.

17. Watson PD, Denny SJ, Adair V. Adolescents' perceptions of a health survey using multimedia computer-assisted self-administered interview. Aust N Z J Public Health 2001;25(6):520–4.

18. Stevens J, Kelleher KJ, Gardner W, et al. Trial of computerized screening for adolescent behavioral concerns. Pediatrics 2008;121(6):1099–105.

19. Lightfoot M, Comulada WS, Stover G. Computerized HIV preventive intervention for adolescents: indications of efficacy. Am J Public Health 2007;97(6):1027–30.

20. Saitz R, Palfai TP, Freedner N, et al. Screening and brief intervention online for college students: the ihealth study. Alcohol Alcohol 2007;42(1):28–36.

21. Hamel LM, Robbins LB, Wilbur J. Computer- and web-based interventions to increase preadolescent and adolescent physical activity: a systematic review. J Adv Nurs 2011;67(2):251–68.

22. Applebaum MA, Lawson EF, von Scheven E. Perception of transition readiness and preferences for use of technology in transition programs: teens' ideas for the future. Int J Adolesc Med Health 2013;25(2):119–25.

23. Hanauer DA, Wentzell K, Laffel N, et al. Computerized automated reminder diabetes system (CARDS): e-mail and SMS cell phone text messaging reminders to support diabetes management. Diabetes Technol Ther 2009;11(2):99–106.

24. Franklin VL, Greene A, Waller A, et al. Patients' engagement with "Sweet Talk" - a text messaging support system for young people with diabetes. J Med Internet Res 2008;10(2):e20.

25. Mulvaney SA, Rothman RL, Wallston KA, et al. An internet-based program to improve self-management in adolescents with type 1 diabetes. Diabetes Care 2010;33(3):602–4.

26. Marciel K, Saiman L, Quittel L, et al. Cell phone intervention to improve adherence: cystic fibrosis care team, patient, and parent perspectives. Pediatr Pulmonol 2010;45(2):157–64.

27. Mehta P, Sharma M. Internet and cell phone based smoking cessation programs among adolescents. Acta Didactica Napocensia 2010;3(4):11–24.

28. Malbon K, Romo D. Is it ok 2 txt? Reaching out to adolescents about sexual and reproductive health. Postgrad Med J 2013;89(1055):534–9.

29. Flicker S, Goldberg E, Read S, et al. HIV-positive youth's perspectives on the Internet and e-health. J Med Internet Res 2004;6(3):e32.

30. Saberi P, Yuan P, John M, et al. A pilot study to engage and counsel HIV-positive African American youth via telehealth technology. AIDS Patient Care STDS 2013; 27(9):529–32.

31. Menon-Johansson AS, McNaught F, Mandalia S, et al. Texting decreases the time to treatment for genital *Chlamydia trachomatis* infection. Sex Transm Infect 2006; 82(1):49–51.

32. Lim EJ, Haar J, Morgan J. Can text messaging results reduce time to treatment of *Chlamydia trachomatis*? Sex Transm Infect 2008;84(7):563–4.

33. Allison S, Bauermeister JA, Bull S, et al. The intersection of youth, technology, and new media with sexual health: moving the research agenda forward. J Adolesc Health 2012;51(3):207–12.

Drugs (Substance Use/Abuse)

Adolescent Substance Involvement Use and Abuse

Erica B. Monasterio, MN, FNP-BC[a,b],*

KEYWORDS

- Adolescent • Substance use disorders • Screening • Brief intervention • SBIRT
- Treatment referral

KEY POINTS

- Adolescent substance use is highly prevalent in the United States.
- Adolescence is a vulnerable developmental period for negative impacts of substance involvement and potential development of a substance use disorder (SUD).
- Screening for substance use should be part of the care for every adolescent patient.
- The primary care provider has an essential role in prevention, early intervention, and identification of adolescents in need of a higher level of care for their substance involvement.

INTRODUCTION

Adolescence is a time of normative experimentation that occurs in a context of significant physical, cognitive, psychological, and emotional development. The range of behaviors by which adolescents engage in this normative experimentation are shaped by personal attributes, familial influences, and a social context that includes peers, school, community, and the broader cultural influences in today's society.

Adolescent substance involvement ranges from experimentation to severe SUD. Opportunity to interact on some level with some substance with abuse potential is close to universal in the American society, and substances with abuse potential are ubiquitous, with easy access in many households and most communities in the United States.

Conflict of interest: None.
[a] Family Nurse Practitioner Program, Department of Family Health Care Nursing, University of California, San Francisco, 2 Koret Way, Box 0606, San Francisco, CA 94143-0606, USA; [b] Division of Adolescent and Young Adult Medicine, Department of Pediatrics, 3333 California Street, Suite 245, University of California, San Francisco, San Francisco, CA 94143-0503, USA
* Family Nurse Practitioner Program, Department of Family Health Care Nursing, University of California, San Francisco, 2 Koret Way, Box 0606, San Francisco, CA 94143-0606.
E-mail address: erica.monasterio@ucsf.edu

RISK AND PROTECTIVE FACTORS: VULNERABILITY TO SUDS

There are developmental aspects of adolescence itself that favor some level of substance experimentation, but only a small subset of adolescents engaging is substance experimentation develop an SUD. The vulnerability of the developing adolescent brain to substances of abuse is of great concern. Many substances of abuse result in high levels of dopamine flooding areas of the brain. Early, consistent, repeated exposure to high levels of dopamine in the developing nucleus accumbens may lead to a cascade of effects via pathways between the nucleus accumbens and the amygdala, hippocampus, and frontal cortex, resulting in the development of substance-related cravings and increasing automaticity of the decision-to-use circuit by which substance use becomes a conditioned response rather than a conscious decision.[1] Progression from casual use to an SUD may be affected by the lower threshold of the adolescent brain for experiencing cravings combined with the relative ease of developing automaticity of use. Owing to the heightened vulnerability of the developing adolescent brain to the impact of substance exposure, the younger an individual is when she or he begins to use an addicting substance, the more likely she or he is to develop an addiction. It has been reported that 1 in 4 youth who use any addicting substance before the age of 18 years are at risk of developing an SUD, whereas only 1 in 25 who begin use after the age of 21 years develop an SUD.[2]

Factors that increase adolescent vulnerability to SUDs can be categorized into family, intrapersonal, interpersonal, and social/environmental domains.[3] These domains are not mutually exclusive, and the associations found in the literature do not necessarily imply a causal relationship.

Examples from each risk domain are as follows:

Family
- Weak parent-adolescent attachment[4]
- Parental substance involvement (from both a genetic and an environmental perspective)[5]

Intrapersonal
- Mental health problems, particularly mood and anxiety disorders and untreated attention-deficit/hyperactivity disorder[6,7]
- Temperament characteristics (impulsivity, sensation seeking, behavioral disinhibition)[8]
- History of childhood maltreatment (for tobacco and alcohol use)[9]

Interpersonal
- Associating with a deviant/substance-involved peer group[10]
- Sexual minority identity in a nonaccepting social context[11]

Social/environmental
- Low school engagement and low academic performance[12,13]
- Involvement in the juvenile justice system[13]
- Living in a community with easy access to substances of abuse[10]

Protective factors are equally deserving of attention, particularly from the perspective of prevention. The body of research related to protective factors is smaller and falls into 2 domains: family factors and interpersonal factors.

Examples from each protective factor domain are as follows:

Family
- Parental disapproval of substance use[14]
- Family involvement[15]
- Parental monitoring[16]

Interpersonal factors
- Adult role models[2]
- Positive peer influences[2]
- Youth involvement in prosocial activities[2]
  - Having academic or career goals
  - Participation in school clubs
  - Community involvement
  - Involvement in a religious community/religiosity

In general, aspects of parental, family, and community engagement that mediate against unhealthy risk-taking behaviors such as early sexual debut and early child-bearing and support positive outcomes such as high-school completion are also associated with lower rates of substance involvement.

PREVALENCE/INCIDENCE

Three-fourths of adolescents surveyed in high school report having used addictive substances including tobacco, alcohol, marijuana, and cocaine, and close to half report being current users of these substances.[2] Trends in adolescent substance use vary by drug, with levels of marijuana use having increased and levels of alcohol use and illicit substance use (other than marijuana) being stable or having decreased since 1991.[17] An emerging issue in adolescent substance use is the increasing misuse of prescription drugs by adolescents. Nearly a quarter of high-school youth surveyed in 2012 reported misusing a prescription drug including prescription stimulants and prescription pain medications.[18]

Although most substance experimentation and use occurs in middle and late adolescence, use before the age of 16 years is associated with problem use and SUDs in young adulthood.[19] In a nationally representative sample (the National Longitudinal Study of Adolescent Health), 34% of youth reported initiation of tobacco, alcohol, and/or marijuana use before they were 16 years old. The largest group reported early alcohol use (52.4%), followed by marijuana (43.6%), with fewer initiating early cigarette smoking (29.3%).[19] Polysubstance use before the age of 16 years was found to be more common than single substance use, and early combined alcohol and marijuana use was the strongest predictor of both licit and illicit substance involvement and prescription drug misuse in young adulthood.[19]

Fig. 1 summarizes the frequency of reported "ever use" and "current use" (use in past 3 months) from the Centers of Disease Control and Prevention's most recent Youth Risk Behavior Survey.[20]

IMPACT OF SUBSTANCE USE ON ADOLESCENT HEALTH

Substance use not only significantly affects the current level of function of youth but also influences their development and progression in young adulthood. Recent research summarized by the National Center on Addiction and Substance Abuse shows associations between common adolescent substances of abuse and health impairment in adolescence, as listed in **Table 1**.[2]

Even in the absence of long-term use or an SUD, substance intoxication is related to very significant adolescent morbidity and mortality. Increased risk taking in other domains when intoxicated, such as sexual risk taking, can result in unintended pregnancy and sexually transmitted infections including human immunodeficiency virus infection. Driving or operating machinery while under the influence of alcohol or other drugs is associated with motor vehicle accidents resulting in serious injuries and fatalities. The

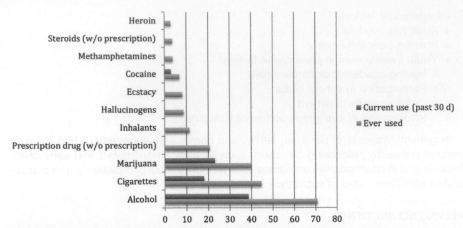

Fig. 1. Percentage of high-school students reporting substance use in 2011. w/o, without. (*From* Centers for Disease Control and Prevention. Youth risk behavior surveillance - United States, 2011. MMWR Surveill Summ 2012;61(4)1–162.)

risk of suicide and homicide, the No. 2 and 3 causes, respectively, of adolescent deaths after unintended injury, is significantly increased in the context of substance use.[2]

In addition to health consequences, adolescent substance use has lasting effects on a young person's trajectory into adulthood. Substance-involved youth are less likely to have academic success with worse grades and poorer school attendance than their non-substance-using peers. They are more likely to drop out of high school and are less likely to graduate from high school, attend college, or obtain a college degree.[21] Those who were substance involved in adolescence have lower levels of occupational attainment, lower wages, and limited employment opportunities in young adulthood.[21]

SUBSTANCES OF ABUSE

Although adolescent substance use covers the entire range of available substances of abuse, tobacco, alcohol, and marijuana are by far the most available and frequently used substances. Adolescent misuse of prescription drugs is also a significant and growing problem, with prescription drugs most commonly acquired from family, friends, peers, or the adolescent's own previous prescriptions.[22]

Periodically, new "designer drugs" emerge, resulting in dangerous fads in adolescent substance use and adverse outcomes related to the use of drugs such as K2 and Spice (synthetic cannabinoids) and bath salts (designer stimulant combinations).[23] Unfortunately, these trends usually come to light after a series of serious or fatal outcomes in a community. Although difficult to foresee, the primary care provider can query patients, clarify responses (if a youth endorses use of a substance that is new to the provider), and stay up to date in community substance use trends to better provide anticipatory guidance and well-informed feedback on the substances a youth may be experimenting with. The National Institute on Drug Abuse maintains an "Emerging Trends" Web page at http://www.drugabuse.gov/drugs-abuse/emerging-trends that is an excellent resource for providers to stay informed regarding new substances and their effects.

Table 2 provides information about common substances of abuse and their effects. The common names listed reflect names used in the local community, and youth may refer to drugs by a wide variety of names. When asking about any substance use, it is essential that the provider clarify what drug the youth is referring to so that she or he can assure that there is a mutual understanding and shared point of reference.

Table 1
Health impairments associated with common substances of abuse

Substance	Associated Health Impairment Found in the Research Literature[2]
Tobacco	Mental Health: • Anxiety disorders • Depressive disorders • Suicidal ideation Medical: • Impaired lung growth and function • Asthma-related symptoms • Shortness of breath and cough • Impaired physical activity tolerance • Nicotine dependence at low levels of exposure • Lower self-ratings of overall physical health than nonsmokers
Alcohol	Mental Health: • Antisocial personality disorder • Depressive disorders • Suicidal ideation Medical: • Benign breast disease (females) • Assault-related injuries • Obesity (long-term heavy drinkers) • Hypertension (long-term heavy drinkers) • More self-reported physical health problems than nondrinkers
Marijuana	Mental Health: • Anxiety disorders (females) • Depressive disorders • Suicidal ideation • Delusional psychosis (including after 1 dose of high-potency marijuana) • Psychotic disorders (in vulnerable individuals) Medical: • Respiratory problems • Acid reflux • Poor attention, planning, and memory
Stimulants (cocaine, methamphetamine)	Mental Health: • Restlessness • Mood disturbance • Anxiety • Paranoia, delusions, and hallucinations (at high levels of use) Medical: • Cardiovascular complications (vasoconstriction, elevated blood pressure, tachycardia, tachyarrhythmia, myocardial infarction [MI], stroke) • Hyperthermia • Extreme weight loss • Insomnia • Dental problems (long-term methamphetamine use)

SCREENING, BRIEF INTERVENTION, AND REFERRAL TO TREATMENT: A FRAMEWORK FOR ADDRESSING ADOLESCENT SUBSTANCE USE

Screening

Assessment for substance use should be incorporated into the standard psychosocial assessment done with every adolescent patient, using a screening tool such as the "HEEADSSS" (Home environment, Education and employment, eating, peer-related

Table 2
Common substances of abuse and their effects

Drug Class	Drug	Common or Brand Name	Dependence Potential Physical	Dependence Potential Psychological	Estimated Detection Time in Urine	Desired or Immediate Effects	Undesired and Long-Term Effects	Overdose Effects
Tobacco	Nicotine	Tobacco, cigarettes, cigars, bidis, squares, stoges	High	High	2–4 d	Relaxation, concentration, stimulation	Chronic withdrawal, chronic bronchitis, asthma, emphysema, lung cancer, exercise intolerance, cardiovascular disease	Anxiety, high blood pressure, tachycardia, nausea
		Smokeless, snuff, dip, chew	High	High				
		Patches, gum, inhaler	Moderate	Moderate				
Alcohol	Ethanol	Beer, 40s	High	High	24 h	Euphoria, reduced inhibitions, impaired judgment, lack of coordination, slurred speech, impaired memory	Liver, brain, heart, and nerve damage; esophageal hemorrhage; pancreatitis; victimization (rape); fetal alcohol syndrome/effects; withdrawal seizures; delirium tremens; accidents	Depressed breathing, abnormal heart beat, amnesia, coma, death
		Wine, wine coolers	High	High				
		Whiskey, liquor, jello shots	High	High				
		Liqueurs	High	High				

		Street names			Detection time	Effects	Consequences	Overdose
Cannabis	Marijuana	Weed, dope, pot, Mary Jane, trees, grapes, purple, dojah, herb, blunts, joints, bud, special brownies, bammer, green, keef, shake, dank, doobie, fade	Low	Moderate	Casual use: 2–7 d	Euphoria, hilarity, altered perceptions, reduced inhibitions, hunger, increased pulse, impaired judgment, red eyes, paranoia, impaired memory, lack of coordination	Accidents; possible respiratory problems: lung damage and asthma; memory impairment; motivation loss; increased heart rate; impaired reaction time	Hallucinations, panic, agitation, delirium
	Hashish, hash oil	Hash	Low	Moderate	Long-term use: Up to 30 d			
Psychostimulants	Cocaine	Coke, crack, rock, yay, chiz, 8 ball, ice, powder, snow, blow, nose candy	High	High	12–72 h	Alertness, increased concentration, excitation, euphoria, appetite loss, headache, jitteriness, increased blood pressure, insomnia, grandiosity, increased activity level, and sexual desire	Tolerance, dehydration, weight loss, itchy and dry eyes/ mouth, blurred vision, CNS damage, anxiety, depression, nausea, abdominal pain, impotence, psychosis, agitated delirium, "crash" withdrawal	Agitation, seizures, paranoia, heart attack, stroke, hallucinations, arrhythmias, respiratory failure, fever, death
	Amphetamine	Dexedrine, adderall, uppers, speed, pep pills	High	High	2–4 d			
	Methylphenidate	Ritalin, pep pills	High	High				
	Methamphetamine	Meth, crystal, tina, speed, chalk, crank, glass	High	High				
	MDMA, MDA, MDEA	Ecstasy, thizz, E, X	Possible	Possible	2–3 d			

(continued on next page)

Table 2
(continued)

| Drug Class | Drug | Common or Brand Name | Dependence Potential | | Estimated Detection Time in Urine | Desired or Immediate Effects | Undesired and Long-Term Effects | Overdose Effects |
			Physical	Psychological				
Opioids	Opium	Chinese molasses, dreams, gong, O	High	High	2–3 d	Euphoric rush, warm flushing of the skin, pain relief, constricted pupils, slowed breathing, sleepiness, heavy feeling in extremities, decreased level of cognitive functioning, nausea, vomiting, and itching	Tolerance, poor appetite, weight loss, pneumonia, constipation, IV use infections: AIDS, Hep B/C, liver disease, collapsed veins, abscesses, and inflammation	Respiratory depression, respiratory arrest, possible coma or death if combined with alcohol or sedatives
	Morphine	Morphine sulfate, M.S., MSO4	High	High	3–4 d			
	Codeine	Tylenol 3	High	High	2–5 d			
	Heroin	H, hey ron, smack, junk, black tar, horse, dope	High	High	3–4 d		Addiction withdrawal: drug craving, nausea, vomiting, abdominal pain, confusion, muscle and bone pain, and restlessness	
	Meperidine	Demerol	High	High	2–4 d			
	Hydromorphone	Dilaudid	High	High				
	Oxycodone	Percocet, percodan, oxycontin	High	High	8–24 h			
	Hydrocodone	Vicodin	High	High				
	Fentanyl	China white, sublimaze	High	High	2–5 d			

Category	Drug	Street names	Physical dependence	Psychological dependence	Duration of detection	Effects	Long-term effects / withdrawal	Effects of overdose
Sedatives/ depressants/ tranquilizers	Barbiturates	Phenobarb, seconal, nembutal, amytal, barbs	High	High	Short acting: 3 d intermediate: 2.5 wk	Relaxation, drowsiness, dizziness, lack of coordination, slurring words, poor concentration, lowered pulse/ breathing	Tolerance, fatigue, memory impairment, delirium, victimization (rape) Addiction withdrawal	Respiratory depression, seizures, possible coma or death if combined with alcohol or opioids
	Benzodiazepines	Valium, ativan, xanax, downers	High	High	Up to 30 d			
	Flunitrazepam	Rohypnol, roofies	High	High	Up to 72 h			
	Methaqualone	Quaalude, ludes, sopor	High	High	4–6 d			
	γ-hydroxybutyrate	GHB, G, liquid E	Unknown	Unknown	Up to 24 h			
	Chloral hydrate	Knockout drops, Mickey	Moderate	Moderate	2–7 d			
Hallucinogens/ dissociative anesthetics	LSD	Acid, blotter, doses	None	None	2 d	Sense of insight, integration or detachment, altered perceptions, visual hallucinations, delusions, jitteriness, fast or slow pulse, chills, intense fear, anxiety, paranoia, panic, euphoria, dizziness, insomnia	Flashbacks, unpredictable behavior, delirium, violence, tolerance, depressed mood, impaired memory, persistent psychosis, mood swings, disorientation, impaired judgment, nausea, hot flashes, rigid motor tone	PCP lethal in overdose especially combined with alcohol or sedatives, muscle contractions, fatal heart rhythms, convulsions, coma, hyperthermia, death
	Psilocybin	Shrooms, magic mushrooms	None	Possible	2–4 d			
	Mescaline	Peyote, buttons, mescalito, mesc	None	Possible	2–3 d			
	PCP	PCP, angel dust, dust	Moderate	Unknown	2–7 d			
	Ketamine	Special K, K, vitamin K, cat tranquilizer	Unknown	Unknown	7–14 d			
	DMT	Businessman special, dimitri	None	None	2–5 d			
	DXM	DXM, syrup, robo, skittles, vitamin D, dex, triple C, CCC	Low	Unknown				

(continued on next page)

Table 2
(continued)

Drug Class	Drug	Common or Brand Name	Dependence Potential Physical	Dependence Potential Psychological	Estimated Detection Time in Urine	Desired or Immediate Effects	Undesired and Long-Term Effects	Overdose Effects
Inhalants	Butyl, cyclohexyl, amyl nitrates	Poppers, rush, aerosols	Low	Unknown	No standard test available	Euphoria, reduced inhibitions, impaired judgment, lack of coordination, slowed reflexes, dizziness, headache	Muscle weakness, disorientation, nerve and brain damage, kidney failure, arrhythmias	Suffocation, coma, heart failure, death
	Nitrous oxide, gases	Laughing gas, whippets, whipped cream	Low	Unknown				
	Petroleum distillates	Glues, solvents, acetone, gasoline	Low	Unknown				
	Chloroalkenes, chloroalkanes	Cleaning agents, adhesives	Low	Unknown				

Abbreviations: AIDS, acquired immunodeficiency syndrome; CNS, central nervous system; DMT, dimethyltryptamine; DXM, dextromethorphan; GHB, γ-hydroxybutyrate; IV, intravenous; LSD, lysergic acid diethylamide; MDA, 3,4-methylenedioxyamphetamine; MDEA, 3,4-methylenedioxy-N-ethylamphetamine; MDMA, 3,4-methylenedioxymethamphetamine; M.S., morphine sulfate; PCP, phencyclidine.

Adapted from Shalwitz J, Sang T, Combs N, et al. Behavioral health: an adolescent provider toolkit. San Francisco (CA): Adolescent Health Working Group; 2007.

Activities, Drugs, Sexuality, Suicide/depression, and Safety from injury and violence) or "SSHADESS" (Strengths, School, Home, Activities, Drugs/substance use, Emotions/depression, Sexuality, and Safety) mnemonic.[24] All youth are in environments, including their homes, where substances may be easily available, and early substance use is associated with greater risk of adverse outcomes. For these reasons, providers should avoid screening based on any profile and assess all youth with whom they interact.

Tobacco Use: Special Considerations

Use of tobacco, the leading preventable cause of disease and death in the United States, is most commonly initiated during adolescence.[25] Youth use a variety of tobacco products, including cigarettes, cigars, and smokeless tobacco (chewing tobacco) as well new tobacco-free nicotine delivery systems such as e-cigarettes. Although high-school students' use of cigarettes has declined since the 1990s, other forms of tobacco use have held steady, and 1 in 5 high-school students use some form of tobacco, with half of those youth using multiple forms.[26]

The American Academy of Pediatrics (AAP) recommends that providers use practice-based systems that reinforce asking every adolescent (and their parent or parents/caregiver) about tobacco product use and second-hand smoke exposure. Electronic health records with prompts that reinforce questioning, cues to promote counseling regarding tobacco cessation, and systems that require documentation of tobacco use and exposure to second-hand smoke are effective supports to assure provider interventions to promote tobacco cessation.[27] Brief primary care interventions (screening and advising not to smoke) have been shown to have a positive impact on adolescents' attitudes, knowledge, intentions to smoke, and quitting behaviors.[28]

Screening for Alcohol and Other Drugs of Abuse

Although the US Preventive Services Task Force (USPSTF) has issued evidence-based recommendations for screening and counseling for alcohol use problems in adults aged 18 years and older (grade B recommendation), they concluded that there is insufficient evidence to assess the efficacy of screening and behavioral counseling interventions in primary care to reduce alcohol misuse in adolescents (I statement).[29] Despite the determination of insufficient evidence by the USPSTF, there is a growing body of research showing both the adverse outcomes associated with adolescent substance use and the efficacy of adolescent-appropriate screening and treatment approaches. In response to this growing body of evidence, the AAP recommends that primary care providers screen all adolescent patients using the Screening, Brief Intervention, and Referral to Treatment (SBIRT) approach championed by the Substance Abuse and Mental Health Services Administration (SAMHSA).[24]

In addition to the question of whether to screen, the questions of how to screen and what screening tool to use must be addressed. Adolescents have indicated a preference for paper- or computer-based screening rather than an oral interview by a nurse or doctor to assess the level of substance use and its impact on function.[30] The reasons for this preference were not queried in the research, but the adolescent subjects did endorse that they were very likely to be honest when responding to paper- or computer-based substance abuse screening questions.[30] The goals of screening are to identify those youth at high risk for an SUD and should in general be followed by a diagnostic, and, as appropriate, an intervention process. Although there are a variety of instruments developed to screen for substance use in adolescence, the CRAFFT has been validated for use in adolescents,[31,32] is the most widely used, and is the only adolescent-appropriate tool with adequate and consistent data to support its use in primary care settings for the range of substances of abuse.[33]

Although the general psychosocial assessment (using either the HEADSSS or SSHADESS mnemonic) can be used to elucidate if the youth has ever used any substances as well as to determine the level of use in the past 12 months, higher detection rates of substance use are reached through the use of a structured substance abuse screening protocol.[34] The Adolescent Substance Abuse Program at Children's Hospital Boston recommends the use of 3 opening questions:[24]

During the past 12 months, did you

- Drink any alcohol (more than a few sips)?
- Smoke any marijuana or hashish?
- Use anything else to get high (anything else includes illegal drugs, over-the-counter and prescription drugs, and things that you sniff or huff)

A positive response to any of these questions, which can be easily asked in the context of the general psychosocial assessment, should trigger the provider (or computerized screening system) to administer the CRAFFT.

The CRAFFT consists of 6 screening questions, preferably administered via paper or computerized screening, each with a yes or no answer. Each question is scored with 1 point for a yes response, and a total score of 2 or more points is considered an indication of risky substance use and a need for further evaluation.[32] The CRAFFT is available in a variety of languages and can be found at www.ceasar.org. **Box 1** describes what the CRAFFT mnemonic stands for.[35]

Brief Intervention

The AAP endorses an adolescent SBIRT algorithm developed by the Massachusetts Department of Public Health Bureau of Substance Abuse Services (their Provider Guide can be found at http://www.mcpap.com/pdf/CRAFFT Screening Tool.pdf) as an efficient, research-informed approach to address adolescent substance use.[24] Using this approach, all adolescents, even those who answer no to the initial 3 screening questions, should receive a brief intervention that includes praise and encouragement for positive behavioral choices and the CRAFFT "Car" question. Any youth who endorses riding in a car driven by someone who was high or had been using alcohol or drugs should additionally receive a message of concern and educational counseling related to the risk to passengers riding with a driver using alcohol or drugs. Discussing a safety plan and eliciting a commitment to avoid future driving/riding risk is an appropriate intervention for youth who are at low risk for substance involvement but answer yes to the "Car" question.[24]

Box 1
CRAFFT screener for adolescent substance use

C	Have you ever ridden in a *Car* driven by someone (including yourself) who was "high" or had been using alcohol or drugs?
R	Do you use alcohol or drugs to *Relax*, feel better about yourself, or fit in?
A	Do you ever use alcohol/drugs while you are by yourself, *Alone*?
F	Do you ever *Forget* things you did while using alcohol/drugs?
F	Do your *Family* or *Friends* ever tell you that you should cut down on your drinking or drug use?
T	Have you gotten into *Trouble* while you were using alcohol or drugs?

From The Center for Adolescent Substance Abuse Research (CeASAR). Available at: www.ceasar.org. Accessed December 19, 2013.

Youth at moderate risk include those who endorse some beginning use of alcohol and/or drugs and score 0–1 on the CRAFFT (CRAFFT-negative youth). These youth may be experimenting with drugs and alcohol but have not yet experienced an impact on function. Despite their low level of substance use, they are still at significant risk for both an adverse outcome related to engaging in other risky behaviors while under the influence and an enhanced vulnerability to developing an SUD. Brief advice to stop all use, with educational counseling about the impact of substances on the developing brain and concerns about risky behavior while under the influence may be of benefit to youth with moderate risk.[24] As with all adolescent behavioral interventions, the youth's strengths and positive behavioral choices should be recognized and supported, and the counseling messages should be tailored to the individual youth's school, work, peer, and family context.

A CRAFFT score of 2 or more indicates a positive result of screening and a youth at high risk for having an SUD. A positive result of CRAFFT does not make a diagnosis of an SUD but is an indication of the need for further directed assessment.[24] Ideally, this assessment includes both open-ended and directed questioning and an opportunity to assess the youth's interest in modifying her or his substance use. A skilled assessment seamlessly moves into a brief intervention based on both adolescents' risk and their motivation to change their substance use behavior.

The Diagnostic and Statistical Manual of Mental Disorders, Fifth Edition, (DSM-V) defines an SUD as "a cluster of cognitive, behavioral, and physiologic symptoms indicating that the individual continues to use a substance despite significant substance-related problems."[36] Specific diagnostic criteria are grouped into the domains impaired control, social impairment, risky use, and pharmacologic criteria. Although each substance of abuse has its own diagnostic criteria, all generally share the following ones (with the exception of withdrawal symptoms, which are not specified for phencyclidine, other hallucinogen use, or inhalant use disorders):[36]

The DSM-V SUD diagnostic criteria are as follows:

- Impaired control
  ○ Substance taken in larger amounts/over longer period than intended
  ○ Desire to cut down or regulate use/unsuccessful efforts to quit use
  ○ Great deal of time taken up by activities involved in use (obtaining/using/recovering from use)
  ○ Craving (intense desire or urge to use)
- Social impairment
  ○ Failure to fulfill major role obligations at home/work/school
  ○ Continued use despite persistent recurring social/interpersonal problems associated with use
  ○ Important social/recreational/occupational activities given up because of use (social/family withdrawal)
- Risky use
  ○ Recurrent use resulting in physically hazardous behavior (eg, driving)
  ○ Continued use despite persistent/recurrent physical or psychological problem likely caused or exacerbated by use
- Pharmacologic
  ○ Tolerance (need for a markedly increased dose to achieve desired effect)
  ○ Withdrawal (physiologic symptoms resulting from decreased blood or tissue concentrations of the substance)

The severity of the SUD is based on the number of symptom criteria endorsed by the youth. A mild SUD is diagnosed with the presence of 2 to 3 symptoms; a moderate

SUD, with 4 to 5 symptoms; and a severe SUD, with 6 or more symptoms.[36] The salience of the DSM-V diagnostic criteria in the primary care environment is that it can serve as a guide to appropriate areas of inquiry to determine if there is an SUD (and assess the level of severity of the disorder) and aids in the determination of the appropriate level of intervention (brief intervention vs referral to treatment) for the primary care clinician.

For those youth with a CRAFFT-positive screen, further assessment is initially orientated toward determining if the youth is in acute danger secondary to substance use or manifests any "red flags" for an SUD. Recommended follow-up questions include:[37]

- Tell me about your alcohol/drug use. When did you begin using? What is your use like now?
- Have you had any problems at school, at home, or with the law?
  ○ If yes, were you drinking or using drugs just before that happened?
- Have you ever tried to quit? Why? How did it go? For how long did you stop? Then what happened?

These recommended questions start with an open-ended approach to gaining an understanding of age of onset of use, range of substances used, pattern of use, and stability or progression of the level of substance involvement (impaired control criteria). Social impairment and risky use are addressed in the second question set, and both impaired control and any experience of tolerance and withdrawal are assessed using the third question set. Allowing the youth to tell their story as it relates to their substance use garners more useful information than rapid-fire, close-ended questioning to quantify and qualify substance use.

Signs of acute danger include use of injection drugs, a drug-related hospital visit, combination sedative use (combining alcohol, benzodiazepines, barbiturates or opioids), consumption of potentially lethal quantities of alcohol ($\geq$14 drinks), or driving/swimming/diving or engaging in other potentially dangerous activities while using drugs or alcohol.[24] Any of these signs warrant an immediate intervention. The intervention must be tailored to the age and developmental stage of the youth and can range from a psychoeducational intervention including information about the risk and advice to modify behavior to engagement with the parent or parents/caregivers in the interest of protecting safety. The provider should carefully consider the decision to breach confidentiality and disclose dangerous substance-related behaviors, weighing maintenance of the provider-youth relationship and the opportunity to support the youth in changing their own behaviors against the immediate threat to health and safety. State laws vary as to whether substance abuse treatment is a minor consent service, and also vary in the latitude the treating professional has in involving the parent/guardian in treatment planning and decisions. The need for disclosure should be discussed with the youth, explaining that the rationale is based on concern for the youth's well-being with the goal of protecting the adolescent patient from harm.

Once immediate risk of harm has been determined, the provider must assess for red flags for addiction. Any of these red flags are a rationale to consider parent/caregiver involvement in counseling and follow-up and referral for in-depth assessment and treatment with a substance abuse specialist/program that works with adolescents.

The red flags for addiction are as follows:[24]

- CRAFFT score of 2 or more in a youth aged 14 years or less
- CRAFFT score of 5 or more in any adolescent
- Daily (or near-daily) use of any substances
- Alcohol-consumption-related blackouts

Again, considerations related to the age and developmental stage of youth, the context of their use, as well as youth's stated intentions to modify use and interest in treatment all contribute to the provider's decision regarding parent/caregiver involvement. Often, the parents of youth with red flags for addiction are already aware of their adolescent's substance use problem and have expressed their concern and distress to both their child and the provider. In these instances, disclosure becomes a nonissue, but still needs to be discussed with the youth before meeting with the youth and family. Framing the intervention in the positive by advising the youth that provider would like to inform their parent or parents/caregiver of their intention to seek care from a substance abuse specialist can be helpful in both allaying fears for the youth and their parents and facilitating the referral to specialty care (see section Referral to Treatment).

Most adolescents might neither be in immediate danger nor have red flags for addiction but may be substance involved with relatively minor current consequences. These youth are candidates for a brief negotiated intervention based on the tenants of motivational interviewing. Motivational interviewing is a collaborative approach of guiding to elicit and strengthen motivation to change.[38] Motivation to change is elicited from the youth, not imposed from without, and it is the youth's task, not the provider's, to articulate and resolve their ambivalence about maintaining or changing their own health-compromising behaviors. A guide to motivational interviewing is beyond the scope of this article, and the interested reader is referred to the excellent handbook by Naar-King and Suarez,[38] *Motivational Interviewing with Adolescents and Young Adults.*

The evidence for the efficacy of brief negotiated interviews (BNI) to affect adolescent substance use has, to this point, centered on alcohol and marijuana use interventions in the emergency department, and findings are inconclusive when looking at the current body of research as a whole.[39] There is not yet a body of research evaluating the impact of BNI in primary care, but the AAP has endorsed this approach as a best practice.[24]

The following are the steps for the primary care provider to take in implementing BNI:

- Summarize findings from the assessment
- List the problems associated with substance use *as identified by the adolescent*
- Ask the youth whether they are interested in changing their approach to substance use

An example of this approach is as follows. AK, a 16-year-old girl, reports "smoking weed" most weekends for fun and to relieve boredom. Her CRAFFT score is 3, with positive responses to the Relax, Family/friends, and Trouble questions. She identifies increased problems managing her asthma and difficulty getting her weekend homework done with a recent "B" on a project that "I should have gotten an 'A' on" as related to her marijuana use. Her best friend recently told her that she acts stupid when she is high and suggested she cut down.

Using BNI, the provider approaches the intervention in the following manner: It sounds like you enjoy getting high on the weekends, and that smoking weed has become something that you do regularly. Even though you find it fun to get high, you are also noticing some problems, like wheezing and having to use your inhaler more, having trouble getting your schoolwork done and your friend telling you that you "act stupid" when you are high. Thinking ahead, is there anything that you want to do about this?

If the youth professes interest in change, specific goals and actions to meet those goals can then be elicited from the youth. These goals and actions may be recorded, and some providers advocate having the youth sign their individualized change plan, although the efficacy of this approach has not been evaluated. Most important to the BNI is the follow-up plan. The youth will need ongoing support and guidance to meet their goals, and follow-up visits should focus on actions taken (or not taken) and goals met. Barriers to change as well as facilitators for change can be explored, goals modified, and actions reevaluated as the youth progresses in efforts to modify the behavior. Praise for any progress, no matter how small, should always be given. For those adolescents with an expressed desire to change but an inability to follow their own plan, a referral to a mental health professional within the practice trained in motivational interviewing, who can engage with the youth on a deeper level and over a longer period, has been shown to be effective in reducing harmful behaviors.[33] Those youth who have made a commitment to modifying their substance use may also be open to involving their parents in the process. If the youth desires parental involvement, the provider can offer to meet with the youth and parents to discuss the change plan. It is important, however, that the provider emphasizes that the locus of control must remain with the youth and that overinvolvement by the parents though monitoring, reminding, correcting, or taking over the recovery process can backfire, leading to withdrawal and secrecy about their use on the youth's part.

Referral to Treatment

Those youth who exhibit signs of acute danger or red flags for an SUD need an intervention that is beyond the scope of a primary care visit.[24] The compounding factors of a condition (substance abuse) characterized by resistance and denial and a developmental stage (adolescence) during which insight is just developing often result in the need for significant engagement from the primary care provider to facilitate a successful referral. Motivational interviewing techniques in these cases focus on moving the youth toward acceptance of a referral for continuing care.

Familiarity with treatment modalities, local resources, and coverage considerations assist the provider in making a successful referral to treatment. SAMHSA maintains a Substance Abuse Treatment Facility Locator at http://findtreatment.samhsa.gov/TreatmentLocator/faces/searchResults.jspx and searches can be sorted by location, type of services, population of focus, forms of payment accepted, and so forth. Although this resource is helpful, it cannot replace personal familiarity with programs and providers. The primary care provider is a known and trusted resource for youth and families, and their referral serves as an endorsement of the treatment provider/program. Generally, the primary care provider refers to a substance abuse specialist for further assessment and determination of the appropriate level of care in the treatment spectrum. Treatment can range from outpatient group therapy to residential treatment options. Common adolescent SUD treatment modalities include:[13]

- Outpatient treatment
  - Psychoeducation/prevention groups (school based or in the community)
  - Group therapy (often using a facilitated alcoholics anonymous/narcotics anonymous [AA/NA] model)
  - Family therapy
  - Intensive outpatient program
    - Usually 2 to 3 h/d, 2 to 5 d/wk, for 1 to 3 months
  - Partial hospital program
    - Usually 8 h/d, 5 d/wk, for 1 to 3 weeks
- Inpatient or residential treatment
  - Detoxification

- Medical management of the symptoms of withdrawal
- Should be followed by outpatient or residential substance abuse treatment program
  - Short-term residential treatment
    - For stabilization of youth in crisis before placement in residential treatment
    - Appropriate for youth with dual diagnoses of mental health and SUD
  - Residential treatment
    - Both short-term (<30 day) and long-term (>30 day) programs available
    - Combination of group and individual therapy and psychological, medical nutritional, educational, and social milieu-based interventions
  - Therapeutic boarding school
    - Highly structured environment
    - Educational institution with specialized classes, individual and group therapy, and social support for recovery

The Facilitated Referral

A commitment to behavior change is difficult to make and harder to maintain, and denial is part of the disease in SUDs. The primary care provider is generally the health care professional who has developed rapport and trust with the youth and family and has a longitudinal relationship with them. Referral to a substance abuse expert for assessment followed by a further referral for treatment is a process with many potential barriers, false starts, and loss to follow-up. It is the responsibility of the primary care provider to facilitate referral to care and actively reach out to the youth and family as they move toward recovery. Providing information, resources, encouragement, and a safety net to loop the youth and family back into care when they encounter barriers are essential components of the facilitated referral. By remaining engaged and supporting youth who are substance involved to evaluate the impact of their own behaviors and move toward behavior change, the primary care provider can have a significant impact on their trajectory into a healthy adulthood.

REFERENCES

1. Duhigg D. Why adolescents use substances of abuse. Adolesc Med State Art Rev 2013;24(2):465–77.
2. National Center on Addiction and Substance Abuse. Adolescent substance use: America's #1 public health problem. New York: National Center on Addiction and Substance Abuse, Columbia University; 2011.
3. Brook JS, Lee JY, Rubenstone E, et al. Longitudinal determinants of substance use disorders. J Urban Health 2013;90:1130–50.
4. Arria AM, Mericle AA, Meyers K, et al. Parental substance use impairment, parenting and substance use disorder risk. J Subst Abuse Treat 2012;43(1): 114–22.
5. Rhee SH, Hewitt JK, Young SE, et al. Genetic and environmental influences on substance initiation, use, and problem use in adolescents. Arch Gen Psychiatry 2003;60(12):1256–64.
6. Conway KP, Compton W, Stinson FS, et al. Lifetime comorbidity of DSM-IV mood and anxiety disorders and specific drug use disorders: results from the national epidemiologic survey on alcohol and related conditions. J Clin Psychiatry 2006; 67(2):247–57.
7. Wilens TE, Adamson J, Monuteaux MC, et al. Effect of prior stimulant treatment for attention-deficit/hyperactivity disorder on subsequent risk for cigarette

smoking and alcohol and drug use disorders in adolescents. Arch Pediatr Adolesc Med 2008;162(10):916–21.

8. Mezzich AC, Tarter RE, Kirisci L, et al. Reciprocal influence of parent discipline and child's behavior on risk for substance use disorder: a nine-year prospective study. Am J Drug Alcohol Abuse 2007;33(6):851–67.

9. Mersky JP, Topitzes J, Reynolds AJ. Impacts of adverse childhood experiences on health, mental health, and substance use in early adulthood: a cohort study of an urban, minority sample in the U.S. Child Abuse Negl 2013;37(11):917–25.

10. Gillespie NA, Kendler KS, Prescott CA, et al. Longitudinal modeling of genetic and environmental influences on self-reported availability of psychoactive substances: alcohol, cigarettes, marijuana, cocaine and stimulants. Psychol Med 2007;37(7):947–59.

11. Ryan C, Huebner D, Diaz RM, et al. Family rejection as a predictor of negative health outcomes in white and Latino lesbian, gay, and bisexual young adults. Pediatrics 2009;123(1):346–52.

12. Bryant A, Schulenberg E, O'Malley P, et al. How academic achievement, attitudes, and behaviors relate to the course of substance use during adolescence: a 6-year, multiwave national longitudinal study. J Res Adolesc 2003;13(3):361.

13. Center for Substance Abuse Treatment. Treatment of adolescents with substance use disorders. Chapter 2-tailoring treatment to the adolescent's problem. Rockville (MD): Substance Abuse and Mental Health Services Administration; 1999. Treatment Improvement Protocol (TIP) Series; No. 32.

14. van der Vorst H, Engels RC, Meeus W, et al. The role of alcohol-specific socialization in adolescents' drinking behaviour. Addiction 2005;100(10):1464–76.

15. Schlauch RC, Levitt A, Connell CM, et al. The moderating effect of family involvement on substance use risk factors in adolescents with severe emotional and behavioral challenges. Addict Behav 2013;38(7):2333–42.

16. Kosterman R, Hawkins JD, Guo J, et al. The dynamics of alcohol and marijuana initiation: Patterns and predictors of first use in adolescence. Am J Public Health 2000;90(3):360–6.

17. Centers for Disease Control. Youth risk behavior surveillance system (YRBSS). Adolescent and school health: alcohol and other drug use web site. 2012. Available at: http://www.cdc.gov/healthyyouth/alcoholdrug/. Accessed December 12, 2013.

18. The Partnership at Drugfree.org. PATS KEY FINDINGS: 2012 partnership attitude tracking study, sponsored by MetLife foundation. The Partnership at Drugfree.org Web site. 2013. Available at: http://www.drugfree.org/wp-content/uploads/2013/04/PATS-2012-KEY-FINDINGS.pdf. Accessed December 12, 2013.

19. Moss HB, Chen CM, Yi HY. Early adolescent patterns of alcohol, cigarettes, and marijuana polysubstance use and young adult substance use outcomes in a nationally representative sample. Drug Alcohol Depend 2014;136:51–62.

20. Eaton DK, Kann L, Kinchen S, et al, Centers for Disease Control and Prevention. Youth risk behavior surveillance - United States, 2011. MMWR Surveill Summ 2012;61(4):1–162.

21. Griffin BA, Ramchand R, Edelen MO, et al. Associations between abstinence in adolescence and economic and educational outcomes seven years later among high-risk youth. Drug Alcohol Depend 2011;113(2–3):118–24.

22. Ross-Durow PL, McCabe SE, Boyd CJ. Adolescents' access to their own prescription medications in the home. J Adolesc Health 2013;53(2):260–4.

23. Seely KA, Patton AL, Moran CL, et al. Forensic investigation of K2, spice, and "bath salt" commercial preparations: a three-year study of new designer drug

products containing synthetic cannabinoid, stimulant, and hallucinogenic compounds. Forensic Sci Int 2013;233(1–3):416–22.

24. Committee on Substance Abuse, Levy SJ, Kokotailo PK. Substance use screening, brief intervention, and referral to treatment for pediatricians. Pediatrics 2011;128(5):e1330–40.

25. U.S. Department of Health and Human Services. Preventing tobacco use among youth and young adults: a report of the surgeon general. Atlanta (GA): Center for Disease Control and Prevention; 2012.

26. Arrazola RA, Kuiper NM, Dube SR. Patterns of current use of tobacco products among U.S. high school students for 2000-2012–findings from the national youth tobacco survey. J Adolesc Health 2014;54(1):54–60.e9.

27. Committee on Environmental Health, Committee on Substance Abuse, Committee on Adolescence, Committee on Native American Child. From the American Academy of Pediatrics: policy statement–tobacco use: a pediatric disease. Pediatrics 2009;124(5):1474–87.

28. Hum AM, Robinson LA, Jackson AA, et al. Physician communication regarding smoking and adolescent tobacco use. Pediatrics 2011;127(6):e1368–74.

29. Moyer VA, Preventive Services Task Force. Screening and behavioral counseling interventions in primary care to reduce alcohol misuse: U.S. Preventive Services Task Force recommendation statement. Ann Intern Med 2013;159(3):210–8.

30. Knight JR, Harris SK, Sherritt L, et al. Adolescents' preference for substance abuse screening in primary care practice. Subst Abus 2007;28(4):107–17.

31. Cook RL, Chung T, Kelly TM, et al. Alcohol screening in young persons attending a sexually transmitted disease clinic. comparison of AUDIT, CRAFFT, and CAGE instruments. J Gen Intern Med 2005;20(1):1–6.

32. Knight JR, Sherritt L, Shrier LA, et al. Validity of the CRAFFT substance abuse screening test among adolescent clinic patients. Arch Pediatr Adolesc Med 2002;156(6):607–14.

33. Pilowsky DJ, Wu LT. Screening instruments for substance use and brief interventions targeting adolescents in primary care: a literature review. Addict Behav 2013;38(5):2146–53.

34. Stevens J, Kelleher KJ, Gardner W, et al. Trial of computerized screening for adolescent behavioral concerns. Pediatrics 2008;121(6):1099–105.

35. Knight JR, Shrier LA, Bravender TD, et al. A new brief screen for adolescent substance abuse. Arch Pediatr Adolesc Med 1999;153(6):591–6.

36. American Psychiatric Association. Diagnostic and Statistical Manual of Mental Disorders. 5th edition. Arlington (VA): American Psychiatric Association; 2013.

37. Massachusetts Department of Public Health Bureau of Substance Abuse Services. Providers guide: adolescent screening, brief intervention, and referral to treatment for alcohol and other drug use: using the CRAFFT screening tool. Boston(MA): Massachusetts Department of Public Health; 2009.

38. Naar-King S, Suarez M. Motivational interviewing with adolescents and young adults. New York: Guilford Press; 2010. p. 224. Available at: https://ucsf.idm.oclc.org/login?url=http://search.EBSCOhost.com/login.aspx?direct=true&scope=site&db=nlebk&db=nlabk&AN=347760.

39. Newton AS, Dong K, Mabood N, et al. Brief emergency department interventions for youth who use alcohol and other drugs: a systematic review. Pediatr Emerg Care 2013;29(5):673–84.

Depression (Mental Health)

Mood Disorders in Adolescents

Diagnosis, Treatment, and Suicide Assessment in the Primary Care Setting

Marilia G. Neves, PsyD[a],*, Francesco Leanza, MD[b]

KEYWORDS

- Mood disorders • Adolescent suicide • Screening • Assessment
- Psychosocial interventions • Pharmacologic interventions

KEY POINTS

- Undetected and untreated early onset mood disorders can lead to more serious mental health problems, including suicide. The primary care setting is the typical entry point of youths with mental health issues and an ideal place to screen, assess, and triage to determine initiation of treatment in primary care and referral to mental health services.
- Evidence-based treatment modalities for adolescents with mood disorders include both psychosocial and pharmacologic therapies. However, selecting one or both of these depends on numerous variables, including the severity of symptoms and their level of impact on the adolescent's psychosocial functioning.
- Treating adolescent mood disorders in primary care requires a comprehensive assessment, a multidisciplinary treatment approach, and close monitoring.

INTRODUCTION

Four million children and adolescents in the United States suffer from a serious mental illness that causes significant impairments at home, at school, and with peers.[1] Moreover, half of all lifetime cases of mental disorders begin at 14 years of age.[1] Despite effective treatments, only 20% of youths with mental illnesses are identified and receive mental health services.[2] Undiagnosed mental illness can progress to more severe, difficult-to-treat illness and to the development of comorbid mental health disorders.[3]

Compared with their peers, youths with mental illness are more likely to be high utilizers of primary care services.[4] Hence, primary care providers are strategically poised

Disclosures: The author has nothing to disclose.
[a] Department of Oncological Sciences, Icahn School of Medicine at Mount Sinai, Box 1130 1 Gustave L. Levy Place, New York, NY 10029, USA; [b] Department of Family Medicine and Community Health, Icahn School of Medicine at Mount Sinai, New York, NY, USA
* Corresponding author.
E-mail address: Marilia.Neves1@mssm.edu

to screen, assess, and treat adolescents for common mental health problems frequently encountered in primary care. This article outlines mood disorders, primary care screening tools and assessment, early treatment options, and decision making regarding treating adolescents with mood disorders in a primary care setting versus referral to mental health treatment.

EPIDEMIOLOGY AND COMORBIDITY

The prevalence of major depressive disorder (MDD) is estimated to be approximately 4% to 8% in adolescents,[5] with a female-to-male ratio of 2:1.[6] The risk for depression increases by a factor of 2 to 4 after puberty, particularly in females.[7] The lifetime prevalence of MDD is less than 1.0% in children younger than 12 years and increases to 17.4% at 19 years of age and older.[8]

Approximately 5% to 10% of children and adolescents have depressive symptoms that do not meet the criteria of MDD.[9] However, these youth have considerable psychosocial difficulties, significant family depression, and an increased risk for suicide and developing MDD.[10–13] The few epidemiologic studies on dysthymic disorder, renamed persistent depressive disorder (PDD) in the *Diagnostic and Statistical Manual of Mental Disorders* (Fifth Edition) (*DSM-5*), have reported 1.6% to 8.0% prevalence in adolescents.[9,14]

Both MDD and PDD are often accompanied by other psychiatric and medical conditions, and they often co-occur; depression also increases the risk of non–mood-related psychiatric problems, such as conduct and substance abuse disorders.[9,15,16] Forty percent to 90% of youths with MDD have other psychiatric disorders, with at least 20% to 50% having 2 or more comorbid disorders (**Table 1**).[9,15] Psychiatric comorbidity is associated with poor academic performance, poor adherence to mental health treatment, prior suicide attempts, and a strained parent-child relationship.[16]

Because of the lack reliable bipolar disorder (BD) epidemiologic studies and the controversy over using the diagnosis in youths, prevalence rates of BD in adolescents are difficult to accurately identify.[17] However, estimates in adolescents are thought to be approximately between 1% and 3%.[18] Although overall BD affects both sexes, early onset cases are predominantly in boys, especially in cases with an onset before 13 years of age.[19] Common psychiatric comorbidities in youths with BD are attention-deficit/hyperactivity disorder (ADHD), conduct disorder, and oppositional defiant disorder.[20]

RISK FACTORS

Risk factors for adolescent depression include genetic, environmental, and cognitive factors as well as comorbid disorders (**Box 1**).[9] Of youths who experience depression, 2% to 50% have a family history of depression or other mental health problems.[21] A family history of depression is the single most predictive factor associated with the risk for developing MDD.[22,23]

Table 1	
Comorbid psychiatric disorders of youth MDD	
Anxiety disorder (%)	30–80
Disruptive behavior disorder (including attention-deficit/hyperactivity disorder) (%)	10–80
Substance use disorders (%)	20–30
Persistent depressive disorder (%)	30–80
Eating disorders (%)	10

Box 1
Risk factors of adolescent depression

Genetic

- Family psychiatric history

Environmental

- Parental modeling of depressive affect, behaviors, and thinking patterns
- Increased family conflict
- Low socioeconomic status
- Neglect, sexual and/or physical abuse
- Poor peer relationships
- Early death of a parent or of a loved one
- Loss of a friendship
- Inadequate support system

Cognitive

- Poor coping skills

Comorbid disorders

- Anxiety disorders
- Disruptive disorders
- Substance use disorders
- ADHD
- Eating disorders
- Medical illness

Furthermore, adolescents with first-degree relatives with BD have a 4- to 6-fold increased risk of developing this disorder.[24] Offspring of parents with BD display more episodic symptoms suggestive of risk for the disorder than those of normal controls, including mood lability, anxiety, attention difficulties, hyperarousal, depression, somatic complaints, and school problems.[25,26] In addition, traumatic experience can trigger an episode of BD in individuals who are genetically vulnerable.[27]

RECOGNIZING SYMPTOMS OF MOOD DISORDERS IN ADOLESCENTS

It is developmentally normal for all adolescents to go through periods when their mood fluctuates[28]; however, a persistently abnormal mood for an extended period of time resulting in a significant change in psychosocial functioning and impairment may indicate a mood disorder.[29] Furthermore, it is important to rule out symptoms of mood disorders induced by alcohol and substance use, medical illness, medication side effects, or other psychiatric disorders.[29] **Table 2** includes a brief list of selected medical problems that mimic symptoms of mood disorders.[30]

Table 3 provides a comparison of mood episodes found in mood disorders.[29] MDD and PDD are specified as mild, moderate, or severe. The greater the number of symptoms and the higher their intensity, the greater the impact of these symptoms on the adolescent's psychosocial functioning. Bipolar I disorder is characterized by discrete episodes of mania and major depression, whereas bipolar II disorder includes distinct episodes of hypomania and major depression.

Table 2 Medical conditions that mimic symptoms of mood disorders	
NEUROLOGIC	• Migraine • Multiple sclerosis • Brain neoplasm • Epilepsy • Head trauma
ENDOCRINE	• Hypothyroidism • Hyperthyroidism • Pheochromocytoma
INFECTIONS	• Human immunodeficiency virus/AIDS • Infectious mononucleosis • Brain abscess • Systemic bacterial infection
METABOLIC AND SYSTEMIC	• Hepatic encephalopathy • Hepatolenticular degeneration • Hypoxemia
TOXIC	• Drug or alcohol intoxication or withdrawal • Adverse effects of medications • Environmental toxins
AUTOIMMUNE	• Systemic lupus erythematosus

Data from Singh T. Pediatric bipolar disorder: diagnostic challenges in identifying symptoms and course of illness. Psychiatry (Edgmont) 2008;5:35–42.

Although the clinical presentation of depression in adolescents is similar to that of adults, there are some differences that can be attributed to the physical, cognitive, social and emotional developmental stages of these youth.[10,31,32] **Box 2** includes common symptoms of depression symptom present in adolescents.[21,33–36] Of note, adolescents often report internalizing symptoms, such as sadness, suicidal thinking, and sleep disturbances; whereas their parents report externalizing symptoms, such as irritability, moodiness, and loss of interest.[33]

Mania in adolescent BD is frequently associated with psychotic symptoms, marked labile moods, and/or mixed manic and depressive features.[37–40] Hypersexuality, a criterion for adult bipolar disorder, is seen in approximately 40% of BD in youths.[41] Increased talkativeness with pressure speech and "affective storms", which are severe and dramatic mood eruptions, are also very prominent symptoms in these adolescents.[42]

Mental Status Examination

Although the diagnosis of mood disorder is primarily made based on criteria obtained during a thorough history, the Mental Status Examination (MSE) (**Box 3**)[43] provides observable, objective information and gathers further subjective data, which can support the diagnosis. The components of the MSE can be gathered readily throughout the medical encounter. Primary care providers should be familiar with the components of MSE and document appropriately.[33]

SCREENING AND ASSESSMENT
Depression Screening

The US Preventive Services Task Force (2009) recommends that primary care providers screen adolescents for depression annually at greater than 12 years old

Table 3
Mood episodes of mood disorders

Major Depression	Persistent Depression (Dysthymia)
2 wk of persistent change in mood manifested by either depressed or irritable mood and/or anhedonia plus 4 of the following symptoms: • Appetite disturbance • Sleep disturbance • Psychomotor retardation or agitation • Decreased energy level/fatigue • Feelings of worthlessness or excessive guilt • Difficulty concentrating • Thoughts of death, suicidal ideation, or attempt	1 y of persistent depressed or irritable mood with 2 or more of the following symptoms: • Appetite disturbance • Sleep disturbance • Decreased energy level/fatigue • Low self-esteem • Poor concentrating • Feelings of hopelessness

Mania	Hypomania
1 wk or more of abnormal and persistent elevated, expansive, or irritable mood plus 3 or more of the following symptoms: • Inflated self-esteem or grandiosity • Decreased need to sleep • More talkative than usual • Flight of ideas • Distractibility • Increase in goal-directed activities • Excessive involvement in pleasurable activity • Severe symptoms that cause marked psychosocial impairment	4 consecutive days or more of persistent elevated, expansive, or irritable mood plus 3 or more of the following symptoms: • Inflated self-esteem or grandiosity • Decreased need to sleep • More talkative than usual • Flight of ideas • Distractibility • Increase in goal-directed activities • Excessive involvement in pleasurable activity • Symptoms are not severe to cause marked psychosocial impairment

Data from American Psychiatric Association (APA). Diagnostic and statistical manual of mental disorders. 5th edition. Washington, DC: American Psychiatric Publishing; 2013.

Box 2
Symptoms of depression in adolescents

Vague physical complaints without a definable cause

Sleep disturbance

Changes in appetite

Boredom

Hopelessness

Loss of interest in pleasurable activities

Low self-esteem

Sadness

Suicidal thoughts and/or attempts

Irritability and moodiness

Interpersonal problems

Social isolation

Box 3
MSE components and descriptors

- Appearance: Hygiene, facial expression, head size, stature, nutritional state
- Attitude: Cooperativeness, friendliness, trust, maturity, seductiveness, hostility, evasiveness, defensiveness, guardedness
- Behavior: Gross and fine motor coordination, gait, mannerisms, restlessness, twitches, agitation, retardation, combativeness
- Speech rate, tone, volume and rhythm: Pressured, rapid, slow, incoherent, profanity
- Thought process: Paucity or overabundance of ideas, goal directed, loosing of associations, tangentially, circumstantiality, evasiveness, perseveration, blocking
- Thought content: Self-image, future goals, preoccupation, delusions, ideas of reference such as thought broadcasting and thoughts insertion, suicidal and homicidal ideation
- Attention/concentration: Capacity to focus attention, distractibility, difficulty to follow conversation/information
- Perceptual disturbances: Visual and auditory hallucinations
- Mood described by the adolescent: Happy, down, depressed, anxious, nervous
- Affect observed by the examiner: Mood congruent or mood incongruent
- Insight: Poor, fair, or good degree of awareness and understanding of the nature of the problem
- Judgment: Poor, fair, or good age-appropriate decision making about the problem

Data from Snyderman D, Rovner BW. Mental status examination in primary care: a review. Am Fam Physician 2009;80(8):809–14.

---

when systems are in place to ensure adequate treatment.[44] Although not recommended exclusively as a screening method for depression, the HEADSSS (Home Education Activity Drugs Sexuality Safety Suicide) interview can help identify areas that need further assessment.[45,46] To screen for depressive symptoms, primary care providers should use psychometrically reliable and practical checklists derived from the *DSM-5* or the *International Classification of Diseases, Tenth Revision* criteria for depressive disorders, clinician-based instruments, and/or youth and parent depression self-reports **(Table 4)**.[47,48]

The US Preventive Service Task Force (2009) considers the Beck Depression Inventory II (BDI-II) and Patient Health Questionnaire-Adolescent Version (PHQ-A) to have good sensitivity and specificity in screening adolescents in primary care settings.[44] These screening self-report measures evaluate and rank depression symptom severity in a time-efficient manner. The Pediatric Symptom Checklist is a parent-report measure that screens for general adolescent mental health problems. It does not identify specific mental health disorders; however, it alerts the provider that further assessment is needed.[59] Many primary care practices use the nonadapted version of the PHQ-9, which is validated for 13 years of age and older.[21]

In contrast to asymptomatic screening, adolescents who present to primary care offices with symptoms of depression should be screened using the same validated tools previously discussed. Primary care providers should screen adolescents who present the following:

- Multiple primary care and/or emergency room visits with vague physical symptom complaints

Table 4
Screening tools for depression in adolescents

Name	Age Range (y)	Number of Items	Reading Level (Grade)	Spanish Version	Time to Complete (min)	Test–Retest Reliability
Beck Depression Inventory II[49,50]	13–18	21	Sixth	Yes	5–10	0.93–0.94
Patient Health Questionnaire–Adolescent Version[51]	13–18	9	Sixth	Yes	5–10	0.76
Children's Depression Inventory[52]	7–17	27	First	Yes	10–15	0.71–0.89
Pediatric Symptom Checklist[53]	4–16	35	Fifth–sixth	Yes	2–12	0.84–0.91
Center for Epidemiologic Studies–Depression Scale for Children[54]	12–18	20	Sixth	Yes	5–10	0.84–0.90
Reynolds Adolescent Depression Scales-2[55]	11–20	30	Third	No	10–15	0.89
Mood and Feelings Questionnaire[56,57]	8–18	33	Third	No	10–15	0.80
Mood and Feelings Short Form[58]	6–17	13	Third	No	5–10	0.75

- Symptoms of mood disorders including psychosomatic complaints
- Poor psychosocial functioning
- Parental concerns regarding the adolescent's mood or behaviors
- Family history of depression and/or BD
- Alcohol and/or substance use

BD Screening

Although it is the standard of care for BD to be diagnosed by a mental health provider, it is crucial for primary care providers to know about BD and be aware of it as a diagnosis in the differential of unipolar depression and other mood disorders. Screening for manic symptoms should follow depression screening, especially when there is a family psychiatric history and/or the adolescent presents symptoms suggestive of history of mania, such as hypersexuality, pressured speech, psychomotor agitation, and excessive irritability. The American Academy of Child and Adolescent Psychiatry Child workgroup on BD and primary care parameters recommends clinicians to use the following acronym *FIND* to assess manic symptoms once they are recognized (**Box 4**).[60]

In addition, it is also helpful to ask families to keep a daily log for at least 2 weeks that tracks mood, activity level, energy and sleep, frequency, intensity, and duration of these symptoms as well as triggers of temper tantrums.[33]

Assessment of Mood Disorders

Because emotional and behavioral difficulties in youths are often context dependent, it is important to assess symptoms and behaviors in perspective given family, school, peers, sociocultural background, and other psychosocial factors rather than just simply relying on a checklist to identify psychopathology.[19] Interviews can be time consuming; however, they are more personable and make it easier to engage adolescents in self-disclosure and gather detailed psychosocial information necessary for a diagnostic impression (**Box 5**). Open-ended questions (eg, How are things at home? How are things at school?) are very useful for initiating the conversation with a teen.[17] Clinical interviewing also facilitates primary care decision making regarding initiating treatment and referral to mental health services.

Adolescents and their parents should be screened and interviewed separately to facilitate self-disclosure in a confidential manner. However, it is also important to notify teens about any restrictions on the confidential nature of the interview, particularly if they disclose situations of abuse and of intent to harm self and/or others. In these circumstances, the provider may need to communicate with the adolescents' guardians and possibly other providers who work in collaboration with the primary care provider

---

Box 4
Manic symptoms assessment

*F*requency (symptoms occur most days in a week)

*I*ntensity (severity of symptoms is enough to significantly impact one psychosocial domain or moderately impact 2 or more domains)

*N*umber (symptoms occur 3 or more times each day)

*D*uration (symptoms occur 4 or more hours per day)

From Kowatch RA, Fristad M, Birmaher B, et al. Treatment guidelines for children and adolescents with bipolar disorder. J Am Acad Child Adolesc Psychiatry 2005;44(3):213–35.

Box 5
Areas of assessment

History of presenting symptoms and behaviors

- Symptoms onset, duration, and frequency
- Attempts made to treat the symptoms
- Suicidality, homicidality, and psychosis
- Context of symptoms
- Adolescent's perspective on the symptoms
- How symptoms affect the adolescent's level of functioning
- Adolescent's coping with symptoms
- Family's perspective on and coping with symptoms
- Adolescent's and family's perspective on how to treat the symptoms

Adolescent's psychiatric history

- Past psychiatric diagnosis
- Psychiatric treatment, admissions, and their outcome
- Suicidality, homicidality, and psychosis

Family psychiatric history

- Family psychiatric diagnoses
- Family psychiatric treatment
- Impact of family psychiatric diagnoses on family functioning
- Family coping with psychiatric illness

Medical history

- Medical illnesses that affect the central nervous system
- Traumatic brain injury
- Adverse effects of prescribed and over-the-counter medications

Substance abuse history

- Onset, duration, frequency, and amount of drug or alcohol use
- Context of drug or alcohol use
- Past substance or alcohol abuse treatment and its outcome
- How drug or alcohol use affects the adolescent's level of functioning
- Intoxication or withdrawal associated with drug or alcohol abuse

Developmental history

- Age-appropriate versus developmental delays in physical, sexual, cognitive, emotional, and social development

Social history

- Sociocultural background
- Family structure, functioning, and dynamics
- Support system
- Activities of daily living
- School history
- Sexuality
- Abuse and trauma history

to promote adolescents' safety and well-being. These other providers might be a primary care social worker and/or mental health providers, child protection services, or a local emergency department.

SUICIDE

Youth suicide represents a serious health problem for the nation and a clinical challenge for health care providers.[61] As the third leading cause of death among adolescents, suicide accounts for more deaths than the top 7 non–injury-based medical conditions combined.[62] Nearly 90% of suicidal youth had primary care visits during the prior 12 months.[63,64] By identifying at-risk youth, primary care providers can play a very significant role in adolescent suicide prevention.

Demographics

Although completed suicide rates are higher among adolescent boys than girls, girls have the highest rates of suicidal ideation and attempted suicide.[65] American Indian and Alaskan Native youths have the highest rate of attempted and completed suicide followed by Hispanic and non-Hispanic white males.[66,67] Among US adolescents, the leading method of completed suicide is self-inflicted gunshot wounds, followed by suffocation by hanging or use of plastic bags and self-poisoning.[68]

Risk Factors

Psychopathology is a very significant risk factor in youth suicide. Eighty percent to 90% of adolescent suicide victims and attempters from both community and clinical settings have a psychiatric disorder.[68] The most common psychiatric conditions in completed and attempted suicide are mood, anxiety, conduct, alcohol or substance abuse disorders,[65] with 60% of adolescent suicide victims having a depressive disorder at the time of death.[69–71] Forty percent to 80% of adolescents meet the diagnostic criteria for depression at the time of the suicide attempt.[72,73]

Adolescents who may be at risk for suicide include those with early onset BD; a history of previous suicide attempts; severe depression; mixed episodes; rapid cycling; psychosis; a family history of suicide attempts; availability of methods; exposure to stressful events; and comorbid disorders, such as alcohol or substance abuse, disruptive behavior, and anxiety.[74]

Of note, alcohol and substance abuse disorders are highly correlated with the risk of suicide, especially in older adolescent boys when co-occurring with mood disorder or disruptive disorders.[69–71] Family factors, including parental psychopathology, family history of suicidal behavior, family discord, loss of a parent to death or divorce, poor quality of the parent-child relationship, and sexual and physical abuse, are associated with an increased risk of adolescent suicide and suicidal behavior.[68]

Adolescents who identify as lesbian, gay, bisexual, and transgender are at greater risk than their peers to have attempted suicide; this risk persists even after controlling for other suicide risk factors.[75] Data suggest that family rejection of an adolescent who is gay, lesbian, or bisexual is associated with greater likelihood of attempted suicide compared with adolescents who experience minimal or no family rejection.[76]

Bullying behavior in youth is associated with depression, suicidal ideation, and suicide attempts.[77] Moreover, victims of bullying consistently exhibit more depressive symptoms than nonvictims; they have high levels of suicidal ideation and are more likely to attempt suicide than nonvictims.[77] Cyberbullying has become an increasing public concern in light of the recent cases associated with youth suicides that have been reported in the mass media.[78]

Change of residence is also a risk factor for adolescent suicide behaviors. Change of residence may result in the discontinuation of personal life in a familiar environment as well as a breakdown of the social network,[79] which may lead to stress and adjustment problems.[80] Regardless of the reasons for frequent change of residence, it may be traumatic or psychologically distressing and it may affect the physical, mental, social, and emotional well-being of the adolescent.[80] Therefore, the more often the adolescent moves, the greater the risk for a suicide attempt and completion.[80]

Suicide Warning Signs and Assessment

In contrast to risk factors, warning signs are indicators of more acute suicide risk.

The American Association of Suicidology developed the following mnemonic to identify key warning signs for adolescent suicide: IS PATH WARM (**Box 6**).[61,81]

When an adolescent reports suicidal ideation, the primary care provider should remind the adolescent of confidentiality parameters previously discussed, do a suicide risk assessment, and document it thoroughly (**Box 7**).[82]

In the case of passive suicidal ideation whereby the adolescent reports contemplating suicide but does not have a plan, the primary care provider should engage the adolescent in creating a safety plan. The suicide safety contract is a written agreement not to harm oneself that includes safe behavioral alternatives to manage suicidal ideation, such as relaxation techniques or physical activity. It also includes names and contact information of individuals the adolescent identifies as a source of support and with whom the adolescent feels safe and can contact for help. The safety contract is also discussed with the adolescent's guardians who participate in reinforcing it. The adolescent is asked to sign the safety contract; a copy is given to the adolescent, and the original is placed in the medical record. The adolescent's participation in establishing this safety plan is essential. Readily agreeing to or resisting a suicide safety contract should be interpreted as an inability to adhere to the contract, and a same-day mental health evaluation should be considered.[82]

An adolescent presenting with suicidal ideation and a well thought-out plan should be considered an emergency and referred to appropriate suicide crisis services; his or her guardians should be contacted and informed about the primary care safety plan for the adolescent. Primary care providers should also have a low threshold for referring adolescents who report suicidal ideation without a plan to the emergency department in the following situations:

Box 6
Key warning signs for adolescent suicide

*I*deation	Talking about or threatening to kill or hurt oneself; looking for ways to kill oneself; talking or writing about death, dying, or suicide
*S*ubstance abuse	Increased substance use
*P*urposelessness	Feeling that there is no purpose in life and future
*A*nxiety	Anxiety, agitation, or changes in sleep pattern
*T*rapped	Feeling like there is no way out
*H*opelessness	Feeling that nothing will be helpful or change
*W*ithdrawal	Withdrawing from friends, family, and society
*A*nger	Easily irritated
*R*ecklessness	Increase in risk-taking behaviors
*M*ood changes	Subjective report or observed by others

From American Association of Suicidology. Available at: http://www.suicidology.org/c/document_library/get_file?folderId=231&name=DLFE-598.pdf. Accessed November 15, 2013.

Box 7
Areas of suicide risk assessment

Suicide plan including method, time, place, and available means

History of suicide attempts

Psychiatric disorders including alcohol and substance abuse disorders

History of impulsivity, violence, and aggression

Interpersonal conflict

History of physical or sexual abuse

Accessibility of firearms in the home

Recent suicide completed by someone the adolescent knows

Family history of suicide attempts

Environmental or family stress

Family violence

- There is a history of previous suicide attempts.
- There is current or past psychosis and/or manic symptoms.
- The adolescent presents agitated, angry, or impulsive.
- There is current or past alcohol or substance use.
- The adolescent's support system is inadequate.

It is also best practice to provide all adolescents who endorse suicidal ideation and their guardians emergency contact numbers, such as the National Suicide Prevention Lifeline's toll-free number, 1-800-273-TALK (8255), which is available 24 hours a day, 7 days a week.[82]

TREATMENT

Treatment of mood disorders in youths consists of psychotherapy, pharmacotherapy, or a combination of both. The choice of treatment depends on symptom severity, presence of developmental delays and/or psychiatric and medical comorbidities, associated risk factors, patient preferences, and availability of services.[21]

The American Academy of Child and Adolescent Psychiatry's guidelines and expert opinion agree that, unless the depression is severe or recurrent, the use of medication is generally unwarranted,[9,83] and psychosocial interventions are the first-line treatment approaches.[59]

Psychosocial Interventions

Cognitive-behavioral therapy (CBT) is considered to be an effective treatment of mood disorders in youths. It focuses on helping adolescents identify thinking patterns underlying psychological distress, become aware of associations between these cognitive patterns and negative feelings, and how both reflect on behaviors to promote cognitive-behavioral change. CBT includes educating adolescents about their mood disorder and teaching them techniques to dispute problematic thinking patterns and modulate emotions. It assists them in developing skills to cope with stress, solve problems, and build social skills. CBT is used in both individual or group treatment formats. The intensity of symptoms, level of psychosocial impairment, and the cognitive resources of the adolescent should determine the use of CBT alone or as an adjunct to pharmacotherapy.[84] For individuals with BD, CBT promotes adherence to psychiatric treatment and reduces the chance of relapse.[85]

Interpersonal psychotherapy (IPT) is also effective in the treatment of adolescent depression. IPT focuses on helping the adolescent adapt to changes in relationships, transitioning personal roles, and forming interpersonal relationships.[86] IPT has not been compared with medication, combination treatment, or placebo to treat depression.[35] However, it is considered to be more effective than no therapy and as effective or more effective than CBT.[87,88]

Because families are the main support system of adolescents and are affected by their mental health issues, family therapy is often adjunct treatment in the adolescent's mental health care. Family plays an essential role in ensuring the adolescent's adherence to mental health treatment, promoting his or her development of effective coping and social skills, monitoring symptoms, and intervening to prevent relapse. Therefore, family interventions include educating the family about the adolescent's mental illness; the importance of mental health treatment; and the strategies to facilitate the adolescent's cognitive, social, and emotional development. In addition, family therapy teaches the family about symptom recognition, their warning signs, and emergency planning. Family therapy also addresses family functioning, dynamics, adjustment, and coping with the adolescent's mental illness. CBT family therapy is recommended in the treatment of depression in youths,[37] whereas family focused therapy is the indicated adjunct modality in the treatment of youth BD.[89]

Pharmacologic Interventions

Pharmacologic intervention may be considered as first-line treatment in adolescents who present chronic, disabling, and recurrent depressive symptoms including suicidal ideation or have a family history of depression with good response to medication.[33] Medications may also be added when symptoms persist despite ongoing psychosocial interventions. Selective serotonin reuptake inhibitors (SSRIs) are the most commonly prescribed medication for depression.[90]

Among the various SSRIs, fluoxetine (Prozac) is the only SSRI approved by the Food and Drug Administration (FDA) to treat depression in youths aged 10 years and older.[91] According to the FDA's recommendations, adolescents treated with any SSRI should be monitored closely throughout the duration of treatment (usually about 6–9 months). The prescribing provider should initially see adolescents on SSRIs once a week for 4 weeks in order to evaluate the response to treatment as well as to monitor for potential side effects or adverse reactions. After a month of treatment, adolescents should be seen once every 2 weeks during the second month of treatment and then once a month for the duration of the medication therapy.[91]

Although SSRIs have less side effects than other antidepressants, prescribing providers are urged to assess suicidality in every medication management visit because of the black box warning with this category of medications.[17] In addition, adolescents' weight, height, and blood pressure should be assessed every month.[59]

In order to evaluate the response to treatment across time, the prescribing provider may use the screening tool, such as the PHQ-A or BDI-II, initially given to the adolescent to assess symptoms of depression as a comparison measurement in medication management visits. Moreover, tracking of treatment goals and outcomes should include an evaluation of the adolescent's psychosocial functioning, including familial, social, academic, and interpersonal domains.[92] If improvement is not seen within 6 to 8 weeks of treatment, mental health consultation should be considered.[92]

Further information regarding the use of antidepressants to treat depression in adolescents is found in the Guidelines for Adolescent Depression in Primary Care toolkit.[92]

Pharmacotherapy for adolescents with BD includes mood stabilizers and atypical antipsychotics.[17] A mental health provider usually initiates these medications. On occasion, primary care providers may initiate treatment because of a lack of mental health resources in the community and/or lack of insurance. However, it is the standard of care to treat these patients in consultation with a mental health clinician. Detailed information regarding medication algorithms for the treatment of BD in children and adolescents can be found in "Treatment Guidelines for Children and Adolescents with Bipolar Disorder: Child Psychiatry Workgroup on Bipolar Disorder."[19]

Educating Families and Obtaining Consent

Once a thorough assessment is completed, the primary care provider should educate the adolescent and his or her guardians about the diagnosis and recommended treatment modalities. When prescribing a psychotropic medication, the primary care physician should educate the adolescent and his or her guardian about the risks and benefits, including the expected effect of the medication on target symptoms, duration of treatment, and medication side effects. It is essential to teach the adolescent's guardians how to monitor for medication side effects and document their consent to treatment and follow-up.

Referral to Mental Health Services

Decision making regarding treating adolescent mood disorders in primary care versus referring the adolescent to mental health services should take the following into consideration:

- Primary care provider's knowledge of mood disorders in adolescents and competence in comprehensive assessment and diagnostic skills
- Availability of mental health providers in the primary care setting to provide adjunct psychosocial treatments and supportive approaches
- Availability of child and adolescent psychiatry for consultation
- Chronicity and severity of symptoms as well as level of psychosocial impairment
- Psychiatric and/or substance abuse history, including comorbidities, current or past psychosis, suicidality, homicidality, and/or agitation
- Mental illness and/or substance abuse in primary caregivers
- Mental health treatment waiting lists
- Whether the adolescent presents a psychiatric emergency

The more severe the mental health history and clinical presentation of adolescents and their family, the more difficult it is to treat mood disorders in the primary care setting. Hence, the threshold for referral to mental health services should be lower. In the case of mental health waiting lists and lack of insurance, the primary care provider should consider initiating treatment in consultation with a child and adolescent psychiatrist and monitor the adolescent very closely until he or she begins psychiatric treatment. This approach prevents untreated mood disorders in youths from worsening across time leading to serious consequences, such as suicide. Prompt initiation of treatment may also facilitate engaging these youngsters in mental health care.

CASE

The following case illustrates the integration of an MSE and a brief psychosocial assessment during a walk-in adolescent visit leading to clinical decision making and referral to mental health services.

Aimee is a healthy 18 year old who presented at a primary care clinic for the first time as a walk-in requesting screening for sexually transmitted infections (STI). Throughout the medical interview, her speech was pressured and rapid and her thought process presented racing thoughts, making it difficult for the clinician to follow despite attempts to slow her down. She was also observed to be easily distracted and needed questions to be repeated. Aimee appeared excessively irritated by the clinician's questions and impatient with the medical interviewing. Nevertheless, she spoke openly about having 35 current male sex partners and not using protection. Aimee reported being sexually active since 15 years of age with one partner for an extended period of time. However, in the past week she began being more sexually active on a daily basis and several times a day, leading her to have significantly more sexual partners she meets in different settings, such as school, streets, and with peers. She denied using protection and being forced to have sex. She also denied being a sex worker and using substances, including alcohol. Although her affect was irritable, Aimee described her mood as "feeling great" while attributing it to being very energetic with no need to sleep in the past week and not feeling tired. She said that she has never felt this great before and referred to herself as being superior than her peers, with whom she has had a lot of conflict in the past week because of waking them up with numerous late phone calls and text messages. When asked about her aspirations, Aimee expressed interest in multiple activities in which she has engaged with very little planning. Although she denied feeling depressed, she reported experiencing episodes of depression in the past that were never treated. She denied current and past psychotic symptoms and suicidal and homicidal ideation. Aimee is in her senior year in high school and blamed the school for not graduating her this year. She mentioned attending special classes in the past for unclear reasons. Her medical history was unremarkable. Nevertheless, she reported significant family history of mental illness. Her mother has BD, and her father has depression. Her parents have been in psychiatric treatment in a community mental health clinic. She is the only child, denied child abuse history, and said that she feels safe at home.

Because of Aimee's current mental status, the clinician tactfully discussed STI prevention and engaged Aimee in a conversation regarding the benefits of a referral to mental health services because she presented symptoms highly suggestive of BD. Aimee agreed to be evaluated at an on-site mental health clinic the next morning and to return to see the clinician in a week for the STI screening results. The clinician continued to work on STI prevention with Aimee as her psychiatric symptoms were stabilized with pharmacotherapy and psychotherapy treatments for bipolar I disorder. The clinician also assessed Aimee's adherence to mental health treatment and did a risk assessment in every primary care visit to monitor stabilization of her mental illness. In addition, the clinician and psychiatrist collaborated with one another in Aimee's health maintenance. With her consent, the clinician included her parents in some of her follow-up primary care visits to obtain collateral information as well as to assess family functioning and coping with Aimee's mental illness.

SUMMARY

Primary care recognition of mood disorders and their comorbidities in adolescents is essential to promote health and prevent illness and suicide. However, because of the developmental characteristics of adolescence, symptoms of mood disorders are easily overlooked with problems in social, academic, and interpersonal functioning thought of as being developmentally appropriate. The integration of mental health screening, the MSE, and psychosocial assessment of adolescents, including collateral information obtained from their guardians and school, is an effective strategy to evaluate adolescents who present symptoms of mood disorders. It also facilitates differentiating mood disorders in adolescents from similar clinical or developmentally appropriate presentations. Furthermore, a comprehensive assessment enables the primary care physician to make decisions regarding evidenced-based treatment modalities and initiating treatment. The delivery of treatment of mood disorders in primary care should be carefully considered given the need for clinical resources and systems in place to provide high monitoring and extensive management. Furthermore, collaboration between primary care and mental health providers is essential for a good health outcome of adolescents and their families.

REFERENCES

1. National Alliance on Mental Illness. Facts on children's mental health in America. 2013. Available at: http://www.nami.org. Accessed November 15, 2013.
2. U.S. Department of Health and Human Services. Report of the Surgeon General's conference on children's mental health: a national action agenda. Washington, DC: U.S. Public Health Service; 2000.
3. National Institute of Mental Health release of landmark and collaborative study conducted by Harvard University, the University of Michigan and the NIMH Intramural Research Program. 2005. Available at: www.nimh.nih.gov. Accessed November 15, 2013.
4. Stein R, Zitner L, Jensen P. Interventions for adolescent depression in primary care. Pediatrics 2006;18(2):669–82.
5. Birmaher B, Arbealez C, Brent D. Course and outcome of child and adolescent major depressive disorder. Child Adolesc Psychiatr Clin N Am 2002;11:619–37.
6. Angold A, Costello EJ. Puberty and depression. Child Adolesc Psychiatr Clin N Am 2006;15(4):919–37.
7. Angold A, Costello EJ, Worthman CM. Puberty and depression: the roles of age, pubertal status and pubertal timing. Psychol Med 1998;28:51–61.
8. Glowinski AL, Madden PA, Bucholz KK, et al. Genetic epidemiology of self reported lifetime DSM-IV major depressive disorder in population-based twin sample of female adolescents. J Child Psychol Psychiatry 2003;44(7): 988–96.
9. Birmaher B, Brent D, AACAP Work Group on Quality Issues. Practice parameter for the assessment and treatment of children and adolescents with depressive disorders. J Am Acad Child Adolesc Psychiatry 2007;46:503–26.
10. Fergusson DM, Horwood LJ, Ridder EM, et al. Subthreshold depression in adolescence and mental health outcomes in adulthood. Arch Gen Psychiatry 2005;62:66–72.
11. Gonzalez-Tejera G, Canino G, Ramirez R, et al. Examining minor and major depression in adolescents. J Child Psychol Psychiatry 2005;46:888–99.
12. Lewinsohn PM, Solomon A, Seeley JR, et al. Clinical implications of "subthreshold" depressive symptoms. J Abnorm Psychol 2000;103:345–51.
13. Pine DS, Cohen P, Gurley D, et al. The risk for early adulthood anxiety and depressive disorders in adolescents with anxiety and depressive disorders. Arch Gen Psychiatry 1998;55:56–64.

14. Birmaher B, Ryan ND, Williamson DE, et al. Childhood and adolescent depression: a review of the past ten years. Part I. J Am Acad Child Adolesc Psychiatry 1996;35:1427–39.
15. Angold A, Costello EJ, Erkanli A. Comorbidity. J Child Psychol Psychiatry 1999; 40(1):57–87.
16. Lewinsohn PM, Rohde P, Seeley JR. Major depressive disorder in older adolescents: prevalence, risk factors, and clinical implications. Clin Psychol Rev 1998; 18:765–94.
17. Yearwood EL, Meadows-Oliver M. Mood dysregulation disorders. In: Yearwood EL, Pearson GS, Newland JA, editors. Child and adolescent behavioral health. West Sussex (United Kingdom): Wiley-Blackwell; 2012. p. 165–86.
18. Merikangas K, He J, Burstein M, et al. Lifetime prevalence of mental disorders in U.S. adolescents: results from the national comorbidity survey replication adolescent supplement. J Am Acad Child Adolesc Psychiatry 2010;49(10):980–9.
19. McClellan J, Kowatch R, Findling RL, et al, AACAP Work Group on Quality Issues. Practice parameter for the assessment and treatment of children and adolescents with bipolar disorder. J Am Acad Child Adolesc Psychiatry 2007; 46(1):107–25.
20. Rockhill C, Hlastla S, Myers K. Early onset bipolar disorder. In: Cheng K, Myers K, editors. Child and adolescent psychiatry: the essentials. Philadelphia: Lippincott Williams & Wilkins; 2005. p. 191–210.
21. Richardson L, Katzenellenbogen R. Childhood and adolescent depression: the role of primary care providers in diagnosis and treatment. Curr Probl Pediatr Adolesc Health Care 2005;35:1–24.
22. Nomura Y, Wickramarante PJ, Warner V, et al. Family discord, parental depression, and psychopathology in offspring: ten-year follow-up. J Am Acad Child Adolesc Psychiatry 2002;41:402–9.
23. Weissman MM, Wichramaratne P, Nomura Y, et al. Families at high and low risk for depression: a 3-generation study. Arch Gen Psychiatry 2005;62:29–36.
24. Nurnnerger JI Jr, Foroud T. Genetics of bipolar affective disorders. Curr Psychiatry Rep 2000;2:147–57.
25. Chang K, Steiner H, Ketter T. Studies of offspring of parents with bipolar disorder. Am J Med Genet 2003;123:226–35.
26. Egeland JA, Shaw JA, Edicott J, et al. Prospective study of prodromal features for bipolarity in well Amish children. J Am Acad Child Adolesc Psychiatry 2003; 42:786–96.
27. Etain B, Henry C, Belliever F, et al. Beyond genetics: childhood affective trauma in bipolar disorder. Bipolar Disord 2008;10(8):867–76.
28. Lack CW, Green AL. Mood disorders in children and adolescents. J Pediatr Nurs 2009;24(1):13–25.
29. American Psychiatric Association (APA). Diagnostic and statistical manual of mental disorders. 5th edition. Washington, DC: American Psychiatric Publishing; 2013.
30. Singh T. Pediatric bipolar disorder: diagnostic challenges in identifying symptoms and course of illness. Psychiatry (Edgmont) 2008;5:35–42.
31. Klein DN, Taylor EB, Dickstein S, et al. Primary early-onset dysthymia: comparison with primary nonbipolar nonchronic major depression on demographic, clinical, familial, personality, and socio-environmental characteristics and short-term outcome. J Abnorm Psychol 1988;97:387–98.
32. Yorbik O, Birmaher B, Axelson D, et al. Clinical characteristics of depressive symptoms in children and adolescents with major depressive disorder. J Clin Psychiatry 2004;65:1654–9.

33. Jeffrey D, Sava D, Winters N. Depressive disorders. In: Cheng K, Meyers K, editors. Child and adolescent psychiatry: the essentials. Philadelphia: Lippincott Williams & Wilkins; 2005. p. 169–89.
34. American Academy of Child and Adolescent Psychiatry (AACAP). Practice parameters for the assessment and treatment of children and adolescents with depressive disorders. J Am Acad Child Adolesc Psychiatry 1998;37: S63–83.
35. Clark MS, Jansen KL, Cloy JA. Treatment of childhood and adolescent depression. Am Fam Physician 2012;86(5):442–8.
36. Bailey M, Zauszniewski J, Heinzer M, et al. Patterns of depressive symptoms in children. J Am Acad Child Adolesc Psychiatry 2007;20(2):86–95.
37. Pavuluri MN, Graczyk PA, Henry DB, et al. Child- and family-focused cognitive-behavioral therapy for pediatric bipolar disorder: development of preliminary results. J Am Acad Child Adolesc Psychiatry 2004;43:528–37.
38. Pavuluri MN, Henry DB, Carbray JA, et al. Open-label prospective trial of risperidone in combination with lithium or divalproex sodium in pediatric mania. J Affect Disord 2004;82(Suppl):S103–11.
39. Pavuluri MN, Henry DB, Devineni B, et al. A pharmacotherapy algorithm for stabilization and maintenance of pediatric bipolar disorder. J Am Acad Child Adolesc Psychiatry 2004;43:859–67.
40. Pavuluri MN, Herbener ES, Sweeney JA. Psychotic symptoms in pediatric bipolar disorder. J Affect Disord 2004;80:19–28.
41. Kowatch RA, Youngstrom E, Danielyan A, et al. Review and meta-analysis of the phenomenology and clinical characteristics of mania in children and adolescents. Bipolar Disord 2005;7:483–96.
42. Hamrin V, Pachler M. Pediatric bipolar disorder: evidence-based psychopharmacological treatments. J Child Adolesc Psychiatr Nurs 2007;20(1):40–58.
43. Snyderman D, Rovner BW. Mental status examination in primary care: a review. Am Fam Physician 2009;80(8):809–14.
44. U.S. Preventive Task Force. Screening and treatment for major depressive disorder in children and adolescents: U.S. Preventive Services Task Force recommendation statement. Pediatrics 2009;123(4):1223–8.
45. Goldenring JM, Cohen E. Getting into adolescent heads. Contemp Pediatr 1988;5:75–90.
46. Reif C, Warford A. Office practice of adolescent medicine. Prim Care Clin Office Pract 2006;33:269–84.
47. Zuckerbrot R, Maxon L, Pagar D, et al. Adolescent depression screening in primary care: feasibility and acceptability. Pediatrics 2007;119(1):101–8.
48. Klein DN, Dougherty LR, Olino TM. Toward guidelines for evidence-based assessment of depression in children and adolescents. J Clin Child Adolesc Psychol 2005;34:412–32.
49. Beck AT, Steer R, Brown G. Beck depression inventory-II (BDI-II) manual. San Antonio (TX): Psychological Corporation; 1996.
50. Beck AT, Steere RA, Ball R, et al. Comparison of Beck Depression Inventories IA and II in psychiatric outpatients. J Pers Assess 1996;67(3):588–97.
51. Spitzer RL, Kroenke K, Williams JB. Validation and utility of a self-report version of PRIME-MD: the PHQ primary care study. Primary care evaluation and mental disorders. Patient Health Questionnaire. JAMA 1999;282(18): 1737–44.
52. Kovacs M. Children's depression inventory. North Tonawanda (NY): Psychological Assessment Resources, Multi-Health System; 1992.

53. Jellinek M, Murphy JM, Little M, et al. Use of the pediatric symptom checklist (PSC) to screen psychosocial problems in pediatric primary care: a national feasibility study. Arch Pediatr Adolesc Med 1999;153(3):254–60.
54. Fendrich M, Weissman MM, Warner V. Screening for depressive disorder in children and adolescents: validating the Center for Epidemiologic Studies Depression Scale for Children. Am J Epidemiol 1990;131:538–51.
55. Reynolds WM. Reynolds adolescent depression scale. Odessa (FL): Psychological Assessment Resources; 1986.
56. Angold A, Costello EJ. Mood and feelings questionnaire. Durham (NC): Duke University Health System Center for Developmental Epidemiology; 1987.
57. Daviss WB, Birmaher B, Melhem NA, et al. Criterion validity of the mood and feelings questionnaire for depressive episodes in clinic and non-clinic subjects. J Child Psychol Psychiatry 2006;47(9):927–34.
58. Rew IC, Simpson K, Tracy M, et al. Criterion validity of the short Mood and Feelings Questionnaire and one- and two-items depression screens in young adolescents. Child Adolesc Psychiatry Ment Health 2010;4(8):1–11.
59. Hamrin V, Margono M. Assessment of adolescents for depression in the pediatric primary care setting. Pediatr Nurs 2010;36(2):103–11.
60. Kowatch RA, Fristad M, Birmaher B, et al. Treatment guidelines for children and adolescents with bipolar disorder. J Am Acad Child Adolesc Psychiatry 2005; 44(3):213–35.
61. Wintersteen MB, Diamond GS, Fein JA. Screening for suicide risk in the pediatric emergency and acute care setting. Curr Opin Pediatr 2007;19(4):398–404.
62. Centers for Disease Control and Prevention. WISQARS fatal injuries: leading causes of death. Available at: http://webappa.cdc.gov/sasweb/ncipc/leadcaus. html. Accessed November 15, 2013.
63. McCarty CA, Russo J, Grossman DC, et al. Adolescents with suicidal ideation: health care use and functioning. Acad Pediatr 2011;11:422–6.
64. McNeill YL, Russo J, Grossman DC, et al. Fifteen year olds at risk of parasuicide or suicide: how can we identify them in general practice. Fam Pract 2002;19: 461–5.
65. Cash SJ, Bridge JA. Epidemiology of youth suicide and suicidal behavior. Curr Opin Pediatr 2009;21(5):613–9.
66. Eaton D, Kann L, Kinchen S, et al, Centers for Disease Control and Prevention (CDC). Youth risk behavior surveillance-United States, 2009. MMWR Surveill Summ 2010;59(5):1–142.
67. Anderson RN. In: National vital statistics report, vol. 50. Hyattsville (MD): National Center for Health Statistics; 2002. Deaths: leading causes for 2000.
68. Bridge JA, Goldstein TR, Brent DA. Adolescent suicide and suicidal behavior. J Child Psychol Psychiatry 2006;47(3–4):372–94.
69. Brent DA, Baugher M, Bridge J, et al. Age- and sex-related risk factors for adolescent suicide. J Am Acad Child Adolesc Psychiatry 1999;38(12):1497–505.
70. Shaffer D, Gould MS, Fisher P, et al. Psychiatric diagnosis in child and adolescent suicide. Arch Gen Psychiatry 1996;53:339–48.
71. Shafii M, Steltz-Lenarsky J, Derrik AM, et al. Comorbidity of mental disorders in the post-mortem diagnosis of completed suicide in children and adolescents. J Affect Disord 1988;15(3):227–33.
72. Goldston DB, Daniel SS, Reboussin BA, et al. Psychiatric diagnoses of previous suicide attempters, first-time attempters, and repeat attempters on an adolescent inpatient psychiatric unit. J Am Acad Child Adolesc Psychiatry 1998; 37(9):924–32.

73. Gould MS, King R, Greenwald S, et al. Psychophathology associated with suicidal ideation and attempts among children and adolescents. J Am Acad Child Adolesc Psychiatry 1998;37(9):915–23.
74. Faust DS, Walker D, Sands M. Diagnosis and management of childhood bipolar disorder in the primary care setting. Clin Pediatr 2006;45:801–8.
75. Russell ST, Joyner K. Adolescent sexual orientation and suicide risk: evidence from a national study. Am J Public Health 2001;91(8):1276–81.
76. Ryan C, Huebner D, Diaz RM, et al. Family rejection as a predictor of negative health outcomes in white and Latino lesbian, gay and bisexual young adults. Pediatrics 2009;123(1):346–52.
77. Klomek AB, Sourander A, Niemela S, et al. Childhood bullying behaviors as a risk for suicide attempts and completed suicides: a population-based birth cohort study. J Am Acad Child Adolesc Psychiatry 2009;48(3):254–61.
78. Steinhouser J. Verdict in MySpace suicide. The New York Times 2009.
79. Pettit B. Moving and children's social connections. Sociol Forum (Randolph N J) 2004;19:285–311.
80. Quin P, Mortensen PB, Pedersen CB. Frequent change of residence and risk of attempted and completed suicide among children and adolescents. Arch Gen Psychiatry 2009;66(6):628–32.
81. Rudd MD, Berman AL, Joiner TE Jr, et al. Warning signs of suicide: theory, research, and clinical applications. Suicide Life Threat Behav 2006;36:255.
82. Hatcher-Kay C, King C. Depression and suicide. Pediatr Rev 2003;24(11):363–71.
83. Cheung AH, Zuckerbrot RA, Jensen PS, et al. Expert survey for the management of adolescent depression in primary care. Pediatrics 2008;121:101–7.
84. DeFillipis M, Wagner KD. Bipolar depression in children and adolescents. CNS Spectr 2013;18:209–13.
85. Hausmann A, Hortnagl C, Muller M, et al. Psychotherapeutic intervention in bipolar disorder: a review. Neuropsychiatr 2007;21(2):102–9 [in German].
86. David-Ferdon C, Kaslow N. Evidence-based psychosocial treatments for child and adolescent depression. J Clin Child Adolesc Psychol 2008;37(1):62–104.
87. Klomek AB, Mufson L. Interpersonal psychotherapy for depressed adolescents. Child Adolesc Psychiatr Clin N Am 2006;15(4):959–75.
88. Rosselio J, Bernal G. The efficacy of cognitive-behavioral and interpersonal treatments for depression in Puerto Rican adolescents. J Consult Clin Psychol 1999;67(5):734–45.
89. Krieger FV, Stringaris A. Bipolar disorder and disruptive mood dysregulation in children and adolescents: assessment, diagnosis and treatment. Evid Based Ment Health 2013;16:93–4.
90. Ingram RE, Trenary L. Mood disorders. In: Maddux JE, Winstead BA, editors. Psychopathology: foundations for a contemporary understanding. New York: Lawrence Erlbaum Associates; 2005. p. 187–209.
91. U.S. Food and Drug Administration (FDA). Antidepressant use in children, adolescents, and adults. 2004. Available at: http://www.fda.gov/Drugs/DrugSafety/InformationbyDrugClass/ucm096273.htm. Accessed November 15, 2013.
92. Jensen PS, Cheung AH, Zuckerbrot R, et al. Guidelines for adolescent depression in primary care (GLAD-PC) toolkit. Guidelines for adolescent depression in primary care. Reach Institute; 2010. Available at: http://pediatrics.aappublications.org/content/120/5/e1313.full.

Sex (Sexuality/Reproductive Health)

Adolescent Pregnancy and Contraception

Jessica Dalby, MD*, Ronni Hayon, MD, Jensena Carlson, MD

KEYWORDS

• Adolescent • Pregnancy • Contraception • LARC • Confidentiality

KEY POINTS

- Screening for sexual activity and pregnancy risk should be a routine part of all adolescent visits.
- Emphasize confidentiality with adolescent patients. Lack of access to confidential care has been shown to dissuade adolescents from seeking care.
- At current rates of unintended adolescent pregnancy, 1 in 10 US women will have an abortion by age 20.
- Proven reductions in unintended pregnancy in teens are attained by providing access to contraception at no cost and promoting the most effective methods.
- Long-acting reversible contraceptive methods should be considered first-line options in adolescents.
- Counsel teens on the importance of dual-method use: barrier protection against sexually transmitted infections combined with highly effective contraception.

CASE STUDY

An 18-year-old girl presents for evaluation of vaginal spotting. Her last menstrual period was 8 weeks ago. Today in clinic, a urine pregnancy test is positive. This is a surprise to her. She has been with her 21-year-old boyfriend for 3 months and is using condoms intermittently. You review her options with her and she says that she can't imagine having a child at this time. You review the process of having an abortion and she makes an appointment with you later in the week for an office-based uterine aspiration procedure. When she returns for the abortion, you counsel her on contraceptive options and she decides to have an intrauterine device (IUD) placed. You place the IUD immediately after the abortion procedure.

INTRODUCTION

The United States faces high rates of teen pregnancy. Seven percent of US teen women became pregnant in 2008, totaling 750,000 pregnancies nationwide.[1] For

Department of Family Medicine, University of Wisconsin School of Medicine and Public Health, 1100 Delaplaine Court, Madison, WI 53715, USA
* Corresponding author.
E-mail address: Jessica.dalby@fammed.wisc.edu

Prim Care Clin Office Pract 41 (2014) 607–629
http://dx.doi.org/10.1016/j.pop.2014.05.010   **primarycare.theclinics.com**

women ages 15 to 19, 82% of pregnancies are unintended.[2] This is in contrast to 43% for adult women ages 20 and older. One-third of teen pregnancies ended in abortion. At current rates, 1 in 10 US women will have an abortion by age 20.[3]

Substantial differences exist between states and demographics for teen pregnancy rates and outcomes. Teen pregnancy rates are the highest in the south and southwest United States and lowest in the upper midwest and New England, with a range of 33 to 93 per 1000 women ages 15 to 19.[1] Rates are also much higher among black and Hispanic teens compared with whites. Births, miscarriages, and abortions vary widely by state as a result of local access to reproductive health care choices and sociocultural influences. For example, in New York, more than half of teen pregnancies end in abortion, whereas in Kentucky, only 14% of teen pregnancies end in abortion.[1]

US teen pregnancy rates have declined over the past 20 years. In 2008, the pregnancy rate for women in the United States ages 15 to 19 was 68 per 1000, down from 117 per 1000 in 1990.[1] Teens ages 18 to 19 account for most of these pregnancies, making up 64% to 76% of all teen pregnancies while accounting for only 40% of women 15 to 19 years old.[1]

Data indicate that increased contraceptive use and decreased sexual activity accounts for most of this decline. Use of contraception by adolescent girls at first intercourse has increased in the United States from 48% in 1982 to 78% in 2006 to 2010.[4] Decreased rates of teen pregnancy among those 18 to 19 years old appears to be almost entirely attributable to increased use of contraception.[5] Among those 15 to 17 years old, increased contraceptive use likely accounts for about three-quarters of the declining pregnancy rate, with one-quarter of the decline related to decreased sexual activity.[5]

Large percentages of adolescents in the United States (32.9% of 9th graders, 43.8% of 10th graders, 53.2% of 11th graders, and 63.1% of 12th graders) have already had sexual intercourse.[4] Nevertheless, over the past 20 years, fewer high school students report ever having sex, from 51% in 1988 to 43% in 2006 to 2010.[4]

Despite these trends, teen pregnancy in the United States outpaces rates in other developed countries. In 2009, the teen birth rate in the United States reached a historic low of 39 per 1000 women ages 15 to 19.[4] Meanwhile, in Canada, the teen birth rate was 65% lower at 14 per 1000.[4]

Lower use of highly effective contraception is a major factor in the disparity between teen pregnancy rates in the United States compared with other developed countries.

Less effective methods, condoms, and withdrawal are the most commonly used birth control strategies among US teens.[6] Data from the 2011 national Youth Risk Behavior Surveillance System reveal that among all sexually active US high school students, 40% did not use a condom with last sexual intercourse and 77% were not using hormonal birth control.[6]

Preventing unintended and adolescent pregnancies are key public health objectives set forth by the US Department of Health and Human Services in the national campaign, Healthy People 2020 (healthypeople.gov). Each year, publicly funded family planning services prevent 1.94 million unintended pregnancies, including 400,000 teen pregnancies.[7] These services are cost-effective, saving nearly $4 for every $1 spent in Medicaid expenditures for pregnancy-related care.[8] Proven reductions in unintended pregnancy in teens have been attained by providing access to contraception at no cost and promoting the most effective methods.[9] We will therefore review best practices in the contraceptive management of teens and discuss providing care to the pregnant adolescent.

CONFIDENTIALITY, REPRODUCTIVE HEALTH, AND THE ADOLESCENT PATIENT

Promoting confidentiality is essential in obtaining an adolescent sexual history and assessing the risks of pregnancy. Many adolescents will not disclose their sexual history if not asked explicitly. Further, many may not reveal all of their risks because of underestimation of personal risk or desire to provide socially acceptable answers. Lack of access to confidential care has been shown to dissuade adolescents from seeking care. A statewide survey of adolescents in Wisconsin seeking care at Planned Parenthood clinics revealed that more than half (59%) reported that if their parents were notified that they were seeking contraception, they would stop using all sexual health care services, including testing and treatment for sexually transmitted infections (STIs) and HIV.[10] A subsequent national study found that most teenagers seeking care at federally funded family planning clinics had parents who already knew they were receiving services. When examining the subgroup of teenagers whose parents were unaware that they were seeking care at the clinics, the same study found that 70% of teenagers in this group would forego contraceptive services if parental notification were mandated.[11]

The clinician providing care to the adolescent should familiarize himself or herself with the local state laws that delineate to which services a minor can consent. All states and the District of Columbia allow adolescents to consent to STI services, but laws vary significantly from state to state for other services, including prenatal care, reproductive health services, and abortion care. Resources are available with state-specific information on minor-consent laws from organizations such as the Guttmacher Institute (www.guttmacher.org/), the Center for Adolescent Health and the Law (www.cahl.org), and Physicians for Reproductive Health (www.prch.org).

CARING FOR THE PREGNANT ADOLESCENT
Diagnosis and Screening

Adolescents may present for pregnancy screening with classic symptoms of amenorrhea, morning sickness, breast tenderness, and weight gain. However, teens will also often have more subtle presentations of pregnancy, including vague complaints of fatigue, dizziness, or abdominal pain. The variability of the adolescent menstrual cycle and possibility of light spotting at the time of implantation also can make diagnosis challenging. Any complaints of menstrual irregularity should raise concern for the possibility of pregnancy. The most common diagnosis of secondary amenorrhea is pregnancy, but psychological denial may limit the adolescent's consideration of pregnancy as a cause of her symptoms.[12] Adolescent patients also may present to a physician's office under the guise of an unrelated complaint to access care for a pregnancy concern.

Qualitative urine pregnancy test is the gold standard for pregnancy screening. If the urine human chorionic gonadotropin is negative but there is a high suspicion of pregnancy, guidelines recommend repeating the test in 1 to 2 weeks.[12] Physical examination is similar to that of pregnant adults; however, many adolescents have never had a pelvic examination. Providers should be sensitive to this difference and explain both the components and rationale for the elements of the prenatal physical.

Accurate dating of pregnancy, by ultrasound or pelvic examination for uterine size, is essential. Adolescent women frequently present for their first visit later in pregnancy and may have more variable menstrual cycles.[12] Accurate gestational dating is necessary at the time of presentation to guide pregnancy options counseling and further care.

STIs and complications are more common in adolescents.

Adolescents should be screened for STIs at the first pregnancy visit and again in the third trimester.[13] The higher rate of STIs in sexually active adolescents places them at higher risk of pelvic inflammatory disease and ectopic pregnancy.

Pregnancy Options Counseling

Options counseling starts before the positive pregnancy test while awaiting the results (**Box 1**). Open-ended questions begin the discussion about the adolescent's individual risks and also help to explore her feelings about a possible pregnancy. If the test is negative, the clinician can discuss appropriate contraceptive use. However, if the test is positive, these questions begin the discussion about her pregnancy options. Although most adolescent pregnancies are unintentional, this should not be assumed.[2] Adolescents may desire pregnancy for similar reasons as adults, including desire for a family, status within the community, and cultural expectations.

Adolescent women should be offered pregnancy options in an evidence-based, nonjudgmental, and patient-centered manner. If the clinician does not feel comfortable with this discussion because of personal beliefs or knowledge base, he or she should provide an expedited referral to an experienced provider. Although the patient's developmental stage may affect the sophistication of the discussion, there is no evidence that adolescents show poor judgment in the case of pregnancy decision-making when compared with older women.[14]

Adolescents face more barriers to accessing pregnancy options. Many young women present later in gestation for care for reasons that include not recognizing the signs of pregnancy, irregular menstrual cycles, and ambivalence about whether to continue the pregnancy.[14] These factors combined with the limited availability of abortion providers, often limited finances, and logistical difficulties in arranging care often means that adolescents present beyond the gestational age at which termination of the pregnancy is an option.[14] Decisions regarding pregnancy options are complex and may require the adolescent to have several follow-up visits. The clinician should

---

Box 1
Pregnancy options counseling for adolescents

Open-Ended Questions to Initiate Discussion

- Do you have an idea of what the results of your pregnancy test might be?
- What are you hoping the results will be?

Example of Explanation of Options

- You have a decision to make about your pregnancy. Any pregnant woman has 3 options. Alphabetically these options are abortion or pregnancy termination, continuing the pregnancy and arranging for adoption, or continuing the pregnancy and becoming a parent.

Safety Assessment

- Who in your life supports you during difficult times?
- Is there an adult in your life who you'd feel comfortable talking with about this decision?
- Would you like me to help you tell your parents?
- What do you think would happen if you told your parents that you are pregnant?
- Do you feel safe going home?

Data from Aruda MM, Waddicor K, Frese L, et al. Early pregnancy in adolescents: diagnosis, assessment, options counseling, and referral. J Pediatr Health Care 2010;24(1):4–13.

be aware of the local resources and legal restrictions so as to provide the adolescent with the information she needs to make a timely decision.

Counseling should also include consideration of routine prenatal issues. The US Preventive Services Task Force recommends folic acid supplementation for all women of childbearing age to prevent neural tube defects.[15] This is especially important for the newly diagnosed adolescent pregnancy, even while considering options, as folic acid is most critical in early gestation.[16] It is similarly important to address any coexisting medical problems that could impact either continuing or terminating the pregnancy.

All pregnancy options pose potential risks to the adolescent's health. There is a higher risk of complications from childbirth than from termination for all women, including adolescents.[17] The risk of mortality from childbirth in one study was estimated at 14 times greater than termination.[17] Risks of termination include infection, uterine or cervical injury, and hemorrhage and are estimated to be less than 1% to 3%.[14] There is no evidence that having an abortion increases the risk of psychological disorders or decreases fertility when compared with continuing an unintended pregnancy for either adult or adolescent women.[14] There are few data regarding the repercussions of adoption in the setting of adolescent pregnancy.

Safety is an important consideration for pregnant adolescents. Unfortunately, pregnant adolescents are victims of the highest rates of violence, including homicide, of any group of women.[18] Information about her pregnancy should not be shared with others without the patient's consent.[12]

Adolescent women are also at increased risk for coercive sexual activity, especially those with older partners. Population data demonstrate that at least 27% of births to adolescent women are fathered by men 5 to 8 years older than the mother and national data from 1984 showed that 81% of adolescent pregnancies were fathered by men age 20 or older.[19] It is appropriate to inquire about the circumstances surrounding the pregnancy, including who the father is, when diagnosing a pregnancy.[20] Reluctance to reveal the father should alert the clinician to the possibility of sexual abuse or unwanted sexual activity.[12] Physicians should be aware of mandatory reporting laws in their area regarding suspected abuse or statutory rape.

Health Risks of Adolescent Pregnancy

Adolescents have a disproportionate risk of medical complications in pregnancy compared with adult women (**Table 1**). This is especially true in the youngest adolescents, ages 11 to 14.[21] The rate of neonatal death for adolescent pregnancies, which includes stillbirth as well as infant death up to 28 days old, is roughly 3 times that of adult pregnancies.[16] Adolescent women tend to have poor maternal weight gain in addition to poor prepregnancy nutritional status and lower prepregnancy weight and height, all of which predisposes their infants to low birth weight. The risk of maternal death in both adult and adolescent women is low; however, there is a 2 times higher rate of maternal death related to medical complications in adolescent women when compared with adult women.[16]

Psychosocial Consequences

Adolescent parents and their infants are both at increased risk for poor psychosocial outcomes (see **Table 1**). Debate exists as to whether the degree of these outcomes is primarily linked to the pregnant adolescent's age or the circumstances that put the adolescent at risk of pregnancy in the first place. Etiology is likely multifactorial, and teen parents and their infants still fair worse than their age-matched peers.[21]

Table 1	
Increased risks in adolescent compared with adult pregnancies	
Pregnancy complications	Maternal death Anemia Preeclampsia/eclampsia Gastroschisis
Teen parent outcomes	Less likely to graduate from high school Lower earnings Higher rates of substance use Increased prevalence of mood disorders (mothers) Higher rates of legal offenses (fathers)
Neonatal outcomes	Preterm birth Low birth weight Stillbirth Neonatal death
Infant/childhood outcomes	Increased infant death Increased risk of abuse and neglect Decreased academic achievement and cognitive ability Deficits in social development Increased incidence of mental illness and substance abuse Increased risk of incarceration and becoming an adolescent parent

Data from Refs.[15,17,19–22]

Adolescent mothers tend to be less knowledgeable regarding child development, have poorer parenting models, increased maternal stress, and display egocentric behavior typical of adolescent development.[21] Further, adolescent mothers may be less likely to talk with, touch, pick up, and smile at their infant, as well as being less sensitive to and accepting of their infant's behavior.[18] It is presumed that the poor cognitive and social development of these children is, at least in part, due to differences in mother-child interaction.

Improving Outcomes for Pregnant Adolescents

Programs to improve outcomes of adolescent parents and their offspring exist; assessment of their effectiveness is limited by variability in evaluation methods and the minimal evidence for long-term improvement. The primary aims of most of these programs are to improve parent-child interaction, support parental educational achievement, increase social support for teen parents, and decrease rates of repeat pregnancy. These factors seem to be associated with improved outcomes in population studies.[18,21] The best evidence is for a comprehensive adolescent prenatal model, such as CenteringPregnancy programs, which provides prenatal care, support groups, and additional physical resources to the adolescent. These programs seem to be associated with decreased rates of preterm birth and low birth weight infants.[12,22]

Programs for pregnant adolescents can be structured many ways, including in-home visitations, school-based programs, and teen-tot clinics. In general, a multifaceted, multidisciplinary approach seems to show the most sustained and largest impact.[19] Teen-tot programs, which are essentially medical home models for the adolescent mother and her child, can improve parenting skills at least in the short term and are associated with decrease in repeat pregnancies and increased high school completion.[21,22]

Pregnancy Prevention

Screening for sexual activity and pregnancy risk should be a routine part of all adolescent visits (**Box 2**), regardless of the primary complaint. There is good evidence that

Box 2
Predictors of early sexual intercourse

Early pubertal development

History of sexual abuse

Poverty

Lack of parental attention/nurturing

Cultural and family patterns of sexual activity

Lack of educational or career goals

Poor school performance

Dropping out of school

Data from Klein JD. Adolescent pregnancy: current trends and issues. Pediatrics 2005; 116(1):281–6.

these opportunities are frequently missed in primary care.[23] Adolescents may under-estimate their personal risks, especially with regard to sexual activity. Most teens delay visiting a physician to obtain prescription contraception for more than 1 year after initial intercourse.[24] Up to 50% of adolescent pregnancies occur within the first 6 months after initial intercourse.[16,25]

Primary prevention can take place on multiple levels, including in the physician's office, between parents and children, and in schools. The best evidence in primary prevention is for multicomponent programs, which combine comprehensive sexual education, ready access to contraceptive options, and youth development programs.[19,26] Comprehensive sexual education in schools promotes abstinence for pregnancy and STI prevention but also teaches accurate information about contraception. Lack of sex education and abstinence-only programs are both associated with higher rates of unintended pregnancies when compared with comprehensive sex education.[27] Education that discusses contraception has not been shown to increase or hasten the initiation of sexual activity.[27]

The strongest predictor of adolescent pregnancy is a previous pregnancy. Secondary prevention aims to prevent recurrent pregnancies and the associated problems, including low maternal education achievement, increased dependence on governmental assistance, low infant birth weight, and increased infant mortality. Factors associated with increased risk of subsequent adolescent pregnancy include not returning to school within 6 months of delivery, being married to or living with a male partner, receiving significant child care assistance from her mother, not using a long-acting contraceptive within 3 months of delivery, and having peers who are adolescent parents.[18]

FIRST-LINE CONTRACEPTIVES FOR ADOLESCENTS

Helping adolescents plan childbearing can have a significant positive impact on the course of their lives. Adolescence is a time of rapid physical and psychological development; skills such as abstract thinking, impulse control, and delayed gratification vary widely. Not surprisingly, birth control methods that are user-dependent have significantly higher typical-use failure rates than long-acting reversible contraceptives (LARC), which are user-independent, such as the IUD or subdermal implant.

The American College of Obstetricians and Gynecologists (ACOG) supports making LARC available to adolescents. In a recent committee opinion, they stated, "Intrauterine devices and the contraceptive implant are the best reversible methods for preventing unintended pregnancy, rapid repeat pregnancy, and abortion in young women."[28]

There is also evidence that adolescents and young women will choose an LARC method when offered the opportunity. The Contraceptive CHOICE Project was a prospective cohort study in the St. Louis area that enrolled 9256 women of reproductive age (ages 14–45) over 4 years. Participants received counseling on all options for contraception and were provided the method of their choice at no cost. Among young adolescents, ages 14 to 17, 69% chose an LARC method, with most opting for the contraceptive implant. In older adolescents, ages 18 to 20, 61% chose an LARC method, with most choosing an IUD.[29] Not only did adolescents choose LARC methods, but they continued to use them in high numbers. The continuation rates for those 14 to 19 years old who were using LARC methods were 81.8% and 66.5% at years 1 and 2.[30] In a follow-up study, the investigators found a significant reduction in abortion rates, repeat abortions, and teenage birth rates when compared with nearby cities.[9]

When Can LARC Methods Be Initiated?

Traditionally, providers counseled female patients to wait until the onset of their next menses to initiate a new method. New guidelines allow clinicians to provide LARC methods at any time as long as pregnancy can be reasonably excluded (**Box 3**). Routine pelvic examinations are no longer required before initiation of contraceptive methods.

The Center for Reproductive Health Education in Family Medicine has also published a "Quick Start Algorithm" that is accepted as a safe approach (**Fig. 1**) to initiating all methods of contraception.

CONTRACEPTIVE IMPLANT

The contraceptive implant (Nexplanon, Merck & Co, Inc, Whitehouse Station, NJ, USA) is the most effective method of contraception available (**Table 2**).[31] It is also an excellent

---

Box 3
Criteria for reasonable exclusion of pregnancy

Pregnancy can be reasonably excluded if a woman has no symptoms or signs of pregnancy and meets *any one* of the following criteria:

- Is ≤7 days after the start of normal menses
- Has not had sexual intercourse since the start of last normal menses
- Has been correctly and consistently using a reliable method of contraception
- Is ≤7 days after spontaneous or induced abortion
- Is within 4 weeks postpartum
- Is fully or nearly fully breastfeeding (exclusively breastfeeding or the vast majority [≥85%] of feeds are breastfeeds), amenorrheic, and less than 6 months postpartum

These criteria are highly accurate with a negative predictive value of 99%–100% in ruling out pregnancy among women who are not pregnant. However, if a woman does not meet any of these criteria, the clinician cannot be reasonably certain that she is not pregnant, even with a negative pregnancy test.

Data from Division of Reproductive Health, National Center for Chronic Disease Prevention and Health Promotion, Centers for Disease Control and Prevention (CDC). US Selected Practice Recommendations for Contraceptive Use, 2013: adapted from the World Health Organization selected practice recommendations for contraceptive use, 2nd edition. MMWR Recomm Rep 2013;62(RR-05):1–60.

Quick Start Algorithm

Woman requests a new birth control method:

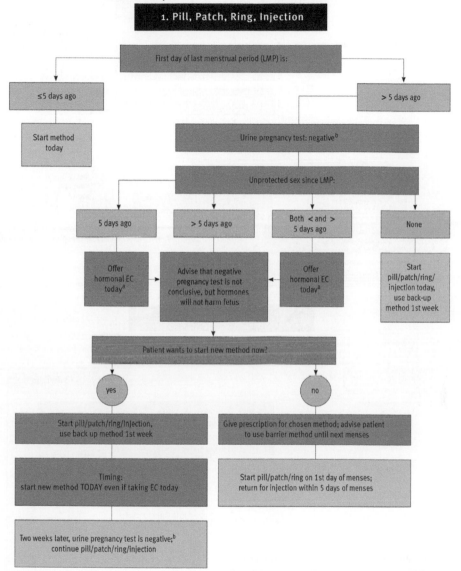

Fig. 1. RHEDI.org quick-start algorithm. (*Adapted from* Hatcher RA, Zieman M, Cwiak C, et al. 2005 pocket guide to managing contraception. Bridging the Gap Communications; 2004. p. 135.)

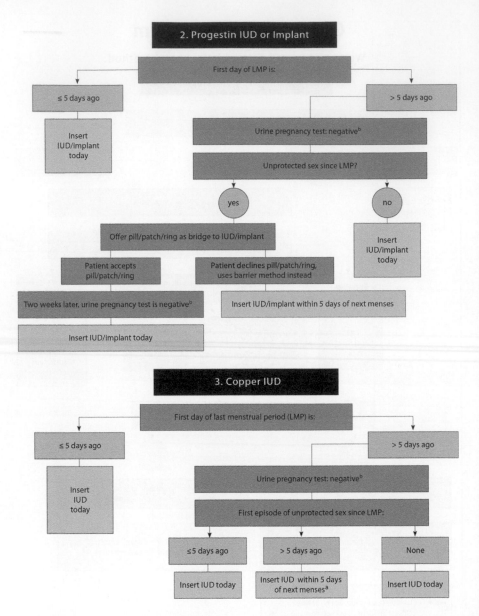

2. Progestin IUD or Implant

First day of LMP is:

≤ 5 days ago

> 5 days ago

Insert IUD/implant today

Urine pregnancy test: negative[b]

Unprotected sex since LMP?

yes

no

Offer pill/patch/ring as bridge to IUD/implant

Insert IUD/implant today

Patient accepts pill/patch/ring

Patient declines pill/patch/ring, uses barrier method instead

Two weeks later, urine pregnancy test is negative[b]

Insert IUD/implant within 5 days of next menses

Insert IUD/implant today

3. Copper IUD

First day of last menstrual period (LMP) is:

≤ 5 days ago

> 5 days ago

Insert IUD today

Urine pregnancy test: negative[b]

First episode of unprotected sex since LMP:

≤5 days ago

> 5 days ago

None

Insert IUD today

Insert IUD within 5 days of next menses[a]

Insert IUD today

[a] Pill/patch/ring may be started as a bridge to copper IUD.
[b] If pregnancy test is positive, provide options counseling.

Fig. 1. (*continued*)

choice because of its ease of use and acceptability to adolescents. Additionally, efficacy is maintained regardless of weight. The Contraceptive CHOICE project evaluated Nexplanon in overweight and obese women and found that failure rates of the implant did not vary by body mass index.[32]

Although the implant is approved by the Food and Drug Administration only for contraception, one randomized controlled trial showed that dysmenorrhea is

Table 2
Summary of prescribed contraceptive methods

Method	Failure Rate (Typical Use)[65]	Description	Mechanism of Action	Advantages	Disadvantages	Absolute Contraindications	Back-Up Method Needed
Implant	0.05	4 cm × 2 mm rod containing 68 mg ENG	Primarily suppression of ovulation. Also thickens cervical mucus and thins endometrium	Long-acting (3 y) Reversible No estrogen No pelvic examination needed May improve dysmenorrhea and acne	Unpredictable, irregular bleeding	Current breast cancer	7 d[a]
LNG IUD	0.2	T-shaped device that releases LNG	Thickens cervical mucus, thins endometrium, inhibits sperm function, inhibits ovulation (Mirena only)	Long-acting (5 y) Reversible No estrogen Reduced menstrual flow (Mirena)	Risk of uterine perforation (0–2/1000), expulsion. If pregnancy occurs, increased risk of ectopic (although overall risk is lowered with this method)[35]	For initiation only: Purulent cervicitis, current PID, cervical cancer (awaiting treatment), endometrial cancer For initiation or continuation: Distorted uterine cavity, malignant gestational trophoblastic disease, immediately after septic abortion, puerperal sepsis, pregnancy, unexplained	7 d[a]

(continued on next page)

Table 2
(continued)

Method	Failure Rate (Typical Use)[65]	Description	Mechanism of Action	Advantages	Disadvantages	Absolute Contraindications	Back-Up Method Needed
						uterine bleeding, pelvic TB	
Copper IUD	0.8	T-shaped device wrapped with copper wire	Prefertilization: inhibition of sperm migration and viability, change in ovum transport speed and damage to or destruction of ovum. Postfertilization: damage to or destruction of a fertilized ovum.	Long-acting (10 y) Reversible No hormones Can be used as EC	Heavier, more painful menses. Risk of uterine perforation, expulsion. If pregnancy occurs, increased risk of ectopic (although overall risk is lowered with this method).	Same as LNG IUD with the addition of Wilson disease	None
DMPA	6	150-mg IM injection every 12 wk (104 mg SQ)	Inhibits ovulation Thickens cervical mucus Causes endometrial thinning	No estrogen Reversible Minimal drug interactions Amenorrhea	Irregular bleeding with initiation Weight gain Bone density decrease Delayed return to fertility	Current breast cancer	7 d[a]
COC	9	Estrogen + progestin	Inhibits ovulation Thickens cervical mucus	Rapidly reversible Reduced bleeding and pain with menses Improved acne	Daily dosing	High DVT risk Migraine with aura Severe HTN Complicated heart disease Active liver disease	7 d[a,b]

Method	%	Description	Mechanism	Benefits	Side effects	Contraindications	Duration
Patch	9	Thin, flexible patch releases 150 µg norelgstromin and 20 µg EE daily	Inhibits ovulation Thickens cervical mucus	Convenience of weekly regimen Easy to verify use Rapidly reversible	Skin reaction Breast symptoms, headaches, nausea	Same as COC	7 d[a,b]
Ring	9	Flexible ring 54 mm in diameter releases 120 µg ENG and 15 µg EE daily	Inhibits ovulation Thickens cervical mucus Endometrial thinning	Convenience of monthly dosing Rapidly reversible Excellent cycle control Fewer systemic side effects	Vaginal symptoms	Same as COC	7 d[a,b]
POP	9	Norethindrone 35 µg	Thickens cervical mucus Inhibits ovulation (variable)	Very safe	Irregular bleeding Lower efficacy possible	Current breast cancer	2 d
EC: UPA		30 mg UPA	Delays ovulation	More effective than LNG EC Effective in obesity up to BMI of 35	Prescription only Safety unknown in breastfeeding – advise "pump and dump" × 36 h	None	
EC: LNG		1.5 mg LNG	Delays ovulation	Available OTC Safe in breastfeeding	Less effective after 72 h and in women with BMI over 26	None	

Abbreviations: BMI, body mass index; COC, combined oral contraceptive; DMPA, depomedroxyprogesterone acetate; DVT, deep vein thrombosis; EC, emergency contraception; EE, ethinyl estradiol; ENG, etonogestrel; HTN, hypertension; IM, intramuscular; IUD, intrauterine device; LNG, levonorgestrel; OTC, over-the-counter; PID, pelvic inflammatory disease; POP, progestin-only contraceptive; SQ, subcutaneous; TB, tuberculosis; UPA, ulipristal acetate.
[a] Unless inserted within first 5 days of menses, immediately postpartum, postabortion, or immediately on switching from another method.
[b] Not recommended immediately postpartum.

improved with the ENG implant (Merck & Co, Inc, Whitehouse Station, NJ, USA).[33] Data were mixed on the implant's effect on acne.[33]

Trouble-Shooting

The most common adverse effect users experience is abnormal bleeding, which accounts for approximately 10% of discontinuations.[34] Adolescents are no more likely than adult women to discontinue implants due to side effects.[34] Other adverse events occurring with the implant include acne, depression, emotional lability, weight gain, and headache. Each of these symptoms accounts for 1% to 2% of discontinuation.[31]

Anticipatory guidance regarding the likelihood of irregular bleeding is essential when counseling patients about the implant. Bleeding with implant use is thought to be caused either by endometrial changes or by ovarian effects. Thus, content experts recommend obtaining a pelvic ultrasound to evaluate the endometrial stripe and ovaries as a way to clarify the etiology of bleeding before attempting medical management.[33] For women with a thick endometrial stripe suggestive of hyperestrogenism, treatment with an oral progestin may help reduce bleeding by thinning the endometrium. On the other hand, women with a thin endometrial stripe are likely bleeding due to an atrophic and unstable endometrium, and treatment with combined oral contraceptives containing 30 μg of ethinyl estradiol (EE) for 1 or 2 cycles may reduce bleeding by stabilizing the endometrium.

LEVONORGESTREL IUD

Like the implant, Levonorgestrel (LNG) IUDs are highly effective and discreet. Additional benefits for adolescents may include increased duration of use and reliably decreased menstrual bleeding and pain. Currently, there are 2 hormone-containing IUDs available for use in the United States: Mirena and Skyla (Bayer HealthCare Pharmaceuticals Inc, Whippany, NJ, USA) (**Table 3**).

Adolescents should be tested for STIs before initiating the IUD; testing also can be done at the time of insertion and need not delay the insertion to await results. If the results of testing are positive, patients can simply be treated with appropriate antibiotics. The IUD does not need to be removed. The IUD also may be left in place in the event an adolescent develops pelvic inflammatory disease while initiating antibiotic treatment.[35] Prophylactic antibiotics at the time of insertion are not indicated.[35]

Table 3 Comparison of levonorgestrel intrauterine devices		
	Mirena	**Skyla**
Size	32 mm across × 32 mm tall, inserter 4.75 mm in diameter	28 mm across × 30 mm tall, inserter 3.8 mm in diameter
Amount of levonorgestrel	52 mg	13.5 mg
Length of Use	5 y	3 y
Mechanism of action	Thickens cervical mucus Thins endometrium Inhibits sperm function Suppresses ovulation	Thickens cervical mucus Thins endometrium Inhibits sperm function
Noncontraceptive uses	Approved to treat menorrhagia and dysmenorrhea	None
Safe to use in nulliparous women	Yes	Yes

Nulliparity is not a contraindication to IUD placement (**Table 4**). According to the World Health Organization (WHO) and Centers for Disease Control and Prevention Medical Eligibility Criteria for Contraception (MEC), the LNG IUD is considered a category 2 for nulliparous women (advantages generally outweigh theoretic or proven risks for women from menarche until 20 years of age).[36]

The main risks to discuss with patients are uterine perforation, IUD expulsion, and ectopic pregnancy. In the first year of use, the reported rates of expulsion range from 2% to 10%. A recent retrospective descriptive study found that rates of expulsion were 4 times higher for women younger than 18 when compared with women aged 18 to 21 years.[37]

COPPER IUD

Currently, there is one copper-containing IUD available for use in the United States, which is the Paragard (TEVA Pharmaceuticals, Sellersville, PA, USA). Adolescent patients may choose the copper IUD because it is hormone-free and menses continue monthly, which provides reassurance that they are not pregnant. An often unrecognized benefit of the copper IUD is the ability to use it as a highly effective method of emergency contraception. There also have been a number of case control studies that show a protective effect against endometrial cancer.[38]

Women often experience an increase in menstrual bleeding and cramping with the copper IUD, and a portion of women will experience intermenstrual bleeding or spotting. Although the menstrual bleeding and cramping usually resolve back to baseline a year after insertion, if a patient has intermenstrual symptoms, those will not likely resolve.[39]

Trouble-Shooting IUDs

Anticipatory guidance is the most important tool a clinician can use when initiating an IUD with an adolescent. Giving developmentally appropriate counseling about risks and benefits, what to expect during a pelvic examination, method of insertion, and bleeding patterns is essential. Discussion about gynecologic examinations is especially salient now that many young women may not experience their first examination until age 21 with new cervical cancer screening guidelines.

Concerns about pain control can cause both patients and clinicians to avoid IUDs in young, nulliparous women. To date, no routine interventions have been shown to be effective at reducing pain with IUD insertion. There is no evidence that preprocedure nonsteroidal anti-inflammatory drugs, paracervical blocks, topical anesthetic, and cervical ripening agents, such as misoprostol, decrease pain or ease insertion in adolescents.[40–48] In fact, misoprostol seems to succeed only in causing unpleasant side effects for the patient, such as nausea and cramping.[44] The best tool providers have for pain control is "verbicaine" or a "vocal local," good counseling, and calm reassurance throughout the procedure.

For a difficult insertion, the practitioner can try gently dilating the cervical os with tapered dilators, or attempting the insertion under ultrasound guidance. If the insertion is still unsuccessful and the patient still wishes to pursue IUD placement, returning for a second visit while the patient is menstruating is also an option.

SECOND-LINE CONTRACEPTIVES
Depo-Medroxyprogesterone Acetate

Depo-medroxyprogesterone acetate (DMPA) is an excellent second-line contraceptive method for adolescents, with lower rates of failure compared with other second-line methods (pill, patch, ring).[49] Although recommended to be given every

Table 4
Long-acting reversible contraceptive methods US Medical Eligibility Criteria for Contraception for common adolescent issues

Condition	Subcondition	ENG Implant Initiate	Continue	LNG IUD Initiate	Continue	Copper IUD Initiate	Continue
Age	Menarche to < 18	1		-		-	
	Menarche to < 20	-		2		2	
Current purulent cervicitis			1	4	2	4	2
Parity	Nulliparous	1		2		2	
	Parous	1		1		1	
PID	History of PID with subsequent pregnancy	1		1	1	1	1
	History of PID with no subsequent pregnancy	1		2	2	2	2
	Current	1		4	2	4	2
Post-Partum and Breast Feeding	< 3 wks postpartum	2					
	3-4 wks postpartum	2		See postpartum IUDs		See postpartum IUDs	
	>4 wks postpartum	1					
Post Partum IUD	< 10 minutes after delivery of the placenta			2		1	
	10 minutes after delivery of the placenta to < 4 wks			2		2	
	≥ 4 wks			1		1	
Tobacco use			1	1		1	

Key

1	Method can be used without restriction
2	Advantages generally outweigh theoretical or proven risks
3	Method not usually recommended unless other, more appropriate methods are not available or not acceptable
4	Method not to be used

Abbreviations: ENG, etonogestrel; IUD, intrauterine device; LNG, levonorgestrel; PID, pelvic inflammatory disease.

Adapted from Center of Disease Control Summary Chart of U.S. Medical Eligibility Criteria for Contraceptive Use. Available at: http://www.cdc.gov/reproductivehealth/unintendedpregnancy/Docs/USMEC-BW-62012.docx. Accessed December 16, 2013.

12 weeks, data support efficacy through 16 weeks, allowing a sizable window period of birth control coverage for adolescents who may present late for follow-up injection.[50] After discontinuing DMPA injections, the return to ovulation is variable, occurring between 15 and 49 weeks from the last injection.[50]

Weight gain can be problematic with DMPA, especially in obese adolescents. For women 18 years or younger who have a body mass index (BMI) of 30 kg/m^2 or more, DMPA is a category 2 due to the risk of weight gain.[36] DMPA remains highly effective in overweight and obese women. However, adolescents who gain more than 5% of their body weight by 6 months are at risk for continued excessive weight gain and should be counseled accordingly.[51]

DMPA use should not be limited in adolescents based solely on concerns for bone mineral density (BMD). WHO, ACOG, and the Society for Adolescent Health and Medicine all recommend that the benefits of DMPA often outweigh the risks. Although adolescents using DMPA have a decrease in BMD, these losses are reversible with a return to baseline BMD within 1 to 2 years of discontinuation.[52] Long-term correlation with osteoporotic fractures has not been clearly established. Many adolescents are vitamin D deficient, thus supplementation with calcium and vitamin D during DMPA use may be beneficial.

Noncontraceptive benefits of DMPA include decreased seizure frequency, decreased sickle cell crises, and reduced pain from menstruation and endometriosis.[53] In addition, DMPA avoids first-pass metabolism, and thus does not interact with most other medications, including antiseizure medicine.[53]

Trouble-shooting

The most common reason for discontinuation of DMPA is changes in bleeding pattern. Appropriate counseling about expected bleeding effects has been shown to improve continuation rates.[54] Up to two-thirds of teenagers using DMPA will be amenorrheic at 6 months.[55] With DMPA initiation, bleeding patterns can be irregular and unpredictable during the first year. There is a decrease in irregular bleeding with each reinjection. Possible interventions to manage bleeding with initial use of DMPA include dual use of combined oral contraceptives containing 30 to 35 mg EE or a short course of exogenous estrogen or mefenamic acid.[56]

Combined Hormonal Contraception (Pills, Patch, Ring)

Contraceptive pills are the most commonly used form of hormonal contraception in adolescents.[4] Combined hormonal contraception (CHC) methods, however, have the lowest rates of satisfaction and continuation at 1 year.[34] Not only will 50% or more of adolescents discontinue use of their prescribed CHC by 1 year, many will not return for clinical follow-up.[30] Only 18% of sexually active adolescents in the United States reported using birth control pills the last time they had sex.[6]

Failure rates of CHC in teens are higher than in older women. For women younger than 21 using the pill, patch, or ring, the risk of unintended pregnancy was 2 times that for older women.[49] Technology offers increasing opportunities for teens to improve adherence to CHC regimens. Several Web sites and smart-phone applications offer reminders and education targeted to adolescents at minimal or no cost. Examples of smartphone applications include myPill for Apple devices and Contraceptive Pill for Androids.[57] Stayteen.org and plannedparenthood.org/info-for-teens are examples of informative and engaging Web sites directed at teens.

Adolescent women are generally more successful in using methods that require less frequent dosing, making the patch and ring plausibly advantageous. However, continuation rates are generally no better than with oral contraceptives, and typical-use failure rates are equivalent.[30] In fact, adolescents using the patch are almost twice as likely to discontinue use by 1 year compared with teens using combined oral contraceptives (COCs), with most discontinuation in the first 4 months.[58] The weekly contraceptive patch causes higher serum estrogen levels than other COCs, which may translate to increased side effects, such as breast tenderness and nausea. This tends to decrease with continued use. There also may be a higher risk of venous thromboembolism (VTE) compared with COCs; however, epidemiologic studies have had variable results and the risk of VTE remains much lower than with pregnancy and the puerperium. Adolescents are more likely to have skin reactions at the site of patch placement and experience the patch detaching more often.[59,60] Teens should receive anticipatory counseling that the skin reaction is transient. The vaginal ring has lower serum levels of estrogen and patients report fewer systemic side effects than with other CHCs. The monthly ring may cause vaginal symptoms, such as increased discharge.

Noncontraceptive benefits of CHCs include improved menstrual cycle regulation, decreased dysmenorrhea and menstrual blood loss, and improvement of acne.

Trouble-shooting

There is a wide selection of pills available on the market. Most pills contain between 20 and 35 µg EE, which is considered low-dose estrogen. Problems with breakthrough bleeding or spotting are typically better controlled with pills containing 30 to 35 µg EE. Side effects of nausea, breast tenderness, or bloating may resolve by transitioning to a 20-µg EE pill. There are several generations of progestin formulations used in combined pills, which vary by potency and half-life as well as androgenic effects. Some pills are marketed specifically for lower androgenic side effects and acne treatment. Concern has been raised about potential for some of the newer progestin forms to increase risk of blood clots. However, absolute risk in adolescents is very low regardless of the formulation chosen. As a general rule, initial prescription of COCs should be for a generic and affordable monophasic pill with low-dose estrogen and a second-generation progestin, such as LNG. Providers are encouraged to use a quick-start method (see **Fig. 1**), as this has been shown to increase adolescents' utilization of the chosen method.[61]

Extended cycling of all CHC methods can improve use and satisfaction with these methods. By reducing the duration of the hormone-free interval, the efficacy is also increased.[62] Increased satisfaction is related to higher rates of amenorrhea, but teens must be counseled about the higher rates of unscheduled bleeding days as well.

Progestin-Only Pills

Progestin-only pills (POPs) can be safely used by almost all adolescents. However, they may be less effective than CHC methods. General guidance emphasizes the need to take pills at the same time every day to improve efficacy. This is because of the waning serum progestin levels that become nearly undetectable by 24 hours. Without any hormone-free intervals during POP dosing, irregular bleeding is a common side effect.[63]

EMERGENCY CONTRACEPTION

Emergency contraception (EC) education should be included in all clinical visits addressing sexual health in adolescents, both male and female. Need for advance prescriptions of EC also should be assessed. Consider providing advance prescriptions for EC at the initiation of any contraceptive method, given high rates of method discontinuation and poor follow-up.

The copper IUD is the most effective form of emergency contraception. A study in China enrolled 2000 women presenting to family planning clinics for EC within 120 hours of unprotected intercourse. There were no pregnancies at the 1-month follow-up visit, making the efficacy rate of the copper IUD 100% in this study.[64] Other studies have found similarly high rates of efficacy. The challenge is how to increase access for adolescents during this 5-day-window period. Updated office protocols can help women needing EC to access this care.[65]

Prescriptions for EC provided in advance of need also improve access. LNG EC has been approved for over-the-counter (OTC) status without age restriction. However, multiple obstacles still exist that limit adolescents' ability to obtain EC. In some states, pharmacists and/or pharmacies may refuse to sell EC based on conscience clauses that protect religious objections to birth control. Cost is another substantial obstacle for teens, with OTC pricing approximately $50 for this 1-time-use medication.

Ulipristal acetate (UPA) is more effective than LNG EC, and can be used up to 120 hours after unprotected intercourse.[66] Alarming research also has shown that LNG EC is ineffective for women with a BMI greater than 26.[67] UPA is more effective than LNG EC in overweight and obese women, up to a BMI of 35. UPA requires a prescription and advance provision is highly recommended.

Teens should be counseled that oral EC works by delaying ovulation. The implication for the adolescent is that subsequent unprotected intercourse in the week following EC use continues to put them at high risk for unintended pregnancy. Despite increasing access to oral EC, there have not been proven reductions in unintended pregnancy rates. Thus, opportunities to provide and discuss EC also should emphasize the importance of highly effective ongoing contraceptive methods.

DUAL METHODS

Dual-method contraception, with the use of barrier contraception in addition to one of the previously discussed methods, increases the efficacy of pregnancy prevention while providing protection from STIs. The availability of condoms, including free condoms in the school setting, does not increase the frequency or initiation of sexual activity.[68] Condom use reported at last intercourse has been increasing from 46.2% in 1991 to 60.2% in 2011.[6] With typical use, condoms alone have an 18% failure rate, which makes concurrent use of hormonal contraception the optimal strategy.[68,69] Currently, dual-method contraception is used by 18% to 29% of adolescent couples.[69] Dual-method use is associated with higher perceived risks of pregnancy and STIs, communication with parents and parental approval of birth control, positive attitudes toward condoms, and partner support and self-efficacy in negotiation of condom use.

SUMMARY

Promoting the most effective methods of contraception in teens and providing access to these methods reduces unintended pregnancies. Educating teens on condom use, providing advance prescriptions for EC, and ensuring adolescent confidentiality are also important patient-centered practices in the care of adolescents. Clinicians can play an active role in preventing unintended adolescent pregnancy and decrease the associated negative consequences for teen parents and their children.

REFERENCES

1. Kost K, Henshaw S. U.S. teenage pregnancies, births and abortions, 2008: state trends by age, race and ethnicity. New York: Guttmacher Institute; 2013.

2. Finer LB, Henshaw SK. Disparities in rates of unintended pregnancy in the United States, 1994 and 2001. Perspect Sex Reprod Health 2006;38(2):90–6.
3. Guttmacher Institute. In brief: facts on induced abortion in the United States. New York: Guttmacher Institute; 2013.
4. Martinez G, Copen CE, Abma JC. Teenagers in the United States: sexual activity, contraceptive use, and childbearing, 2006-2010 national survey of family growth. Vital Health Stat 23 2011;(31):1–35.
5. Santelli JS, Lindberg LD, Finer LB, et al. Explaining recent declines in adolescent pregnancy in the United States: the contribution of abstinence and improved contraceptive use. Am J Public Health 2007;97(1):150–6.
6. Eaton DK, Kann L, Kinchen S, et al. Youth risk behavior surveillance - United States, 2011. MMWR Surveill Summ 2012;61(4):1–162.
7. Guttmacher Institute. In brief: facts on publicly funded contraceptive services in the United States. Washington, DC: Guttmacher Institute; 2010.
8. Gold RB, Sonfield A, Richards C, et al. Next steps for America's family planning program: leveraging the potential of Medicaid and Title X in an evolving health care system. New York: Guttmacher Institute; 2009.
9. Peipert JF, Madden T, Allsworth JE, et al. Preventing unintended pregnancies by providing no-cost contraception. Obstet Gynecol 2012;120(6):1291–7.
10. Reddy DM, Fleming R, Swain C. Effect of mandatory parental notification on adolescent girls' use of sexual health care services. JAMA 2002;288(6): 710–4.
11. Jones RK, Purcell A, Singh S, et al. Adolescents' reports of parental knowledge of adolescents' use of sexual health services and their reactions to mandated parental notification for prescription contraception. JAMA 2005;293(3):340–8.
12. Committee on Adolescence. Counseling the adolescent about pregnancy options. Pediatrics 1998;101(5):938–40.
13. Workowski KA, Berman S. Sexually transmitted diseases treatment guidelines, 2010. MMWR Recomm Rep 2010;59(RR-12):1–110.
14. Dobkin LM, Perrucci AC, Dehlendorf C. Pregnancy options counseling for adolescents: overcoming barriers to care and preserving preference. Curr Probl Pediatr Adolesc Health Care 2013;43(4):96–102.
15. Wolff T, Witkop CT, Miller T, et al, U.S. Preventive Services Task Force. Folic acid supplementation for the prevention of neural tube defects: an update of the evidence for the U.S. Preventive Services Task Force. Ann Intern Med 2009;150(9): 632–9.
16. Klein JD. Adolescent pregnancy: current trends and issues. Pediatrics 2005; 116(1):281–6.
17. Raymond EG, Grimes DA. The comparative safety of legal induced abortion and childbirth in the United States. Obstet Gynecol 2012;119(2 Pt 1):215–9.
18. Pinzon JL, Jones VF. Care of adolescent parents and their children. Pediatrics 2012;130(6):e1743–56.
19. Elfenbein DS, Felice ME. Adolescent pregnancy. Pediatr Clin North Am 2003; 50(4):781–800, viii.
20. Aruda MM, Waddicor K, Frese L, et al. Early pregnancy in adolescents: diagnosis, assessment, options counseling, and referral. J Pediatr Health Care 2010;24(1):4–13.
21. Ruedinger E, Cox JE. Adolescent childbearing: consequences and interventions. Curr Opin Pediatr 2012;24(4):446–52.
22. Grady MA, Bloom KC. Pregnancy outcomes of adolescents enrolled in a CenteringPregnancy program. J Midwifery Womens Health 2004;49(5):412–20.

23. Irwin CE Jr, Adams SH, Park MJ, et al. Preventive care for adolescents: few get visits and fewer get services. Pediatrics 2009;123(4):e565–72.
24. Guttmacher Institute. Sex and America's teenagers. New York: Guttmacher Institute; 1994.
25. Haffner DW. Facing facts: sexual health for America's adolescents: the report of the National Commission on Adolescent Sexual Health. SIECUS Rep 1995;23(6):2–8.
26. Oringanje C, Meremikwu MM, Eko H, et al. Interventions for preventing unintended pregnancies among adolescents. Cochrane Database Syst Rev 2009;(4): CD005215.
27. Kirby D. Emerging answers 2007: research findings on programs to reduce teen pregnancy and sexually transmitted diseases. Washington, DC: National Campaign to Prevent Teen and Unplanned Pregnancy; 2007.
28. Committee on Adolescent Health Care Long-Acting Reversible Contraception Working Group, The American College of Obstetricians and Gynecologists. Committee opinion no. 539: adolescents and long-acting reversible contraception: implants and intrauterine devices. Obstet Gynecol 2012;120(4):983–8.
29. Mestad R, Secura G, Allsworth JE, et al. Acceptance of long-acting reversible contraceptive methods by adolescent participants in the Contraceptive CHOICE Project. Contraception 2011;84(5):493–8.
30. O'Neil-Callahan M, Peipert JF, Zhao Q, et al. Twenty-four-month continuation of reversible contraception. Obstet Gynecol 2013;122(5):1083–91.
31. Stoddard A, McNicholas C, Peipert JF. Efficacy and safety of long-acting reversible contraception. Drugs 2011;71(8):969–80.
32. Xu H, Wade JA, Peipert JF, et al. Contraceptive failure rates of etonogestrel subdermal implants in overweight and obese women. Obstet Gynecol 2012;120(1): 21–6.
33. Palomba S, Falbo A, Di Cello A, et al. Nexplanon: the new implant for long-term contraception. A comprehensive descriptive review. Gynecol Endocrinol 2012; 28(9):710–21.
34. Peipert JF, Zhao Q, Allsworth JE, et al. Continuation and satisfaction of reversible contraception. Obstet Gynecol 2011;117(5):1105–13.
35. Division of Reproductive Health, National Center for Chronic Disease Prevention and Health Promotion, Centers for Disease Control and Prevention (CDC). U.S. Selected Practice Recommendations for Contraceptive Use, 2013: adapted from the World Health Organization selected practice recommendations for contraceptive use, 2nd edition. MMWR Recomm Rep 2013;62(RR-05):1–60.
36. Centers for Disease Control and Prevention (CDC). US medical eligibility criteria for contraceptive use, 2010. MMWR Recomm Rep 2010;59(RR-4):1–86.
37. Alton TM, Brock GN, Yang D, et al. Retrospective review of intrauterine device in adolescent and young women. J Pediatr Adolesc Gynecol 2012;25(3): 195–200.
38. Hartman LB, Monasterio E, Hwang LY. Adolescent contraception: review and guidance for pediatric clinicians. Curr Probl Pediatr Adolesc Health Care 2012;42(9):221–63.
39. Hubacher D, Chen PL, Park S. Side effects from the copper IUD: do they decrease over time? Contraception 2009;79(5):356–62.
40. Allen RH, Bartz D, Grimes DA, et al. Interventions for pain with intrauterine device insertion. Cochrane Database Syst Rev 2009;(3):CD007373.
41. Hubacher D, Reyes V, Lillo S, et al. Pain from copper intrauterine device insertion: randomized trial of prophylactic ibuprofen. Am J Obstet Gynecol 2006; 195(5):1272–7.

42. Mody SK, Kiley J, Rademaker A, et al. Pain control for intrauterine device insertion: a randomized trial of 1% lidocaine paracervical block. Contraception 2012; 86(6):704–9.

43. McNicholas C, Peipert JF. Long-acting reversible contraception for adolescents. Curr Opin Obstet Gynecol 2012;24(5):293–8.

44. Waddington A, Reid R. More harm than good: the lack of evidence for administering misoprostol prior to IUD insertion. J Obstet Gynaecol Can 2012;34(12):1177–9.

45. Espey E, Singh RH, Leeman L, et al. Misoprostol for intrauterine device insertion in nulliparous women: a randomized controlled trial. Am J Obstet Gynecol 2014; 210(3):208.e1–5.

46. Lathrop E, Haddad L, McWhorter CP, et al. Self-administration of misoprostol prior to intrauterine device insertion among nulliparous women: a randomized controlled trial. Contraception 2013;88(6):725–9.

47. Ibrahim ZM, Sayed Ahmed WA. Sublingual misoprostol prior to insertion of a T380A intrauterine device in women with no previous vaginal delivery. Eur J Contracept Reprod Health Care 2013;18(4):300–8.

48. Scavuzzi A, Souza AS, Costa AA, et al. Misoprostol prior to inserting an intrauterine device in nulligravidas: a randomized clinical trial. Hum Reprod 2013;28(8): 2118–25.

49. Winner B, Peipert JF, Zhao Q, et al. Effectiveness of long-acting reversible contraception. N Engl J Med 2012;366(21):1998–2007.

50. Paulen ME, Curtis KM. When can a woman have repeat progestogen-only injectables—depot medroxyprogesterone acetate or norethisterone enantate? Contraception 2009;80(4):391–408.

51. Bonny AE, Secic M, Cromer B. Early weight gain related to later weight gain in adolescents on depot medroxyprogesterone acetate. Obstet Gynecol 2011; 117(4):793–7.

52. Isley MM, Kaunitz AM. Update on hormonal contraception and bone density. Rev Endocr Metab Disord 2011;12(2):93–106.

53. Cullins VE. Noncontraceptive benefits and therapeutic uses of depot medroxyprogesterone acetate. J Reprod Med 1996;41(5 Suppl):428–33.

54. Halpern V, Lopez LM, Grimes DA, et al. Strategies to improve adherence and acceptability of hormonal methods of contraception. Cochrane Database Syst Rev 2013;(10):CD004317.

55. Cromer BA, Smith RD, Blair JM, et al. A prospective study of adolescents who choose among levonorgestrel implant (Norplant), medroxyprogesterone acetate (Depo-Provera), or the combined oral contraceptive pill as contraception. Pediatrics 1994;94(5):687–94.

56. Abdel-Aleem H, d'Arcangues C, Vogelsong KM, et al. Treatment of vaginal bleeding irregularities induced by progestin only contraceptives. Cochrane Database Syst Rev 2013;(10):CD003449.

57. Carvajal DN, Brittner MR, Rubin SE. Can apps reduce rates of teen pregnancy? J Fam Pract 2013;62(10):538,598.

58. Raine TR, Foster-Rosales A, Upadhyay UD, et al. One-year contraceptive continuation and pregnancy in adolescent girls and women initiating hormonal contraceptives. Obstet Gynecol 2011;117(2 Pt 1):363–71.

59. Rubinstein ML, Halpern-Felsher BL, Irwin CE Jr. An evaluation of the use of the transdermal contraceptive patch in adolescents. J Adolesc Health 2004;34(5): 395–401.

60. Bodner K, Bodner-Adler B, Grunberger W. Evaluation of the contraceptive efficacy, compliance, and satisfaction with the transdermal contraceptive patch

system Evra: a comparison between adolescent and adult users. Arch Gynecol Obstet 2011;283(3):525–30.

61. Lara-Torre E, Schroeder B. Adolescent compliance and side effects with Quick Start initiation of oral contraceptive pills. Contraception 2002;66(2):81–5.

62. Dinger J, Minh TD, Buttmann N, et al. Effectiveness of oral contraceptive pills in a large U.S. cohort comparing progestogen and regimen. Obstet Gynecol 2011; 117(1):33–40.

63. Grimes DA, Lopez LM, O'Brien PA, et al. Progestin-only pills for contraception. Cochrane Database Syst Rev 2013;(11):CD007541.

64. Wu S, Godfrey EM, Wojdyla D, et al. Copper T380A intrauterine device for emergency contraception: a prospective, multicentre, cohort clinical trial. BJOG 2010;117(10):1205–10.

65. Dalby J, Hayon R, Paddock E, et al. Emergency contraception: an underutilized resource. J Fam Pract 2012;61(7):392–7.

66. Glasier AF, Cameron ST, Fine PM, et al. Ulipristal acetate versus levonorgestrel for emergency contraception: a randomised non-inferiority trial and meta-analysis. Lancet 2010;375(9714):555–62.

67. Glasier A, Cameron ST, Blithe D, et al. Can we identify women at risk of pregnancy despite using emergency contraception? Data from randomized trials of ulipristal acetate and levonorgestrel. Contraception 2011;84(4):363–7.

68. Committee on Adolescence. Condom use by adolescents. Pediatrics 2013;132: 973–81.

69. Bearinger LH, Resnick MD. Dual method use in adolescents: a review and framework for research on use of STD and pregnancy protection. J Adolesc Health 2003;32(5):340–9.

Common Sexually Transmitted Infections in Adolescents

Erica J. Gibson, MD[a],*, David L. Bell, MD, MPH[a],
Sherine A. Powerful[b]

KEYWORDS

- Sexually transmitted infections • Symptoms • Management • Treatment
- Adolescent • Health

KEY POINTS

- Sexually transmitted infections (STIs) have a significant impact on the health of sexually active young people.
- Medical providers should be alert for both asymptomatic and symptomatic STIs.
- Following screening guidelines and using appropriate diagnostic testing provides for timely and effective treatment of STIs.
- Using effective primary treatment regimens with timely follow-up is essential for the treatment of STIs and prevention of complications.
- Diagnosis of an STI can be substantial for all, and in particular for adolescents. Effective empathy and counseling are essential aspects of diagnosis and treatment.

GENERAL BACKGROUND

Sexually transmitted infections (STIs) are a common cause of morbidity in sexually active adolescents and may be caused by bacteria, viruses, protozoa, parasites, or fungi. The most common viral STI is human papillomavirus (HPV), and the most common bacterial STI is chlamydia.[1] Other common infections in adolescents include gonorrhea, syphilis, trichomonas, and herpes simplex virus (HSV). Some bacterial STIs, such as chlamydia, are curable with antibiotics. Others such as HSV persist in the body in dormant and active states, as there are no currently available curative treatments.

Assorted complications of STIs include:

- Severe infections
- Chronic pain

[a] Columbia University Medical Center, New York Presbyterian Hospital, 60 Haven Avenue, B-3, New York, NY 10032, USA; [b] Department of Population & Family Health, Columbia University Medical Center, 60 Haven Avenue, B-3, New York, NY 10032, USA
* Corresponding author.
E-mail address: eg2446@cumc.columbia.edu

Prim Care Clin Office Pract 41 (2014) 631–650
http://dx.doi.org/10.1016/j.pop.2014.05.011
0095-4543/14/$ – see front matter © 2014 Elsevier Inc. All rights reserved.

- Infertility
- Cancer
- Ectopic pregnancy
- Deleterious effects in utero

Half of the nearly 20 million new STIs every year in the United States occur in youth between 15 and 24 years of age. This percentage is remarkable because 15- to 24-year-olds represent just 25% of the sexually experienced population in the United States.[1] Because of a variety of factors, many adolescents' sexual practices and behaviors put them at risk for acquiring STIs. These risk factors include[2,3]:

- Early age at sexual initiation
- Having multiple sex partners concurrently
- Having sequential sex partners of limited duration
- Having increased biological susceptibility to infection
- Failing to use barrier protection consistently and correctly
- Experiencing multiple obstacles to accessing health care

There are significant disparities in the STI rates for young people of different ages, gender, and sexual orientation. The highest rates of STIs are in young adults and adolescents, but detection of these infections depends greatly on the different screening recommendations for each STI, as many infections are asymptomatic. In the United States, young women have the highest rates of chlamydia and HPV, whereas young men who have sex with men (MSM) are at increased risk for contracting syphilis and human immunodeficiency virus (HIV). Women who engage in sex with other women should still be considered at risk for acquiring STIs, and be offered routine screening as per recommendations for the heterosexual population. African Americans continue to have the highest STI prevalence rates in the United States, although Latinos and American Indian/Alaskan Natives also have higher rates than whites. Asians have lower rates than whites.[1]

Special Considerations

STI prevention programs

A seminal report by Kirby[4] provides a detailed review of the important characteristics of effective curriculum-based sex education programs, and states that the following factors can reduce the probability of a young person contracting an STI:

- Increasing abstinence (both delaying the initiation of sex and increasing the return to abstinence)
- Reducing the number of sexual partners
- Reducing the occurrence of concurrent partners
- Increasing the period of time between sexual partners
- Decreasing the frequency of sex
- Increasing the correct and consistent use of condoms
- Increasing testing and treatment of STIs
- Being vaccinated against STIs for which vaccines are available
- Being circumcised (boys)

Expedited partner therapy

The Centers for Disease Control and Prevention (CDC) emphasizes 5 main areas that need to be addressed in preventing STIs, which include much of the aforesaid but also address the importance of partner evaluation and treatment.[3] Expedited partner therapy (EPT) is one of the newest public health strategies to influence partner treatment, particularly for chlamydia. EPT refers to the ability of a provider to dispense medication for partners to the patient, and has been shown to be as good as or better than standard partner referral options.[5,6] The American Medical Association, the American Academy of Pediatrics (AAP), The American Academy of Family Practitioners, The American College of Gynecologists, and The Society for Adolescent Health and Medicine all support EPT.[7–11] EPT is legal in certain states for certain STIs.[12]

Condom use

More adolescents are using condoms at first intercourse than in the past. Sixty-eight percent of females and 80% of males aged 15 to 19 years reported using condoms at first sex in 2010, representing a significant increase from 2002 to 2010.[13] Other barrier methods, dental dams, and female condoms are infrequently used. Although condom use has increased overall, consistent condom use is still a challenge. The maturation of thinking processes, along with cultural and relationship contexts of condom use, create challenges to influence change in risk-reduction behavior toward more consistent condom use.[14] The contextual challenge to choosing risk-reduction messages is that our culture presents mixed messages related to condom use: irresponsibility for wanting to have sex but responsibility for using condoms. Condoms represent responsibility on one hand and distrust in relationships on the other hand. Influencing consistent condom use will require messaging that supports personal responsibility, safety, and trust in relationships.

Confidentiality

Confidentiality is an important element in providing quality care to adolescents. In primary care settings, this is achieved by structuring portions of the visit with an adolescent without the parent. Frank discussions about confidentiality improve rates of honest disclosures to the provider.[15] It is important to be aware of structural barriers to confidentiality, such as the requirement for private insurance companies to send explanation of benefits (EOBs) so as to be transparent regarding medical costs and billing.[3] Parents might realize that their adolescent was screened for STIs and infer sexual activity. On-site distribution of medications may also help ensure confidentiality. In choosing medication regimens many patients, in particular adolescents, adhere best to the simplest dosing regimens (eg, once-daily dosing) whenever possible, which may also promote greater degrees of confidentiality.

Circumcision

Male circumcision (MC) has been associated with specific decreased risks for STIs and HIV. MC is associated with a lower risk of chancroid and syphilis, but not necessarily HSV-2.[16]

In Africa, where there is a higher incidence of HIV transmission among men who have sex with women, studies indicated that MC is associated with a 60% decreased risk of acquisition of HIV by heterosexual males.[17–19] However, there is no protective effect for women or for MSM.[17–20] Owing to the lack of generalizability of these studies to the United States, an expert panel suggests that heterosexually active noncircumcised adolescent and adult males be informed about the significant but partial efficacy of MC in reducing the risk for HIV acquisition. Condom use is still the most effective means of STI prevention; however, if an uncircumcised male chooses to consider MC, the panel recommends that he be provided with affordable access to voluntary, high-quality surgical and risk-reduction counseling services.[21] Though controversial, the AAP now endorses newborn male circumcision but does not recommend universal MC.[21,22]

Health education
One challenge is to develop and engage adolescents in sexual health discussions appropriate for their developmental level. The younger adolescents are, the more likely their cognitive processing will be more concrete and that they may not be developmentally able to comprehend long-term future consequences. Younger and some older adolescents lack personal life experiences and are unable to abstractly locate themselves in a theoretical future position; or empathetically place themselves in another's experience to influence their own behaviors. Therefore, to be effective, health education messages would need to be as specific as possible, aimed at specific risk behaviors identified. It is important for these discussions to be thorough, genuine, nonjudgmental, and confidential, to increase the likelihood of honest and full disclosures of risk behaviors. In addition, print or electronic educational materials should always be offered, as a young patient may not absorb educational information while in the clinic and/or receiving bad news or treatment. Health literacy should be assessed in all situations.

MOST COMMON BACTERIAL INFECTIONS

See **Table 1** for a summary.

Chlamydia

Organism/Transmission/Epidemiology
Chlamydia trachomatis serovars D to K are transmitted through oral, vaginal, or anal sexual contact.

Female adolescents are especially at risk for contracting chlamydia for a variety of reasons:

- Columnar epithelium of ectocervix is more susceptible to pathogens
- Lower estrogen levels result in a weaker cervical mucus barrier
- Thinner genital tissue is more vulnerable to trauma

Females between 15 and 19 and from 20 to 24 years of age have the highest chlamydia prevalence rates in the United States. Overall rates for males are much lower than for females, but are highest in the 20- to 24-year age group.[1] Higher reporting rates of chlamydia in females might be due to the fact that there is greater surveillance of females.

Screening
The CDC and the US Preventive Services Task Force (USPSTF) recommends that all sexually active females 25 years old or younger be screened annually for chlamydia.[3] Although routine screening of young asymptomatic males is not routinely recommended, it should be considered in those who are at risk for infection.

Symptoms
It is important to bear in mind that most male and female patients infected with chlamydia are asymptomatic.[23,24] Symptoms can include:

- Females:
  - Vaginal discharge or bleeding
  - Dysuria
  - Abdominal/pelvic pain
- Males:
  - Testicular pain
  - Penile discharge
  - Dysuria

Diagnosis

At present, nucleic acid amplification tests (NAATs) are the preferred method for testing for chlamydia. The current NAATs on the market test for chlamydia and gonorrhea simultaneously.

- Females:
  - The best sample is obtained from a patient- or provider-collected vaginal swab or endocervical sample; research has shown that vaginal swabs identify as many infected patients as cervical swabs and that acceptance of self-swabbing by patients is high.[25,26]
  - Urine samples are sensitive and specific; a first void sample of 10 to 30 mL should be obtained 1 hour or later after last void.
- Males:
  - Urine screening is the preferred strategy.[27]

Most NAATs are not cleared by the Food and Drug Administration (FDA) for rectal and pharyngeal specimens. However, some laboratories have met Clinical Laboratory Improvement Amendments (CLIA) requirements, and have validated NAAT testing on rectal and pharyngeal swabs.[28]

Management

If history, physical examination, or laboratory results indicate chlamydia infection, treat with antibiotics as per the CDC sexually transmitted diseases treatment guidelines, 2010.[3] To maximize compliance, directly observed treatment on-site should be provided for STIs whenever possible.

Preferred treatment regimen:

- Azithromycin 1 g by mouth (PO) × 1 or
- Doxycycline 100 mg PO twice daily (BID) × 7 days

Patients should be instructed to abstain from sexual intercourse for 7 days after completion of treatment. Persons who have already had chlamydia and were treated can be reinfected, so it is recommended that all adolescents who test positive for chlamydia be screened again in 3 to 6 months for reinfection. A test of cure is no longer recommended.[3]

EPT for chlamydia is legal in many states and should be provided whenever possible. Chlamydia is a CDC-mandated reportable disease, so reporting is required as per individual state department of health requirements.

Gonorrhea

Organism/Transmission/Epidemiology

Neisseria gonorrhoeae is transmitted through oral, vaginal, or anal sex. Gonorrhea is the second most commonly reported STI, with rates highest among the adolescent and young adult age groups.[3,24]

Screening

Widespread screening for gonorrhea is not recommended.[3] Health care providers should consider local gonorrhea epidemiology when making screening decisions. The CDC supports USPSTF recommendations:

- Females: Target sexually active females 25 years old or younger, including those who are pregnant, who are at increased risk of infection.
  - Among the risk factors to consider are[3]:
    - Previous STI infection

Table 1
Most common STIs in adolescents: quick reference

	Symptoms in Adolescents	Screening Recommendations[3,5]	Preferred Outpatient Diagnostic Tests	Primary CDC Treatment Guidelines[3]
Chlamydia	1. Asymptomatic 2. Discharge 3. Dysuria 4. Pelvic/abdominal pain	Females: ≤25 y, yearly Males: Only those at risk for infection[a]	NAAT	Azithromycin 1 g PO × 1 or Doxycycline 100 mg PO BID × 7 d[b]
Gonorrhea	1. Asymptomatic 2. Discharge 3. Dysuria 4. Pelvic/abdominal pain	Males and females at risk for infection[a]	NAAT	Ceftriaxone 250 mg IM × 1 plus azithromycin 1 g PO × 1 or Doxycycline 100 mg PO BID × 7 d[b]
Syphilis	1. Primary: painless papule/chancre, swollen lymph nodes 2. Secondary: reddish-brown rash, condyloma lata, systemic symptoms 3. Tertiary: infection spreads to various organ systems	MSM: Annual screening Others: selective and based on local epidemiology	VDRL and RPR nontreponemal tests with confirmatory FTA-ABS treponemal test for positives	Primary: benzathine penicillin G 2.4 million units IM × 1[c]
Trichomonas	1. Asymptomatic 2. Diffuse, frothy, yellow-green vaginal discharge	Not routinely recommended[a]	TMA and RAT	Metronidazole 2 g PO × 1 or Tinidazole 2 g PO × 1 dose

	Clinical presentation	Screening/diagnosis	Treatment
HPV	1. Asymptomatic 2. Genital warts	Females: Pap smear for cervical neoplasia at age 21 y	Pap smear, HPV serology should not be sent for patients younger than 30 y
			1. Warts: patient or provider applied topical regimens 2. Cervical neoplasia management[d]
HSV	1. Asymptomatic 2. Blisters/ulcerations 3. Headache, fever, malaise	Not routinely recommended[a]	Viral culture, polymerase chain reaction, antibody-based tests
			Primary episode: Acyclovir 400 mg PO TID × 7–10 d Valacyclovir 1 g PO BID × 7–10 d Recurrence: Acyclovir 800 mg PO BID × 5 d Valacyclovir 500 mg PO BID × 3 d[e]
HIV	1. Asymptomatic 2. Acute retroviral syndrome: fever, malaise, lymphadenopathy, rash	Should be offered at least once to all patients age 13–64 y	Conventional or rapid EIA
			Per-patient status and most recent CDC guidelines

Abbreviations: BID, twice daily; CDC, Centers for Disease Control and Prevention; EIA, enzyme immunoassay; FTA-ABS, fluorescent treponemal antibody–absorbed; HIV, human immunodeficiency virus; HPV, human papillomavirus; HSV, herpes simplex virus; IM, intramuscularly; MSM, men who have sex with men; NAAT, nucleic acid amplification testing; Pap, Papanicolaou; PO, by mouth; RAT, rapid antigen testing; RPR, rapid plasma reagin; TID, 3 times daily; TMA, transcription-mediated amplification assay; VDRL, Venereal Disease Research Laboratory.

[a] See text for situations when screening might be recommended.
[b] See text for pelvic inflammatory disease regimen.
[c] See text for secondary and tertiary treatment regimens.
[d] See text for details of management.
[e] See text for extensive additional primary treatment regimens.

- New or multiple sex partners
- Inconsistent condom use
  - Universal screening for adult females up to the age of 35 years should be conducted at intake in jail facilities or based on local institutional prevalence data.
- Males: Screening should be considered in those who are at risk for infection. MSM who engage in receptive anal or oral sex should be screened for rectal and pharyngeal gonorrhea infection.[3]

Symptoms

Most females with gonorrhea are asymptomatic, so screening is critical. Most men with infection have symptoms. Symptoms can appear 2 to 5 days after infection. Often the infection lies dormant for up to 30 days.[29] Symptoms can include:

- Females:
  - Dysuria
  - Vaginal discharge or bleeding
- Males:
  - Dysuria
  - Purulent discharge
  - Sore throat (rare)

Complications

- Females:
  - Pelvic inflammatory disease
  - Infertility
  - Spontaneous abortion in the first trimester
  - Ectopic pregnancy
- Males:
  - Epididymitis
  - Prostatitis
  - Increased susceptibility to acquiring HIV[29]

Diagnosis

- NAATs represent the preferred approach for testing for oral, urine, vaginal, and anal specimens.[3] As with chlamydia testing, patient- or provider-collected vaginal swabs are the preferred method of collection in women.
- Most NAATs are not FDA-cleared for rectal and pharyngeal specimens. However, some laboratories have met CLIA requirements and have validated NAAT testing on rectal and pharyngeal swabs.[28]
- Cultures and antibiotic sensitivity testing are preferred for subsequent testing for antibiotic resistance.
- Gram stains in symptomatic males with urethral discharge can be considered diagnostic.

Management

If history, physical examination, or laboratory results indicate gonorrhea infection, treat with antibiotics as per the CDC guidelines.
Preferred treatment regimen[3]:

- Ceftriaxone 250 mg intramuscularly (IM) × 1
- Plus: Azithromycin 1 g PO × 1 or doxycycline 100 mg BID × 7 days

Dual therapy has been recommended since 2010 because of the decreased susceptibility of *Neisseria* gonorrhea to cephalosporins.[30] The additional oral therapy also covers chlamydia, which is a frequent coinfection with gonorrhea. On a global level, strains of gonorrhea show resistance to treatments such as ciprofloxacin (Europe, Asia, Central Asia, the South Pacific, California, Hawaii), penicillin, tetracycline, and spectinomycin.[31,32]

Persons who have already had gonorrhea and have undergone treatment can be reinfected, so it is recommended that all adolescents who test positive for gonorrhea be screened again in 3 to 6 months for reinfection.

Given the newer recommendation against oral therapy alone for the treatment of gonorrhea (cefixime plus azithromycin or doxycycline), EPT is not as feasible, even though in certain states it is legal for gonorrhea.[8,10,11]

Gonorrhea is a CDC-mandated reportable disease, so reporting is required as per individual state department of health requirements.

Syphilis

Organism/Transmission/Epidemiology

The spirochete bacterium *Treponema pallidum* is transmitted through unprotected oral, vaginal, or anal sexual contact.[3,33]

The prevalence of syphilis among adolescents is not as high as in other STIs. Rates are higher among young adult men, particularly among the MSM population.[1]

Screening

Routine screening is not recommended except for:

- Persons at increased risk for syphilis, in particular, MSM[3]
- All pregnant women

Screening of other patients should be selective and based on local health department epidemiology.[3]

Symptoms

Early syphilis

- Defined as the stages of syphilis (primary, secondary, and early latent) that tend to occur within the first year of the infection.[3]

Primary syphilis:

- Begins between 14 and 21 days after exposure
- Small painless papule emerges, evolves into small painless ulcer called a chancre, accompanied by swollen lymph nodes[24,25]
- Initial chancre resolves on its own after 3 to 6 weeks

Secondary syphilis:

- Occurs a few weeks to a few months after primary stage
- In untreated patients, occasionally relapses can occur for up to 5 years
- A symmetric reddish-brown rash emerges on abdomen and extremities, including palms and soles
- Condyloma lata; weeping lesions in the genitals and anus might also occur
- Other signs and symptoms such as fever, malaise, weight loss, sore throat, hair loss, weight loss, anorexia, and fever can also occur
- Various signs and symptoms contribute to syphilis being known as the "great imitator"
- Can resolve on its own, even in the absence of therapy

Early latent syphilis:

- Patients are potentially infectious in early latent stage (<1 year)
- This stage is characteristically asymptomatic

Neurosyphilis[34,35]:

- Refers to infection of the central nervous system
- Can occur at any time after initial infection (early or late syphilis)
- Can be classified into early forms involving cerebrospinal fluid, meninges, and vasculature, and late forms that affect the brain and spinal cord parenchyma
- HIV infection may be associated with an increased risk of developing neurosyphilis

Late syphilis Late latent syphilis[3,36]:

- Characteristically asymptomatic
- Not infectious in the late latent stage
- Can last for years before proceeding to the tertiary stage

Diagnosis
Definitive immediate diagnosis of primary or secondary syphilis can be made with dark-field microscopy, which is not traditionally available in primary care offices.[3]

In general office settings, screening nontreponemal tests such as the Venereal Disease Research Laboratory (VDRL) and rapid plasma reagin (RPR) tests are done initially. False positives occur with the VDRL and RPR, sometimes occurring in pregnancy. If the screening nontreponemal test is positive, a reflex treponemal test such as the fluorescent treponemal antibody-absorbed (FTA-ABS) test is performed as the confirmatory test.

Management
If a physical examination or laboratory results indicate syphilis infection, treat with antibiotics as per the CDC guidelines[3]:

- Preferred treatment
  - Early syphilis (primary, secondary, and early latent):
    - Benzathine penicillin G 2.4 million units IM × 1 dose (adult dosing)
  - Late latent syphilis:
    - Benzathine penicillin G 2.4 * million units IM every week × 3 doses for total of 7.2 million units

Patients treated for primary and secondary syphilis should be seen for clinical and serologic follow-up at least at 6 and 12 months.[3]

- Expect at least a 4-fold decrease in titers
- Reinfection is determined by a 4-fold increase in titers

Sexual partners in the 90 days before diagnosis should be treated presumptively. Those partners who were potentially exposed greater than 90 days before diagnosis should be treated presumptively if no testing is available.

In the case of penicillin allergy, it is preferable to desensitize patients allergic to penicillin rather than use alternative medications such as doxycycline.

Syphilis is a CDC-mandated reportable disease, so reporting is required as per individual state department of health requirements.

Special considerations/specific counseling points

- Syphilis and HIV
  - When syphilis is present, the risk of acquiring HIV is increased by 2 to 5 times more than when syphilis is not present.[37,38]
  - Syphilis will increase the viral load of someone who is already infected by HIV.[39]
- Jarisch-Herxheimer reaction
  - An acute febrile reaction frequently accompanied by headache, myalgia, fever, and other symptoms that usually occur within the first 24 hours after the initiation of any therapy for syphilis

Trichomonas Vaginalis

Organism/Transmission/Epidemiology

The pathogenic protozoan *Trichomonas vaginalis* is transmitted through unprotected oral, vaginal, or anal sexual contact.

Trichomonas is the third most common cause of vaginitis after bacterial vaginosis and candida. Vaginitis may be caused by more than 1 infection at a time.

Screening

Routine screening for *T vaginalis* is not recommended, but may be considered in women at high risk for infection.[3]

Symptoms

- Females:
  - Vaginitis characterized by yellow-green odorous, frothy, and diffuse vaginal discharge
  - Urethritis and irritation of the vulva
  - "Strawberry cervix": a cervix remarkable for punctate hemorrhages and tiny ulcerations
  - Patients may also be asymptomatic
- Males:
  - Often asymptomatic
  - Can present with urethritis

Complications

- Females:
  - Preterm labor
  - Rupture of membranes
  - Low birth weight
  - Pelvic inflammatory diseases

Diagnosis

Transcription-mediated amplification assays (TMA) and rapid antigen testing (RAT) are highly sensitive, specific, and far superior to wet mount.[40] RAT is equivalent to culture in sensitivity and specificity; and compares favorably with TMA regarding sensitivity.

Management

If history, physical examination, or laboratory results indicate trichomonas infection, treat as per the CDC Guidelines.[3]

Preferred treatment

- Metronidazole 2 g PO × 1 dose or
- Tinidazole 2 g PO × 1 dose

Topical vaginal treatment is not recommended. Partner treatment of trichomonas is recommended.

All patients treated with metronidazole should be counseled not to drink alcohol while taking the medication and for 24 hours thereafter.

Special considerations

Trichomonas is often transmitted with another STI such as chlamydia or gonorrhea.

MOST COMMON VIRAL INFECTIONS
Human Papillomavirus

Organism/Transmission/Epidemiology

HPV is a DNA virus that has more than 100 identified subtypes, and more than 30 types that infect the genital tract.

- Spread by skin-to-skin contact, mainly sexual contact
- Infects mucous membranes and epithelial tissues
- High-grade types, including 16 and 18, can lead to cervical cancer, whereas low-grade types 6 and 11 are linked to genital warts (condyloma acuminata)

Although the exact prevalence of HPV in adolescents is difficult to assess, several studies have revealed that high-risk types of infection are common in adolescents, although most infections resolve spontaneously within 24 months.[41,42]

Screening

Healthy young women should be screened for HPV with cervical cytology (Papanicolaou smear) starting at age 21 years, and every 3 years thereafter until age 29 assuming results are normal.[43,44] Cotesting for HPV DNA is not recommended for women younger than 30 years because of the high prevalence of HPV infection in this age group.

Symptoms

- Usually asymptomatic
- When present, symptoms include:
  - Genital warts: Raised lesions that are painless and fleshy and usually in moist areas of the body. Most resolve spontaneously through the immune system, clearing the infection
  - Cervical neoplasia: Very rare in young women but may present on routine cervical cytology starting at age 21 years or with abnormal vaginal bleeding

Diagnosis

- Cervical cytology starting at age 21 years to detect subclinical infection and abnormalities
- Recognized clinically from genital warts

Management

- No cure
- Recommended treatment as per CDC guidelines[3]
  - Genital warts: patient-applied

- Podofilox 0.5% solution or gel BID × 3, off × 4 days, repeat as needed for maximum 4 cycles (Note: use 0.5 mL/d maximum, do not cover more than 10 cm^2) or
- Imiquimod 5% cream apply every night at bedtime 3 times a week for up to 16 weeks, wash off with soap and water 6 to 10 hours after treatment or
- Sinecatechins 15% ointment 3 times daily (TID) for maximum of 16 weeks (Note: use 0.5-cm strand of ointment, do not wash off)
  - ○ Genital warts: provider-applied
    - Cryotherapy: liquid nitrogen or cryoprobe every 1 to 2 weeks or
    - Podophyllin resin 10% to 25% in compound with tincture of benzoin, wash off in 1 to 4 hours, repeat weekly or
    - Trichloroacetic acid every week or
    - Bichloroacetic acid 80% to 90% every week or
    - Surgical removal by tangential scissor excision, curettage, electrosurgery, or tangential shave excision[3]

Abnormal cervical cytology results with the advent of screening at age 21 years should be managed as per the guidelines of the American Society for Colposcopy and Cervical Cytology.[44]

Vaccination
The CDC Advisory Committee on Immunization Practices recommends routine vaccination of both females and males aged 11 to 12 years with an initial dose of HPV vaccine.[45] The quadrivalent HPV vaccine is approved for both males and females; the bivalent HPV vaccine is only approved for females. A 3-dose series is recommended for both vaccines, and both vaccines may be administered as early as 9 years of age.

Special considerations
Although high-risk HPV types 16 and 18 are found in approximately 70% of cervical cancers, infection with the virus is not the only causative factor in disease, and many women clear the virus without progressing to cancer.[41]

Genital Herpes

Organism/Transmission/Epidemiology
Herpes simplex virus is a DNA virus with 2 members (HSV-1 and HSV-2) that infect humans.

- Spread through skin-to-skin contact
- Spread by direct contact with mucous membranes, especially sexual contact

The overall age-adjusted HSV-2 seroprevalence is approximately 17% and the overall age-adjusted HSV-1 seroprevalence is 58%.[46]

Screening
Universal screening by serum testing in the general population for HSV-1 and HSV-2 is not recommended.[3,46]

Type-specific HSV serologic assays may be useful if[3]:

- Genital symptoms or atypical symptoms recur with negative HSV cultures
- There has been a clinical diagnosis of genital herpes without laboratory confirmation
- Patient has a known partner with genital herpes

HSV serologic testing should be considered in[3]:

- Persons with multiple sex partners who present for STI evaluation
- Persons with HIV infection
- MSM at increased risk for HIV acquisition

Symptoms
The average incubation period is 4 days for both HSV-1 and HSV-2, with a range of 2 to 12 days.[46]

Classic symptoms[3]:

- Macules and papules
- Vesicles, pustules, and painful ulcers
- Absent in many infected individuals

Many infected individuals have mild or unrecognized infections and shed the virus intermittently. Most are undiagnosed.[3]

Diagnosis
A patient's prognosis and the type of counseling needed depend on the type of genital herpes (HSV-1 or HSV-2) causing the infection. The clinical diagnosis and cytologic detection of cellular changes (ie, Tzanck preparation or Papanicolaou smears) of herpes are both nonsensitive and nonspecific.

Preferred HSV tests:

- For persons with genital ulcers or mucocutaneous lesions
  - Cell culture
  - Polymerase chain reaction
    - Test of choice for detecting HSV in spinal fluid

Management
Medications can be used episodically with outbreaks to decrease the duration of the outbreak.[3] Medications can also be used as suppressive therapy to decrease the frequency, duration, and severity of outbreaks in addition to reducing asymptomatic viral shedding.

First clinical episode:

- Acyclovir 400 mg PO TID × 7 to 10 days or
- Famciclovir 250 mg PO TID × 7 to 10 days or
- Valacyclovir 1 g PO BID × 7 to 10 days

Recurrence: effective treatment should begin within 1 day of lesion or during prodrome[3]

- Acyclovir 800 mg PO BID × 5 days or
- Famciclovir 1 g PO BID × 1 day or
- Valacyclovir 500 mg PO BID × 3 days

Suppressive therapy:

- Acyclovir 400 mg PO BID or
- Famciclovir 250 mg PO BID or
- Valacyclovir 500 mg or 1g PO daily

Adherence is better with once-daily dosing for all patients, in particular with teens.

Management should address the chronic nature of the disease and go beyond the treatment of acute episodes of genital ulcers.[3] Recurrences and subclinical shedding is much less for genital HSV-1 infections than for genital HSV-2 infections. Most persons with a first episode of genital HSV-2 are at risk for frequent recurrences over the next few years.[46]

Therefore, consider suppressive therapy initially for HSV-2 infections because it reduces the likelihood of symptomatic recurrence and the frequency of subclinical (asymptomatic) viral shedding, results in a better quality of life, is safe, and reduces the risk of transmission of HSV to uninfected partners.[3]

Human Immunodeficiency Virus

Organism/Transmission/Epidemiology
HIV is an RNA retrovirus.

Most HIV infections in the United States are caused by HIV-1. HIV-2 infections should be suspected in patients who have lived or whose sex partners have lived in endemic areas or areas of increasing HIV-2 infection (West Africa and Portugal), whose partners are positive for HIV-2, and those who have received blood transfusions in an endemic area.[3]

HIV is spread by

Sharing of certain bodily fluids
- Blood
- Semen
- Vaginal fluids
- Breast milk

Mainly through
- Sexual contact
- Exposure to contaminated blood
- Perinatal contact

Adolescents and young adults are at an increased risk for HIV infection.

- The estimated incidence of HIV in adolescents and young adults, 13 to 24 years of age, is 26% of the new infections
  - 80% of those infections occurring in males[47]
    - Comparing 2008 with 2010, the number of new HIV infections among MSM increased by 12%[47]

Screening

- CDC recommends HIV screening for patients, starting in adolescents 13 years and older in all health care settings.[3,48]
- Screening begins with sensitive screening tests:
  - Conventional enzyme immunoassay (EIA)
  - Rapid EIA

Symptoms

- Acute retroviral syndrome develops in 50% to 80% of acutely infected patients.[49,50]
  - Signs and symptoms include:
    - Fever
    - Malaise
    - Lymphadenopathy
    - Rash

- Initially or subsequent to the acute retroviral syndrome, some patients can remain asymptomatic for up to 15 years.

Diagnosis

- Serologic tests detect antibodies against HIV-1 and HIV-2[3]
  - Western blot
  - Indirect immunofluorescence assay
- Virologic tests detect HIV antigens or RNA
  - Can be used to identify acute infection in persons who are negative for HIV antibodies

Management

- Detailed management considerations are not within the scope of this article.[51]
- Important counseling points[3]:
  - Prompt initiation of medical care
  - The effectiveness of HIV treatments
  - What to expect on entering medical care for HIV infection

Special considerations
Assent/consent[52]

- Adolescents 13 years and older can assent to testing confidentially.
- Adolescents should be informed that testing will be performed.
- Adolescents may opt to decline or defer testing.
- Local laws and regulations may preclude routine opt-out testing.
    Further information is available through the National Clinicians Consultation Center (http://www.nccc.ucsf.edu).

Care and transitions to adult care

- Adolescents may take several months to accept their diagnosis and return for treatment owing to[53]:
  - Difficulty accepting their diagnosis
  - Lack of adequate support
  - Engagement in other risk behaviors
- With the evolution of HIV infection from a terminal to a chronic illness, transition of care can be challenging.
  - Models of transition protocols have been proposed.[53]

Postexposure prophylaxis[54]

- A prevention strategy for the use of antiretroviral drugs after a single high-risk event
- Designed to stop HIV from replicating
- Must be started as soon as possible to be effective, always within 72 hours of a possible exposure

Preexposure prophylaxis[55–58]

- A prevention strategy for people who are at high risk of contracting HIV
- Meant to be used
  - Consistently/daily
  - In conjunction with other prevention options

SUMMARY

STIs can have a significant impact on the health of sexually active young people. It is incumbent on medical providers who care for adolescents to be alert for both asymptomatic and symptomatic STIs. Anticipatory guidance, close adherence to screening guidelines, knowledge of presenting symptoms, and use of appropriate diagnostic testing can provide for timely and effective treatment of infections. In addition, the use of effective primary treatment regimens with timely follow-up is essential for adequate treatment and prevention of complications. The emotional impact of STI diagnosis on young persons and their relationships must also be acknowledged; effective empathy and counseling are essential aspects of education, diagnosis, and treatment.

REFERENCES

1. Sexually transmitted disease surveillance 2011. CDC Division of STD Prevention, 2012. Available at: http://www.cdc.gov/std/stats11/Surv2011.pdf. Accessed February 12, 2014.
2. Forhan SE, Gottlieb SL, Sternberg MR, et al. Prevalence of sexually transmitted infections among female adolescents aged 14 to 19 in the United States. Pediatrics 2009;124:1505–12.
3. Center for Disease Control and Prevention. Sexually transmitted diseases treatment guidelines. MMWR Morb Mortal Wkly Rep 2010;59:1–116.
4. Kirby D. Emerging answers 2007: research findings on programs to reduce teen pregnancy and sexually transmitted diseases. Washington, DC: National Campaign to Prevent Teen and Unplanned Pregnancy; 2007.
5. Golden MR, Whittington WL, Handsfield HH, et al. Effect of expedited treatment of sex partners on recurrent or persistent gonorrhea or chlamydial infection. N Engl J Med 2005;352:676–85.
6. Kissinger P, Hogbon M. Expedited partner treatment for sexually transmitted infections: an update. Curr Infect Dis Rep 2011;13:188–95.
7. American Academy of Family Practitioners (AAFP), 2012. Expedited Partner Therapy. Available at: http://www.aafp.org/about/policies/all/partner-therapy.html. Accessed February 18, 2014.
8. American Academy of Pediatrics. Statement of endorsement—expedited partner therapy for adolescents diagnosed with chlamydia or gonorrhea. Pediatrics 2009;124:1264.
9. Opinion 8.07 - Expedited partner therapy. American Medical Association. 2008. Available at: http://www.ama-assn.org//ama/pub/physician-resources/medical-ethics/codemedical-ethics/opinion807.page. Accessed February 18, 2014.
10. Burstein GR, Eliscu A, Ford K, et al. Expedited partner therapy for adolescents diagnosed with chlamydia or gonorrhea: a position paper of the Society for Adolescent Medicine. J Adolesc Health 2009;45:303–9.
11. Expedited partner therapy in the management of gonorrhea and chlamydia by obstetrician-gynecologists. American College of Obstetricians and Gynecologists (ACOG), 2011. Available at: https://www.acog.org/Resources_And_Publications/Committee_Opinions/Committee_on_Adolescent_Health_Care/Expedited_Partner_Therapy_in_the_Management_of_Gonorrhea_and_Chlamydia_by_Obstetrician-Gynecologists. Accessed February 18, 2014.
12. Legal status of expedited partner therapy (EPT). Center for Disease Control, 2014. Available at: http://www.cdc.gov/sTd/ept/legal/default.htm. Accessed February 18, 2014.

13. Martinez G, Copen C, Agma J. Teenagers in the United Sates: sexual activity, contraceptive use, and childbearing, 2006-2010 National Survey of Family Growth. Vital Health Stat 23 2011;(31):1–35.
14. Matson PA, Adler NE, Millstein SG, et al. Developmental changes in condom use among urban adolescent females: influence of partner context. J Adolesc Health 2011;48:386–90.
15. Ford CA. Partnerships between parents and health care professionals to improve adolescent health. J Adolesc Health 2011;49:53–7.
16. Weiss H, Thomas S, Munabi S, et al. Male circumcision and risk of syphilis, chancroid, and genital herpes: a systematic review and meta-analysis. Sexually transmitted infections 2006;82:101–10.
17. Auvert B, Taljaard D, Lagarde E, et al. Randomized, controlled intervention trial of male circumcision for reduction of HIV infection risk: the ANRS 1265 Trial. PLoS Med 2005;2:e298.
18. Gray RH, Kigozi G, Serwadda D, et al. Male circumcision for HIV prevention in men in Rakai, Uganda: a randomised trial. Lancet 2007;369:657–66.
19. Bailey RC, Moses S, Parker CB, et al. Male circumcision for HIV prevention in young men in Kisumu, Kenya: a randomised controlled trial. Lancet 2007;369:643–56.
20. Millett GA, Flores SA, Marks G, et al. Circumcision status and risk of HIV and sexually transmitted infections among men who have sex with men: a meta-analysis. JAMA 2008;300:1674–84.
21. Smith DK, Taylor A, Kilmarx PH, et al. Male circumcision in the United States for the prevention of HIV infection and other adverse health outcomes: report from a CDC consultation. Public Health Rep 2010;125:72.
22. Blank S, Brady M, Buerk E, et al. Circumcision policy statement. Pediatrics 2012;130:585–6.
23. Coyne KM, Barton SE. Epidemiology of sexually transmitted infections. Expert Rev Obstet Gynecol 2007;2:803–16.
24. Risser WL, Bortot AT, Benjamins LJ, et al. The epidemiology of sexually transmitted infections in adolescents. Semin Pediatr Infect Dis 2005;16:160–7.
25. Chernesky MA, Hook EW III, Martin DH, et al. Women find it easy and prefer to collect their own vaginal swabs to diagnose *Chlamydia trachomatis* or *Neisseria gonorrhoeae* infections. Sex Transm Dis 2005;32:729–33.
26. Schachter J, Chernesky MA, Willis DE, et al. Vaginal swabs are the specimens of choice when screening for *Chlamydia trachomatis* and *Neisseria gonorrhoeae*: results from a multicenter evaluation of the APTIMA assays for both infections. Sex Transm Dis 2005;32:725–8.
27. Association of Public Health Laboratories. Laboratory diagnostic testing for *Chlamydia trachomatis* and *Neisseria gonorrhoeae*. Report: Expert Consultation Meeting Summary. 2009.
28. Schachter J. Nucleic acid amplification tests in the diagnosis of chlamydial and gonococcal infections of the oropharynx and rectum in men who have sex with men. Sex Transm Dis 2008;35:637–42.
29. Gewirtzman A, Bobrick L, Conner K, et al. Epidemiology of sexually transmitted infections. In: Gross G, Tyring S, editors. Sexually transmitted infections and sexually transmitted diseases. Houston (TX): Springer; 2011. p. 13–34.
30. Center for Disease Control and Prevention. Update to CDC's sexually transmitted diseases treatment guidelines, 2010; oral cephalosporins no longer a recommended treatment for gonococcal infections. MMWR Morb Mortal Wkly Rep 2012;61:590–4.

31. Center for Disease Control and Prevention (CDC). Report: Sexually transmitted disease surveillance 2004 supplement: Gonococcal Isolate Surveillance Project (GISP) annual report - 2004. In: US Department of Health and Human Services, editor. Atlanta (GA): CDC; 2005. p. 1–31.
32. Center for Disease Control and Prevention (CDC). Report: Sexually transmitted disease surveillance 2007 supplement, Gonococcal Isolate Surveillance Project (GISP) annual report 2007. In: US Department of Health and Human Services, editor. Atlanta (GA): Center for Disease Control and Prevention; 2009. p. 1–120.
33. Hicks CB, Sparling PF. Pathogenesis, clinical manifestations, and treatment of early syphilis. In: Basow D, editor. UpToDate. Waltham (MA): UpToDate; 2013.
34. Marra CM. Neurosyphilis. In: Basow D, editor. UpToDate. Waltham (MA): UpToDate; 2013.
35. Flood JM, Weinstock HS, Guroy ME, et al. Neurosyphilis during the AIDS epidemic, San Francisco, 1985–1992. J Infect Dis 1998;177:931–40.
36. Sparling PF, Hicks CB. Pathogenesis, clinical manifestations, and treatment of late syphilis. In: Basow D, editor. UpToDate. Waltham (MA): UpToDate; 2013.
37. Greenblatt RM, Lukehart SA, Plummer FA, et al. Genital ulceration as a risk factor for human immunodeficiency virus infection. AIDS 1988;2:47–50.
38. Cameron DW, D'Costa L, Maitha G, et al. Female to male transmission of human immunodeficiency virus type 1: risk factors for seroconversion in men. Lancet 1989;334:403–7.
39. Buchacz K, Patel P, Taylor M, et al. Syphilis increases HIV viral load and decreases CD4 cell counts in HIV-infected patients with new syphilis infections. AIDS 2004;18:2075–9.
40. Huppert JS, Mortensen JE, Reed JL, et al. Rapid antigen testing compares favorably with transcription-mediated amplification assay for the detection of Trichomonas vaginalis in young women. Clin Infect Dis 2007;45:194-8.
41. Moscicki AB. The natural history of human papillomavirus infection as measured by repeated DNA testing in adolescent and young women. J Pediatr 1998;132:277–84.
42. Moscicki AB. Human papillomavirus disease and vaccines in adolescents. Adolesc Med 2010;21:347–63, x–xi.
43. ACOG Committee on Practice Bulletins–Gynecology. ACOG practice bulletin no. 109: cervical cytology screening. Obstet Gynecol 2009;114:1409–20.
44. Massad LS, Einstein MH, Huh WK, et al. 2012 updated consensus guidelines for the management of abnormal cervical cancer screening tests and cancer precursors. J Low Genit Tract Dis 2013;17:S1–27.
45. Center for Disease Control and Prevention. FDA licensure of quadrivalent human papillomavirus vaccine (hpv4, gardasil) for use in males and guidance from the Advisory Committee on Immunization Practices (ACIP). MMWR Morb Mortal Wkly Rep 2010;59:630–2.
46. Kimberlin DW, Rouse DJ. Genital herpes. N Engl J Med 2004;350:1970–7.
47. Center for Disease Control and Prevention. Estimated HIV incidence in the United States, 2007-2010. HIV Surveillance Supplemental Report. 2012. Available at: http://www.cdc.gov/hiv/pdf/statistics_hssr_vol_17_no_4.pdf. Accessed February 21, 2014.
48. Center for Disease Control and Prevention. Revised recommendations for HIV testing of adults, adolescents, and pregnant women in health-care settings. MMWR 2006;55:1–17.
49. Kahn JO, Walker BD. Acute human immunodeficiency virus type 1 infection. N Engl J Med 1998;339:33–9.

50. Kassutto S, Rosenberg ES. Primary HIV type 1 infection. Clin Infect Dis 2004;38: 1447–53.
51. Aber JA, Kaplan JE, Libman H, et al. Primary care guidelines for the management of persons infected with human immunodeficiency virus: 2009 update by the HIV medicine Association of the Infectious Diseases Society of America. Clin Infect Dis 2009;49:651–81.
52. Centers for Disease Control and Prevention. Persons tested for HIV–United States, 2006. MMWR Morb Mortal Wkly Rep 2008;57:845–9.
53. Maturo D, Powell A, Major-Wilson H, et al. Development of a protocol for transitioning adolescents with HIV infection to adult care. J Pediatr Health Care 2011; 25:16–23.
54. Smith DK. Antiretroviral postexposure prophylaxis after sexual, injection-drug use, or other nonoccupational exposure to HIV in the United States: recommendations from the US Department of Health and Human Services. MMWR Recomm Rep 2005;54:1.
55. Grant RM. Preexposure chemoprophylaxis for HIV prevention in men who have sex with men. N Engl J Med 2010;363:2587–99.
56. Choopanya K, Martin M, Suntharasamai P, et al. Antiretroviral prophylaxis for HIV infection in injecting drug users in Bangkok, Thailand (the Bangkok Tenofovir Study): a randomised, double-blind, placebo-controlled phase 3 trial. Lancet 2013;381:2083–90.
57. Baeten J, Celum C. Antiretroviral pre-exposure prophylaxis for HIV-1 prevention among heterosexual African men and women: the Partners PrEP Study. 6th IAS Conference on HIV Pathogenesis, Treatment and Prevention. Rome, July 17-20, 2011.
58. Thigpen M, Kebaabetswe P, Smith D, et al. Daily oral antiretroviral use for the prevention of HIV infection in heterosexually active young adults in Botswana: results from the TDF2 study. 6th IAS Conference on HIV Pathogenesis, Treatment and Prevention. Rome, July 17-20, 2011.

Sexual Minority Youth

John Steever, MD*, Jenny Francis, MD,
Lonna P. Gordon, MD, PharmD, Janet Lee, MD

KEYWORDS

- LGBT or GLBT youth • Sexual minority youth • Adolescent sexuality
- Adolescent mental health • Transgender youth
- Lesbian, gay, bisexual, and transgender youth • Homophobia • Health disparities

KEY POINTS

- Lesbian, gay, bisexual, and transgender (LGBT) youth are a diverse population that faces a unique set of challenges to their health and well-being.
- Medical personnel need to be culturally sensitive to these youth in order to provide high-quality medical and mental health care.
- Sexual minority youth are at a higher risk for depression, family rejection, sexually transmitted infection acquisition, poor school performance, substance use, and other threats to physical health.
- Homophobia and minority stress status are the main threats to LGBT youth mental health.
- Providers caring for sexual minority youth should not make assumptions about behaviors and risks based only on youth stated sexual or gender orientation.
- Despite challenges to their mental and physical health, most LGBT youth are able to overcome these challenges and lead rich and productive lives.

INTRODUCTION

Lesbian, gay, bisexual, and transgender (LGBT) individuals have been present in human society as far back as recorded history.[1–3] References to same-sex relationships can be found on ancient Japanese and Chinese pottery. Ancient Greek artwork often depicts same sex couples. Certain cultures acknowledge the presence of a *third gender*, or transgendered individuals, in their histories. Several Native American tribes use the term *Two Spirited* to refer to individuals whose gender identity does not match their physical body.[4]

Disclosures: None.
Department of Pediatrics, Mount Sinai Adolescent Health Center, Icahn School of Medicine at Mount Sinai, Second Floor, 312-320 East 94th Street, New York, NY 10128, USA
* Corresponding author.
E-mail address: john.steever@mountsinai.org

LGBT TERMINOLOGY

Sexual orientation refers to an individual's pattern of emotional and physical attraction to others (**Tables 1–3**). *Homosexuality*, commonly known as *gay*, refers to a persistent sexual and emotional attraction to members of one's own gender. *Gay* can be an umbrella term for both homosexual men and women, but the term *lesbian* refers to women only. *Bisexuals* represent those individuals attracted to both men and women in varying degrees. The term *LGBT* refers to lesbian, gay, bisexual, and transgender. Sometimes a *Q* is added to represent either *questioning* or *queer*. The term *sexual minority youth* (SMY) is an alternative to LGBT and includes those that decline categorization. The term *queer*, previously a derogatory term, refers to both sexual

Table 1
Common terms used to describe LGBTQ youth

Term	Definition
Sexual minority	Lesbian, gay, bisexual, transgender, questioning, queer
Sexual orientation	An individual's pattern of emotional attractions to others that involve complex components of fantasies, feelings, and cultural affiliations
Gender identity	Inner knowledge of being male or female, usually established by the time an individual is aged 3 to 4 y
Gender role	Outward expression of maleness or femaleness
Gender variance	Behavioral pattern not typical of one's assigned gender based on biological sex
Lesbian	Female who identifies her primary sexual and loving attachments as being predominantly female
Gay male	Male who identifies his primary sexual and loving attachments as being predominantly male
Bisexual	Female or male who identifies her or his primary sexual and loving attachments as being with both sexes
Homosexual	An individual whose patterns of sexual and emotional arousal are toward members of the same sex (eg, gay, lesbian)
Heterosexual	An individual whose pattern of sexual and emotional arousal is toward members of the opposite sex (eg, straight)
Heterosexism	The societal construct that equates heterosexuality as the expected normal
Transgender male	An individual, born female, whose internal gender identity is male
Transgender female	An individual, born male, whose internal gender identity is female
Transvestite	An individual who derives sexual pleasure or comfort from dressing in clothing of the opposite sex; behavior often independent of the individual's sexual orientation
MTF	Male to female, also called transfemale
FTM	Female to male, also called transmale
WSW	A female who has sexual contact with other females, whether or not she identifies as lesbian or has sexual contact with males
MSM	A male who has sexual contact with other males, whether or not he identifies as gay or has sexual contact with females
Butch	Masculine in appearance and manner
Femme	Feminine in appearance and manner
Queer	Originally derogatory, now reclaimed to describe individuals who reject mainstream cultural norms of sexuality and gender

Table 2
Routine care for adolescent well visits, including LGBTQ items

Health Care Maintenance	Items to Address (All Youth)	Special Focus for LGBT Youth
Physical growth and development	Physical and oral health, body image, healthy eating, physical activity	Eating habits, weight perceptions, and supplements
Risk reduction	Tobacco, alcohol, other drugs; pregnancy; STIs (annual urine for GC/CT and rapid HIV test)	Anal GC/CT swabs and oral GC swabs as indicated per risk behavior; focus on substance use; condom use
Emotional well-being	Coping, mood regulation and mental health, sexuality	Depression, strength building, suicide risk
Violence and injury prevention	Safety belt, helmet use, substance abuse and riding in vehicle, guns, interpersonal violence, bullying	Assess for victims of homophobia, heterosexism, transphobia; asses for bullying
Social and academic competence	Connectedness with family, peers, community, interpersonal relationships, school performance	Assess for victims of abuse, school failure/future plans; family connection, disclosure status with family and friends; connections with peer group
Vaccines	Tdap, MCV4, HPV, annual flu	Hep A, B series; HPV meningococcal vaccine
Vision	Once in early, mid, and late adolescence	Same
Selective screening	If risk factors: hearing, anemia (CBC), TB (PPD), dyslipidemia (lipid screen), pregnancy (urine hCG), cervical dysplasia (once at 21 y of age), STI (screen annual CT and GC, and HIV/RPR if risky)	May screen for STI every 6 mo if high-risk behavior

Abbreviations: CBC, complete blood count; GC/CT, gonorrhea/chlamydia swabs and oral gonorrhea swabs; hCG, human chorionic gonadotropin; Hep, hepatitis; HIV, human immunodeficiency virus; HPV, human papillomavirus; MCV4, meningococcal conjugate vaccine 4; PPD, purified protein derivative; RPR, rapid plasma reagin test; STI, sexually transmitted infection; TB, tuberculosis; Tdap, tetanus toxoid, reduced diphtheria toxoid, and acellular pertussis vaccine.

orientation and/or gender identity.[5] Finally, many youth may not identify with any one term but instead prefer the use of *questioning* or the use of multiple identities for themselves.[6]

Homophobia refers to an irrational fear, prejudice, and hatred of gay individuals.[7] *Heterosexism* denotes the belief that heterosexuality is a superior orientation and fails to value alternative sexual identities.[8] *Men who have sex with men* (MSM) and *women who have sex with women* (WSW) reflect research terms and refer to sexual behavior, not sexual orientation.

Gender identity refers to the knowledge of oneself as male or female. *Transgender*, an overall term, references those individuals who feel that their internal gender identity does not match their natal gender assignment (their biologic sex at birth). *Transgender* is more encompassing and has replaced the term *transsexual*. *Transgender* includes other terms, such as *gender nonconforming*, *gender queer*, *bigendered*, and other

Table 3	
LGBT focused HEADSS	
Home	• Who do you live with? • How out are you and to which family members? • Does your family accept your sexual and gender orientation? • Do you feel supported or rejected by family/friends? • Do you feel safe at home? • Assess risk of homelessness
Education	• Are you in school and at an appropriate grade level? • What are your future plans for education? • Do you feel safe at school? Have you missed school days because of safety concerns? • Are you supported at school by teachers, peers, and/or staff? • Is there a presence of the Gay-Straight Alliance or coming out groups? • Is there bullying at school?
Activities	• What activities do you do for fun? • Who are your peers? Are they the same age or older? Is there a LGBT peer group? • Are you working? What are your future work plans? • What sports or hobbies are you interested in? Investigate strengths of the youth.
Drugs	• Do you use tobacco? How much do you use? Have you attempted to quit? • Do you use alcohol? How much do you use? Does the youth meet the criteria for binge drinking? Does the youth drink with a peer group or with older people? • Do you use marijuana? How much do you use? • Do you use cocaine, crystal methamphetamines, amyl nitrite? • Do you use other substances? Do you use club drugs? Do you attend raves? • What are the circumstances of use? When and why do you use substances? • Do you have blackouts or loss of consciousness? • Do you want help to cut down or quit?
Sex	Natal males • Do you have sexual attractions? Do you have crushes? Are you dating? • What are your sexual activities? Ask about specific behaviors. • What is the age of your partners? What is your partners' HIV status? • Do you use condoms? Are there STI risks? HIV risk factors • Are you aware of HIV postexposure prophylaxis? • Do you use substances before sex? • STI testing based on risk behaviors Natal females • Do you have sexual attractions? Do you have crushes? Are you dating? • What are your sexual activities? Ask about specific behaviors. • Is there a risk of pregnancy? Are you aware of emergency contraception? • Are you aware of the risks of STD? Do you use condoms? • Are you aware of HIV postexposure prophylaxis? • Do you use dental dams and finger cots? • Do you use substances before sex? • STI testing based on risk behaviors
Suicide	• Are there depression, sadness, or self-injury behaviors? • Have there been prior suicide attempts? Current ideation • Are there mental health resources/support? • Is there support from family and friends? • Is there support at school?

Abbreviations: HEADSS, Home, Education, Activities, Drugs, Sex and Suicide; HIV, human immuno-deficiency virus; STD, sexually transmitted disease; STI, sexually transmitted infection.

transidentities that reject the traditional binary description of gender identity. Even though multiple terms can describe a transgendered person, using the simplest explanation to describe the transgender individual often works best for clinicians. For example, the terms *female-to-male* and *male-to-female* easily describe the individual and provide information about them. Other terms may include *transman* for an individual who desires to transition to a male gender. *Transwoman* describes an individual who desires to transition to a female gender. These terms regarding gender identity should not convey information about sexual orientation, surgical status, or the use of hormones. The adjective *cis-gendered* refers to someone whose gender identity reflects his or her natal sex assignment. Gender dysphoria is the discontent/anxiety felt when a person does not agree with his or her assigned gender.

SEXUALITY CONSTRUCTS

Several independent domains seem to compose an individual's overall sexual identity. The primary domains include sexual orientation, sexual behavior, gender identity and expression, biological sex, relationships, and sexual attraction (**Fig. 1**). Although the tendency is to think of each domain as a binary variable (eg, gay or straight), the reality is that sexuality exists as a continuum with variable states. Kinsey,[9] the first investigator to describe sexual orientation as a fluid state, also reported that sexual behavior does not predict sexual orientation.[9] No matter how a teen *currently* self-identifies,

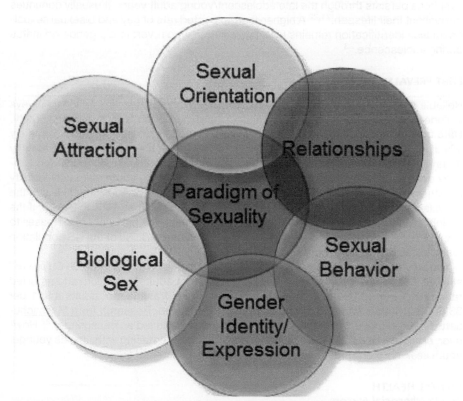

Fig. 1. Domains that compose an individual's overall sexual identity. (*From* Physicians for Reproductive Health. Available at: http://prh.org/teen-reproductive-health/arshep-downloads/. Accessed December 27, 2013.)

their identity may change throughout adolescence.[10,11] Consequently, sexual identities and behaviors, the 2 most fluid constructs, should be assessed regularly; based on the youth's sexual behavior, proper screening questions and tests should follow. Assumptions about behavior based on gender identity or sexual orientation should be avoided.

CAUSE OF SEXUAL ORIENTATION AND GENDER IDENTITY

How an individual's personal experience specifically influences his or her sexuality remains unclear.[12] Sexual orientation and gender identity do *not* reflect a choice by an individual.[13,14] Instead, domains of sexuality likely reflect the impact made by a combination of genetics, environment, and personal experiences.[2,4,12,13] Gender identity develops from a child's cognitions and emotions rather than genitalia and other external sex characteristics and is usually established between 3 to 4 years of age.[4,15,16] Awareness of sexual orientation occurs later in a child's life, often occurring between 9 and 10 years of age.[17] Self-identification (to come out) as lesbian or gay usually happens around 16 years of age.[18–20] Sexual *behavior*, unlike orientation or gender identity, may be influenced by multiple factors, including parenting, previous sexual experience, child physical or sexual abuse, and other life circumstances.

Many young children who have dysphoria regarding their gender identity will spontaneously resolve their gender variant concerns at puberty.[21] However, if gender dysphoria persists through the late adolescent/young adult years, it usually continues throughout their lifespan.[21,22] A higher-than-expected rate of gay and bisexual sexual-orientation identification remains for those children who revert to cis-gendered status during adolescence.[23]

LGBT PREVALENCE

Reliable data on the prevalence of LGBT youth remain sparse. Few national surveys include questions about sexual orientation, and none ask about gender identity. Data from almost 35,000 Minnesotan high school students report that approximately 1% of 9th to 12th graders identify predominately as gay or bisexual[24] and 10% identify as un-sure.[24] As these youth mature, their uncertainty about sexual orientation typically decreases with increasing maturity.[24] Most, but not all, youth ultimately identify as either straight or gay. In the National Longitudinal Survey of Adolescent Health, the prevalence for those with same-sex attraction ranges as high as 14% to 21%.[10] If the definition only focuses on behavior, or same-sex contact, the prevalence decreases to 2% to 7%.[10] From analysis of adult surveys, approximately 3.5% of the US population identifies as gay or lesbian.[25]

The prevalence of transgender individuals is more difficult to evaluate. De Cuypere[26] studied the prevalence of male-to-female transgender adults in Belgium and reported ranges of 1 per 12,000 individuals for male-to-female transgender adults and 1 per 33,800 individuals for female-to-male transgender adults. Research from Massachusetts reported that 0.5% of the surveyed population identified as transgender.[27] However, estimates of transgender prevalence seem to be increasing with time as younger youth seek care and treatment of gender identity dysphoria.[14,28]

MENTAL HEALTH
The Psychosocial Factors

The developmental phases for LGBT adolescents are essentially the same as heterosexual youth. However, LGBT youth also hold the additional tasks of realization, acceptance of their identity, and determination of when and how to disclose this information to others.[29–32] Accomplishing this task often requires confronting challenges posed by homophobia in society as well as pervasive and subtle heterosexism. Alternative gender and sexual identities should not be considered a mental disorder that requires reparative therapy, the discredited theory that sexual orientation is alterable through intense psychotherapy.[29,32]

The concept known as *minority stress* describes a cumulative burden of being reminded that one is different from the majority.[33–35] Minority stress can be caused by external sources, such as being targeted or victimized by others (ie, external homophobia), and also by internal stressors, such as a sense of not fitting in or shame (internalized homophobia). This minority stress can be felt in youth who have not yet acted on or disclosed their same-sex attraction.[36] An initial response to a homophobic society may be to conceal one's sexual identity, leading to what psychologists call a "divided self."[37,38] Concealment over time, however, creates psychological distress.[37] Minority stress and divided self are thought to be the mechanisms mediating the increased vulnerability of LGBT youth to mental health concerns. Through a strengths-based approach, clinicians can play a key role in supporting the adolescent in this process.[33] These concepts apply to both gay/lesbian youth as well as gender variant youth.

Coming Out

Coming out, or disclosure of one's sexual orientation or gender identity, can become an emotionally charged experience. LGBT youth experience an immense amount of anxiety around the timing and mechanism of disclosure. If disclosure goes well and they receive support, coming out decreases the risk of depression, suicide, and illicit drug use and improves resilience.[39] Disclosures that go poorly can lead to social isolation, homelessness, and increased stigma.[40] Regardless of outcome, disclosures can eliminate the divided self, thus leaving a positive impact on mental health.[37] The coming out milestone is another opportunity for the primary care provider to provide support to LGBT youth. Clinicians can counsel youth around the timing and circumstances of the disclosure. Additionally, by presenting themselves as a supportive resource for both youth and families, the provider can give LGBT youth a feeling of security around disclosure.[41]

The biggest fears surrounding disclosure include rejection and possibly disappointing parents or other influential adults.[38] LGBT youth often disclose in a pattern: first to a close peer, followed by a sibling, and finally a parent.[38,42,43] This pattern follows a least threatening to most threatening progression in case rejection occurs as an outcome.[43] Siblings often become the first test to see how the family may react to disclosure. A positive response speeds up the decision to disclose to parents.[43] Usually the mother, deliberately chosen as the first parent, is made aware directly by the youth. Fathers subsequently become an accidental disclosure.[38] Although teens typically view coming out in the context of how it impacts their immediate well-being, evidence suggests the process is formative for future romantic attachments beyond adolescence.[35,40]

The Environmental Factors

The social environment that a youth engages with predicts the ability to thrive despite challenging circumstances. This concept is known as resilience. Even though the impact of family relationships on resilience entails a complex interplay, the overall impact becomes protective.[32] Family relationships with parental closeness and high levels of parental involvement often result in decreased depressive symptoms. Youth in these protective family situations also display higher self-confidence and handle rejection and stigma better.[36,44] Importantly, these factors become protective even if a youth has chosen not to come out yet to the family.[30,36,44]

A combination of poor family support and mental health threats can create a unique set of circumstances in vulnerable youth. Up to 40% percent of homeless youth are LGBT teens.[45] Homelessness places youth at an increased risk for sexual exploitation and risky sexual practices.[33] Others may experience abuse and neglect at the hands of their family members and then become involved with child welfare systems. Gender-nonconforming youth experience problems when placed in group homes based on their genetic sex and not their gender identity.[46] Laws such as the newly enacted California Assembly Bill 1266, allowing students to participate in gender-segregated activities based on their gender identity rather than genetic sex, are a step toward resolving these challenges.[47]

Peers, another component of a youth's environment, play an important role in dealing with minority stress by providing a sense of belonging. LGBT youth who lack a consistent peer group often become bullied in higher proportions, display higher rates of suicide, and use substances more frequently.[33] The lack of same-age peer groups is associated with increased rates of human immunodeficiency virus (HIV) in racial minority groups because of a higher prevalence of older partners.[46,48]

Gender Variant Youth

The experience of minority stress is amplified in transgender youth in comparison with LGB youth because their nonconforming gender expression frequently occurs at a younger age. Transgendered youth experience an increased risk for life stressors, including incarceration, homelessness, commercial sex work, sexual coercion, and difficulties finding a job.[49] In transgender youth, alcohol and marijuana are the most commonly used substances.[49] Transgender youth also display high rates of depression and life-threatening behaviors.[49] Research is underway to evaluate the influences of a supportive family and social environment on transgender youth mental health. By analogy to work done with LGB youth, it is expected that emotionally supported transgender youth will experience less mental health issues than those who are not supported.

MEDICAL PRIMARY CARE

Research shows that SMYs value the same qualities that signify competence to all adolescents seeking health care[50]:

- Clean environment
- Informative, attentive clinician
- Respectful exchanges with clinic staff

When surveyed, youth report they often do not feel safe disclosing their same sex attractions or activities unless broached first by the clinician. This point holds especially true for adolescents who engage in sexual activity with the same gender but who may not publicly identify as gay or lesbian.[51]

Having LGBT-oriented educational materials readily available makes discussing sexuality easier for patients. When asked what a physician could do to help LGBT clients be more comfortable, 64% of participants responded with "Just ask me."[51] The presence of LGBT symbols (eg, the rainbow flag) in the waiting room and offices is reassuring to youth.[52] Further, having private unisex bathrooms, well-trained staff who use nondiscriminatory language consistently, and private triage areas leaves patients feeling more comfortable to disclose their sexual attractions and behaviors to clinicians.[52,53] Intake forms should reflect a greater diversity in options regarding gender and relationship status.[52] Medical confidentiality, a cornerstone of effective adolescent health care, becomes especially important for primary care providers dealing with LGBT youth.[53] Teens should be reminded in every encounter that their personal information will never be shared except in life-threatening circumstances.[50] In some communities, a medical clinic may be the only place that adheres to these messages of respect.[54] If a provider feels inexperienced or uncomfortable with the LGBT community, then referral to another provider may be warranted.[52]

Health Maintenance

The general health maintenance recommendations as noted in guidelines, such as Guidelines for Adolescent Preventative Services (GAPS) and Bright Futures, does not differ much between SMYs and heterosexual youth.[55] The clinician must address the usual components of an adolescent well visit but must also evaluate LGBT patients through the lens of known health risks that these youth face.

The medical history should use language congruent with the cognitive development of patients. Clinicians can demonstrate their comfort with discussing same-sex attraction and behavior by using straightforward language that is inclusive and sensitive.[52] The review of systems should not omit questions on the genital-urinary system. The discussion of sexual behaviors should drive investigations about medical testing. For example, ask about anorectal symptoms in youth who engage in receptive, anal intercourse, and then offer appropriate testing for disease. Clinicians should also inquire about hobbies and other interests, as it is important to approach all youth through their strengths and not simply see them as high-risk patients.[56]

Body Image

Lesbian and bisexual girls are more content with their bodies and less likely to report trying to look like images of women in the media than their heterosexual counterparts.[57] In contrast, gay and bisexual boys were more likely than their heterosexual peers to report trying to look like men in the media.[38]

Young gay males have a higher risk for weight misperception and unhealthy weight control behaviors.[58] Gay males are more likely to use steroids to alter their body appearance in pursuit of a muscular ideal.[58,59] Bisexual- and heterosexual-identified males with same-sex experiences perceive themselves as overweight despite being normal or underweight. Youth risk behavior survey (YRBS) data from Vermont showed that 25.6% of youth reporting bisexual behaviors also reported unhealthy weight-control practices compared with 12.3% of those reporting homosexual practices versus 7.1% of those reporting heterosexual practices. Inquiring about body image, disordered eating, and exercise behaviors becomes paramount during the interview.

Lesbians, in contrast, often perceive themselves at a healthy weight or underweight despite being overweight or obese. When compared with their sisters, lesbians tend to have higher body mass indices and exercise fewer times per week.[60] Furthermore, unhealthy weight-control behaviors (fasting >24 hours, using diet pills and vomiting or using laxatives) became significantly more prevalent among sexual minority females (35%) relative to exclusively heterosexual females (18%).[61] Adult weight-control issues often start in the adolescent years.

Emotional Well-Being

As noted before, clinicians must question sexual minority adolescents about depressive symptoms and suicidal ideation. Those who experience victimization are 2.6

times more likely to report depression and 5.6 times more likely to attempt suicide than those who do not experience victimization. More than 66% of LGBT youth experience verbal abuse from their parents or peers, and 20% to 33% experienced physical abuse.[62] Providers should also understand that current practice acknowledges reparative therapy as inappropriate and psychologically damaging.[32,33] Therapies to adjust a gender identity, gender expression, or sexual orientation only serve to suppress an authentic sexual identity and cause real psychological symptoms.[32] Familiarity with outreach agencies and hotlines can connect at-risk youth with positive role models.[35]

Academic Concerns

School, another component of the social environment, becomes a potential source of stress.[63,64] Alarmingly, 33% of adolescents report that students within their school feel harassed because of their perceived sexual orientation.[33,64] Students who identify or are perceived as LGBT remain more likely to be threatened or injured with a weapon at school.[64] They also skip school because of safety reasons, thus starting a dangerous trajectory of poor academic performance.[65] They also tend to make lower grades in school and perceive their teachers to be less supportive, increasing rates of high school dropouts.[65] Those schools that have policies to not tolerate bullying and minimize heterosexist practices through gay-straight alliances stand protective.[64]

Substance Use

The clinician should inquire about specific substances, including amphetamines, cocaine, and alky nitriles (poppers), when obtaining a history from LGBT youth.[66] Many LGBT youth use drugs, often leading to high-risk sexual behaviors, which can then lead to an increase in transmission of sexually transmitted infections (STIs), including HIV.[66] LGBT youth tend to initiate substances at younger ages and rapidly increase their use over time. They use cigarettes at higher rates and consume alcohol in increased quantities than their heterosexual peers.[14,67] Lesbian and bisexual young women are more than 5 times as likely to use substances than their heterosexual counterparts.[46,68] Tobacco use in MSM remains higher than other LGBT youth.[69]

Violence and Injury Prevention

Bullying, a problem within the general adolescent population, also plays a particularly important role when working with LGBT youth. Clinicians should inquire about bullying and help to coordinate care for additional support.[57] Bullying can occur at home, with peers, and at school.[65] Verbal and physical harassment should be discussed and safety plans made if youth are found to be the target of bullying.

GAY AND BISEXUAL MEN'S SEXUAL HEALTH

Screening for STIs in asymptomatic young men who have sex with men should be based on the recommendations as described in the Morbidity and Mortality Weekly Report (MMWR). These recommendations are based on behavior (men who have sex with men) and not simply sexual orientation (eg, gay). The most common sexual practices in MSM are oral sex and digital (finger) stimulation of the partner's penis and anus, and many, but not all, MSM report experience with penile-anal intercourse as well. Clinicians should also routinely ask sexually active MSM about symptoms consistent with STIs. These include oral, penile and rectal/anal symptomatology.

Common STI symptoms may include penile discharge, sores, rashes, inguinal lymphadenopathy and pain with urination or defecation. Unusual systemic symptoms such as fevers, chills, and body aches should be investigated.[70]

Providers should tailor STI screening to the specific sexual behavior that an MSM patient participates in. If patients participate in receptive oral sex, they can be at risk for contracting pharyngeal STIs, such as gonorrhea or syphilis. If one performs the insertive role during anal intercourse, gonorrhea and Chlamydia screening can be completed by performing a urine nucleic acid amplification test (NAAT) or a urethral NAAT swab.[71] If an individual participates in the receptive role, rectal culture swabs should be performed for the same pathogens.[70] Gonorrhea and Chlamydia are often asymptomatic in the rectal and pharyngeal reservoirs.[72] NAATs can only be used on genital sites; laboratories may only process non–genital site NAATs if they have met all regulatory requirements for an off-label procedure.[70,72]

Oral-anal sex (rimming) can put young gay men at risk for acquiring an enteric pathogen. This infection has the potential to cause proctocolitis or symptoms of diarrhea, abdominal cramps, and inflammation of the rectal mucosa. In healthy patients, Giardia is the most commonly implicated organism; but other enteric pathogens, such as Salmonella and Shigella, should be considered.[70] Hepatitis A can also be spread via oral-anal contact. Saliva is sometimes used as a lubricant during anal intercourse, which can transmit salivary pathogens, such as cytomegalovirus, hepatitis A and B virus, and herpes simplex virus (HSV).[73]

It is important to remember that receptive anal sex is associated with a higher risk of HIV transmission than vaginal intercourse.[74] Seroadaptive behavior has been described in MSM. With seroadaptive behavior, 2 sexual partners of the same HIV status agree to have unprotected sex with each other but not others of a different HIV status.[23] Providers should encourage their HIV-positive gay male patients to disclose their status to their partners and strongly encourage condom use. Education regarding pre-HIV and post-HIV exposure prophylaxis should be provided. HIV acquisition rates in youth aged 13 to 24 years are the second highest age group after 25- to 34-year-old men.[75] There are also concerns about syphilis coinfection accelerating HIV-associated immunosuppression.[76,77]

HSV type 2 is also more common in the MSM population and can facilitate HIV transmission.[78] Frequent screening should be recommended to individuals with multiple sexual partners; those who participate in anonymous sex; and those who abuse substances, such as amphetamines, when engaging in intercourse.[70] Hepatitis C, although often thought of as a blood-borne pathogen, may be transmitted via sexual activity.[79] Syphilis, more common in the MSM population, can increase the risk of acquisition of HIV[70] as well as make HIV more difficult to treat, as noted previously.

Vaccines play an important role in adolescent health in general but have specific relevance in young gay men who have been noted to have a higher prevalence of certain infections in their demographic. This recommendation regarding vaccinations is based on community prevalence, not just individual behavior. Human papillomavirus (HPV) is a major cause of vaccine-preventable anal neoplasia and anogenital warts in the gay male population; thus, vaccination should be strongly encouraged.[80] Hepatitis A is transmitted via the fecal-oral route, and transmission is possible in gay men who practice oral-anal sex. Hepatitis B has been noted in MSM via sexual transmission. For these reasons, hepatitis A, B, and HPV vaccines should be strongly encouraged for young gay adolescents.[80,81]

LESBIAN SEXUAL HEALTH

These recommendations are based on behavior (WSW) and not simply an identity (eg, lesbian). Woman-to-woman STI transmission has been documented for HIV, HPV, syphilis, HSV, gonorrhea, and chlamydia.[70] Bacterial vaginosis can be considered an STI in WSW.[70] Treating bacterial vaginosis should include partner notification, treatment, and counseling.[70,82] Unprotected anilingus, oral-vaginal sex, and the use of sex toys provide a transmission mechanism of cervicovaginal secretions and may result in the transfer of gonorrhea and/or chlamydia.[70] Dental dams, finger cots, and condoms to use on sex toys should be promoted to serve as barriers to protect transmission from infections.

Large, national, cross-sectional surveys clearly demonstrate that many lesbian-identified adolescents have had penile-vaginal intercourse.[82,83] When compared with their heterosexual counterparts, self-identified lesbians report being younger at heterosexual debut, less likely to use hormonal contraception, higher rates of teen-aged pregnancy, and more male and female sexual partners.[84,85] Further, bisexual young women report the earliest sexual debut, highest numbers of male partners, greatest use of emergency contraception, and highest frequency of pregnancy termination.[84] These statistics highlight the importance of reviewing sexual behaviors and not simply sexual identification. Future contraception issues should be addressed even though a lesbian patient may only report sexual contact with same-sex partners currently.

Higher rates of teenage pregnancy for lesbian and bisexual girls may be caused by deliberate attempts to get pregnant in an effort to define and strengthen an identity for themselves.[86] Unlike their heterosexual peers, LGB youth face pressures to deny or reject their same-sex attraction feelings and, therefore, may pursue heterosexual behaviors as a way to explore their emerging sexual identity.[86] Discussing contraception, especially provisional emergency contraception, must be introduced clearly and sensitively for all. Further, lesbian and bisexual youth also report more experiences of being forced to have sex by a male partner than their heterosexual peers, which should prompt a discussion about using nondiscoverable forms of contraception as well as sexual violence prevention and screening.[83]

GENDER VARIANT YOUTH
Primary Care

Practitioners who care for gender variant youth must do so with the conviction that these are normal children and are not mentally ill.[14,15,87] Medical treatments for trans-gendered individuals aim to align the body to one's gender identity. All practitioners can, with some training, provide gender-affirming therapies to youth who desire them. Practitioners should make no assumptions about the extent that youth wish to transition toward masculinization or feminization with either medical treatments or surgical interventions.[14] Of course, those providers who feel uncomfortable with gender variant youth have an ethical obligation to refer to providers who are knowledgeable and comfortable with this population.

General primary care should be based on patients' biology. Transgendered men should be offered appropriate STI and cancer screenings as dictated by their gynecologic history. Contraception, for those who engage in penile-vaginal sex, must be sensitively discussed. Transgender men on testosterone must be made aware that testosterone is contraindicated in pregnancy and may have significant effects on a developing fetus. Transgender women should be offered all the usual screening tests and immunizations that are offered to MSM patients.

Gender-Affirming Therapies for Transgender Youth

Prepubertal children

The Endocrine Society[15] and the World Professional Association for Transgender Health (WPATH)[88] publish widely used guidelines for diagnosing and treating gender dysphoria in transgender youth. For prepubertal youth, clothing, hair, makeup styling, and role changes are the current treatment recommendations. Name and gender documentation may be considered for change on official identification papers at school. A qualified mental health specialist should evaluate the child for gender dysphoria and to exclude disorders of psychotic thinking, but actual medical treatment above and beyond routine medical care is not required.

Puberty blocking agents

At the onset of puberty, if the transgender identity is still present, the use of gonadotropin-releasing hormone (GnRH) agonists is recommended. The diagnosis of gender identity dysphoria should be made by a qualified mental health professional before initiation of any type of medical hormonal therapy.[14,21] Because many children who feel a discrepancy between their gender identity and their physical body spontaneously resolve their dysphoria, an evaluation is important in the adolescent years before the initiation of medical treatments. Both WPATH and The Endocrine Society recommend puberty suppression with GnRH analogues starting at Tanner stage 2 to 3.[14] The use of high-dose medroxyprogesterone has been used to suppress puberty as an alternative, but the results showed only partial suppression.[21]

The therapeutic goal of GnRH agonists is the prevention of difficult-to-correct secondary sexual characteristics.[21] Physical benefits for transmen (natal females) include menstrual cessation, reduction in the need/extent of mammoplasties, prevention of epiphyseal closure for increased height, and the return of ovulatory function for those who discontinue the agonists. For transwomen (natal males), pubertal suppression prevents masculinizing of the facial bones, the development of a prominent Adam's apple, the induction of masculine facial hair patterns, a slowed penis growth, and a decrease in spontaneous erections.

Cross-gender hormones

Based on expert opinion, cross-gender hormones are recommended at 16 years of age.[15,88] When considering hormonal therapy, a mental health professional should reconfirm the diagnosis of gender dysphoria at Tanner stage 2 (or greater) and exclude other diagnoses, such as schizophrenia or delusional disorder,[21] before the initiation of irreversible medical treatments.

For transwomen (natal men), estrogens with a testosterone receptor blocker are the mainstays of therapy. Ideally, these treatments would start early enough to change the trajectory of the natal puberty; once certain pubertal milestones, such vocal pitch dropping, bone fusion, and facial hair, have been reached, estrogen therapy will not reverse these features. The current recommended regiments include oral estradiol, transdermal estrogens in creams and patches, and the injectable estrogens. Ethinyl estradiol is no longer recommended, as it induces a clinically relevant prothrombotic state and predisposes patients to thromboembolism side effects as compared with other forms of estrogen.[89,90] There is no definitive evidence that a particular estrogen regiment improves breast shape or development. There is also no evidence that any medically approved type or method of administration is more effective than any other in producing the desired physical changes.[88]

Common antiandrogens include spironolactone, cyproterone acetate, 5-alpha reductase inhibitors (finasteride and dutasteride), and GnRH agonists (leuprolide acetate). These antiandrogens are used to decrease testosterone levels and are frequently used with estrogen as a part of feminizing regiments. They are used to decrease the doses of the estrogen and, therefore, decrease the risk of side effects from the estrogen.[88]

The use of progesterones in transgender women is controversial. There are no clinical trials to support its use in transwomen. There is, however, evidence that exogenous progestins can induce a proinflammatory profile in healthy men.[29] The common side effects noted in genetic women include depression, weight gain, and lipid changes. Future research will need to be done to assess the role, if any, that progesterones may play in medical management of transgender women.

For transmen (natal women), the mainstay of treatment is testosterone. Ideally, this is started before significant breast development occurs and early enough to suppress regular menstruation. The use of testosterone will cause the vocal pitch to drop, facial hair to grow, a body fat distribution to a more masculine body habitus, and a cessation of regular menstruation. Testosterone will also alter the hematologic and lipid profiles to match genetic males. Un-desired side effects usually include acne, increased body odor, rage/anger issues and male pattern balding. The most commonly used testosterones are transdermal or injectable testosterone. Masculinized secondary sexual characteristics may be noted in 1 month, but full effects may take 3 to 5 years for pubertal completion.

Surgical treatments

Surgical treatments are the most irreversible treatments for gender dysphoria.[14,15,88] These procedures are designed to create a more masculine or more feminine appearance in the individual. For transgender men, the procedures include mastectomy, phalloplasty, construction of a scrotum, and metoidioplasty (surgical release of the clitoris from the labia). Transgendered women may get breast augmentation, vaginoplasty, labioplasty, tracheal shave, and jaw reconstruction. Other procedures may include electrolysis or laser hair removal for transwomen. Transidentified people may or may not have surgery. This decision depends on the individual and their interests in pursing gender-affirming surgeries.

To reduce the dosing of the cross-gender hormones, transgender individuals may elect to have their native gonads removed.[15] Natal males may undergo orchiectomy, and natal females may undergo hysterectomy and oophorectomy later in life. Most surgeons require that patients be at least 18 years of age, have a mental health clearance, and be in medical care before any surgical procedures.

SUMMARY

LGBT youth are a diverse and vibrant group who deserve high-quality health care and praise for standing up against a history of threats and discrimination from society. Although there are many challenges that youth face, emotional support from their families helps to mitigate mental health stressors and, therefore, decrease health-compromising behaviors. Many of the physical and social developmental milestones are the same as heterosexual youth but have the added complexity of coming to terms with their sexual minority status. The role of the health practitioner provides assistance to the family as a navigator through a complex, confusing, and socially challenging period of their child's life. Despite the increased health disparities among the LGBT adolescent community, most retain fun and refreshing personalities that all clinicians should enjoy.

REFERENCES

1. Steever JB. A review of gay, lesbian, bisexual, and transgender youth issues for the pediatrician. Pediatr Ann 2013;42(2):34–9.
2. Friedman RC. Homosexuality. N Engl J Med 1994;331(14):923–30.
3. Frankowski BL. Sexual orientation and adolescents. Pediatrics 2004;113(6): 1827–32.
4. Stieglitz KA. Development, risk, and resilience of transgender youth. J Assoc Nurses AIDS Care 2010;21(3):192–206.
5. Morgan SW. Transgender identity development as represented by a group of transgendered adults. Issues Ment Health Nurs 2012;33(5):301–8.
6. Russell ST. Are teens "post-gay"? Contemporary adolescents' sexual identity labels. J Youth Adolesc 2009;38(7):884–90.
7. Weinberg G. Society and the healthy homosexual. New York: St Martens Press; 1972.
8. Chesir-Teran D. Heterosexism in high school and victimization among lesbian, gay, bisexual, and questioning students. J Youth Adolesc 2009;38(7):963–75.
9. Kinsey AC. Sexual behavior in the human male. Bloomington (IN): Indiana University Press; 1948.
10. Savin-Williams RC. Prevalence and stability of sexual orientation components during adolescence and young adulthood. Arch Sex Behav 2007;36(3):385–94.
11. Diamond LM. Female bisexuality from adolescence to adulthood: results from a 10-year longitudinal study. Dev Psychol 2008;44(1):5–14.
12. Savin-Williams RC. Theoretical perspectives accounting for adolescent homosexuality. J Adolesc Health Care 1988;9(2):95–104.
13. American Academy of Pediatrics Committee on Adolescence: homosexuality and adolescence. Pediatrics 1993;92(4):631 4.
14. Olson J, Forbes C, Belzer M. Management of the transgender adolescent. Arch Pediatr Adolesc Med 2011;165(2):171–6.
15. Hembree WC. Endocrine treatment of transsexual persons: an Endocrine Society clinical practice guideline. J Clin Endocrinol Metab 2009;94(9):3132 54.
16. Grossman A, D'Augelli A, Salter N. Male to female transgender youth: gender expression milestones, gender atypicality, victimization and parents' responses. J GLBT Fam Stud 2006;71–92.
17. Calzo JP, Antonucci TC. Retrospective recall of sexual orientation identity development among gay, lesbian, and bisexual adults. Dev Psychol 2011;47(6): 1658–73.
18. Savin-Williams RC. Sexual identity trajectories among sexual-minority youths: gender comparisons. Arch Sex Behav 2000;29(6):607–27.
19. Grov C. Race, ethnicity, gender, and generational factors associated with the coming-out process among lesbian, and bisexual individuals. J Sex Res 2006;43(2):115–21.
20. Riley BH. GLB adolescent's "coming out". J Child Adolesc Psychiatr Nurs 2010; 23(1):3–10.
21. Hembree WC. Guidelines for pubertal suspension and gender reassignment for transgender adolescents. Child Adolesc Psychiatr Clin N Am 2011;20(4): 725–32.
22. Drummond KD. A follow-up study of girls with gender identity disorder. Dev Psychol 2008;44(1):34–45.
23. De Vries A, Cohen-Kettenis P, Delemarre-van de Waal H. Clinical management of gender dysphoria in adolescents. Int J Transgenderism 2007;83–94.

24. Remafedi G. Demography of sexual orientation in adolescents. Pediatrics 1992; 89(4):714–21.
25. Gates GJ. Demographics and LGBT health. J Health Soc Behav 2013;54(1):72–4.
26. De Cuypere G. Prevalence and demography of transsexualism in Belgium. Eur Psychiatry 2007;22(3):137–41.
27. Conron KJ. Transgender health in Massachusetts: results from a household probability sample of adults. Am J Public Health 2012;102(1):118–22.
28. Spack NP. Children and adolescents with gender identity disorder referred to a pediatric medical center. Pediatrics 2012;129(3):418–25.
29. Committee On Adolescence. Office-based care for lesbian, gay, bisexual, transgender, and questioning youth. Pediatrics 2013;132(1):198–203.
30. Bonet L. A positive look at a difficult time: a strength based examination of coming out for lesbian and bi-sexual women. J LGBT Health Res 2007;3(1):7–14.
31. Troiden RR. Homosexual identity development. J Adolesc Health Care 1988; 9(2):105–13.
32. Society for Adolescent Health and Medicine. Recommendations for promoting the health and well-being of lesbian, gay, bisexual, and transgender adolescents: a position paper of the Society for Adolescent Health and Medicine. J Adolesc Health 2013;52(4):506–10.
33. Coker TR, Austin SB, Schuster MA. The health and health care of lesbian, gay, and bisexual adolescents. Annu Rev Public Health 2010;31:457–77.
34. Bjorkman M, Malterud K. Lesbian women coping with challenges of minority stress: a qualitative study. Scand J Public Health 2012;40(3):239–44.
35. The health of lesbian, gay, bisexual, and transgender people: building a foundation for better understanding. Institute of Medicine 2011(4):141–84.
36. Pearson J, Wilkinson L. Family relationships and adolescent well-being: are families equally protective for same-sex attracted youth? J Youth Adolesc 2013; 42(3):376–93.
37. Sedlovskaya A, Purdie-Vaughns V, Eibach RP, et al. Internalizing the closet: concealment heightens the cognitive distinction between public and private selves. J Pers Soc Psychol 2013;104(4):695–715.
38. Rossi NE. "Coming out" stories of gay and lesbian young adults. J Homosex 2010;57(9):1174–91.
39. Ryan C. Family rejection as a predictor of negative health outcomes in white and Latino lesbian, gay, and bisexual young adults. Pediatrics 2009;123(1):346–52.
40. Reitman D. Sexual orientation. 2013. Available at: http://emedicine.medscape. com/article/917792. Accessed December 27, 2013.
41. Rothman EF, Sullivan M, Keyes S, et al. Parents' supportive reactions to sexual orientation disclosure associated with better health: results from a population-based survey of LGB adults in Massachusetts. J Homosex 2012;59(2):186–200.
42. Carnelley KB. Perceived parental reactions to coming out, attachment, and romantic relationship views. Attach Hum Dev 2011;13(3):217–36.
43. Toomey RB, Richardson RA. Perceived sibling relationships of sexual minority youth. J Homosex 2009;56(7):849–60.
44. Ryan C. Family acceptance in adolescence and the health of LGBT young adults. J Child Adolesc Psychiatr Nurs 2010;23(4):205–13.
45. Garofalo R. Health care issues of gay and lesbian youth. Curr Opin Pediatr 2001;13(4):298–302.
46. Arrington-Sanders R, Leonard L, Brooks D, et al. Older partner selection in young African-American men who have sex with men. J Adolesc Health 2013; 52(6):682–8.

47. California Assembly Bill 1266. 2013.
48. Joseph HA, Marks G, Belcher L, et al. Older partner selection, serial risk behavior and unrecognized HIV infection among black and Latino men who have sex with men. Sex Transm Dis 2011;87(5):442–7.
49. Garofalo R. Overlooked, misunderstood and at-risk: exploring the lives and HIV risk of ethnic minority male-to-female transgender youth. J Adolesc Health 2006; 38(3):230–6.
50. Ginsburg KR. How to reach sexual minority youth in the health care setting: the teens offer guidance. J Adolesc Health 2002;31(5):407–16.
51. Meckler GD. Nondisclosure of sexual orientation to a physician among a sample of gay, lesbian, and bisexual youth. Arch Pediatr Adolesc Med 2006;160(12): 1248–54.
52. Coren JS. Assessing your office for care of lesbian, gay, bisexual, and transgender patients. Health Care Manag (Frederick) 2011;30(1):66–70.
53. Allen LB. Adolescent health care experience of gay, lesbian, and bisexual young adults. J Adolesc Health 1998;23(4):212–20.
54. Ragg DM. Slamming the closet door: working with gay and lesbian youth in care. Child Welfare 2006;85(2):243–65.
55. Hagan JF, Shaw JS, Duncan PM, editors. Bright futures: guidelines for health supervision of infants, children, and adolescents. 3rd edition. Elk Grove Village (IL): American Academy of Pediatrics; 2008.
56. Taliaferro LA. Beyond prevention: promoting healthy youth development in primary care. Am J Prev Med 2012;42(6 Suppl 2):S117–21.
57. Berlan ED. Sexual orientation and bullying among adolescents in the growing up today study. J Adolesc Health 2010;46(4):366–71.
58. Blashill AJ. Elements of male body image: prediction of depression, eating pathology and social sensitivity among gay men. Body Image 2010;7(4):310–6.
59. Austin SB. Disordered weight control behaviors in early adolescent boys and girls of color: an under-recognized factor in the epidemic of childhood overweight. J Adolesc Health 2011;48(1):109–12.
60. Zaritsky E. Risk factors for reproductive and breast cancers among older lesbians. J Womens Health (Larchmt) 2010;19(1):125–31.
61. Hadland SE, Austin SB, Goodenow CS, et al. Weight misperception and unhealthy weight control behaviors among sexual minorities in the general adolescent population. J Adolesc Health 2014;54(3):296–303.
62. Grossman AH, D'Augelli AR, Frank JA. Aspects of psychological resilience among transgender youth. J LGBT Youth 2011;8:103–15.
63. Kosciw JG. Who, what, where, when, and why: demographic and ecological factors contributing to hostile school climate for lesbian, gay, bisexual, and transgender youth. J Youth Adolesc 2009;38(7):976–88.
64. McGuire JK. School climate for transgender youth: a mixed method investigation of student experiences and school responses. J Youth Adolesc 2010; 39(10):1175–88.
65. Kosciw JG, Greytak EA, Bartkiewicz MJ, et al. The 2011 National School Climate Survey: The experiences of lesbian, gay, bisexual and transgender youth in our nation's schools. New York: GLSEN; 2012. p. 1–168.
66. Mayer KH. Comprehensive clinical care for men who have sex with men: an integrated approach. Lancet 2012;380(9839):378–87.
67. Schauer GL, Berg CJ, Bryant LO. Sex differences in psychosocial correlates of concurrent substance use among heterosexual, homosexual and bisexual college students. Am J Drug Alcohol Abuse 2013;39(4):252–8.

68. Herrick AL. Health risk behaviors in an urban sample of young women who have sex with women. J Lesbian Stud 2010;14(1):80–92.
69. Greenwood GL. Tobacco use and cessation among a household-based sample of US urban men who have sex with men. Am J Public Health 2005;95(1): 145–51.
70. Center for Disease Control. Sexually transmitted diseases treatment guidelines, 2010. MMWR Recomm Rep 2010;59(RR-19):1–110.
71. Jin F. Incidence and risk factors for urethral and anal gonorrhoea and chlamydia in a cohort of HIV-negative homosexual men: the Health in Men Study. Sex Transm Infect 2007;83(2):113–9.
72. Schachter J. Nucleic acid amplification tests in the diagnosis of chlamydial and gonococcal infections of the oropharynx and rectum in men who have sex with men. Sex Transm Dis 2008;35(7):637–42.
73. Butler LM. Use of saliva as a lubricant in anal sexual practices among homosexual men. J Acquir Immune Defic Syndr 2009;50(2):162–7.
74. Jin F. Per-contact probability of HIV transmission in homosexual men in Sydney in the era of HAART. AIDS 2010;24(6):907–13.
75. CDC. Estimated HIV incidence in the United States, 2007-2010. HIV surveillance supplemental report. 2012;17(4). Available at: http://www.cdc.gov/hiv/topics/surveillance/resources/reports/#supplemental. Accessed December 27, 2013.
76. Heffelfinger JD. Trends in primary and secondary syphilis among men who have sex with men in the United States. Am J Public Health 2007;97(6): 1076–83.
77. Buchacz K. Syphilis increases HIV viral load and decreases CD4 cell counts in HIV-infected patients with new syphilis infections. AIDS 2004;18(15):2075–9.
78. Glynn JR. Herpes simplex virus type 2: a key role in HIV incidence. AIDS 2009; 23(12):1595–8.
79. Fierer DS. Epidemic of sexually transmitted hepatitis C virus infection among HIV-infected men. Curr Infect Dis Rep 2010;12(2):118–25.
80. Makadon HJ. Optimizing primary care for men who have sex with men. JAMA 2006;296(19):2362–5.
81. Gunn RA. Hepatitis B vaccination of men who have sex with men attending an urban STD clinic: impact of an ongoing vaccination program, 1998-2003. Sex Transm Dis 2007;34(9):663–8.
82. Evans AL. Prevalence of bacterial vaginosis in lesbians and heterosexual women in a community setting. Sex Transm Infect 2007;83(6):470–5.
83. Saewyc EM. Sexual intercourse, abuse and pregnancy among adolescent women: does sexual orientation make a difference? Fam Plann Perspect 1999; 31(3):127–31.
84. Tornello SL. Sexual orientation and sexual and reproductive health among adolescent young women in the United States. J Adolesc Health 2014;54(2): 160–8.
85. Charlton BM. Sexual orientation differences in teen pregnancy and hormonal contraceptive use: an examination across 2 generations. Am J Obstet Gynecol 2013;209(3):204.e1–8.
86. Rotheram-Borus MJ, Fernandez MI. Sexual orientation and developmental challenges experienced by gay and lesbian youths. Suicide Life Threat Behav 1995; 25(Suppl):26–34.
87. Edwards-Leeper L, Spack NP. Psychological evaluation and medical treatment of transgender youth in an interdisciplinary "Gender Management Service" (GeMS) in a major pediatric center. J Homosex 2012;59(3):321–36.

88. Coleman E, Brockting W, Butzer M. Standards of care for the health of trans-sexual, transgender, and gender-nonconforming people. Int J Transgenderism 2011;13(4):165–232.
89. Seal LJ. Predictive markers for mammoplasty and a comparison of side effect profiles in transwomen taking various hormonal regimens. J Clin Endocrinol Metab 2012;97(12):4422–8.
90. Toorians AW. Venous thrombosis and changes of hemostatic variables during cross-sex hormone treatment in transsexual people. J Clin Endocrinol Metab 2003;88(12):5723–9.

Safety

Adolescent Interpersonal Violence

Implications for Health Care Professionals

Naomi Nichele Duke, MD, MPH[a],*, Iris Wagman Borowsky, MD, PhD[b]

KEYWORDS

- Adolescent violence • Bullying involvement • Adolescent dating/relationship violence
- Adolescent health screening • Adolescent health counseling

KEY POINTS

- Violence involvement represents a significant burden affecting the health and positive development of youth.
- As in other forms of adolescent violence and violence-related behaviors, bullying involvement and dating/relationship violence have immediate and long-term health consequences.
- Health care providers in the primary office setting have a pivotal role in the prevention, identification, and management of adolescent violence involvement.
- Screening and counseling of all youth and parents on violence involvement is recommended. Resources are available to support primary care providers in assessment and intervention on behalf of youth.

INTRODUCTION

The problem of adolescent violence is particularly troubling because each act is preventable. Each year, the number of lives lost and youth potential destroyed by disability related to violence serves as a reminder that adolescent violence prevention is a responsibility for all individuals involved in the care of youth. In the primary care setting, health providers have a pivotal role to play in the detection of adolescent violence involvement and in mitigating health consequences related to youth violence. This review provides a summary of the burden of adolescent violence and violence-related behavior, risk, and protective factors for violence outcomes, the importance

Disclosures: None.
[a] Division of General Pediatrics and Adolescent Health, Department of Pediatrics, University of Minnesota, 3rd Floor, #385, 717 Delaware Street Southeast, Minneapolis, MN 55414, USA;
[b] Division of General Pediatrics and Adolescent Health, Department of Pediatrics, University of Minnesota, 3rd Floor, #389, 717 Delaware Street Southeast, Minneapolis, MN 55414, USA
* Corresponding author.
E-mail address: duke0028@umn.edu

Prim Care Clin Office Pract 41 (2014) 671–689
http://dx.doi.org/10.1016/j.pop.2014.05.013   **primarycare.theclinics.com**

of screening for violence involvement in the primary care setting, and examples of on-line resources to support providers in advocating, assessing, and intervening on behalf of youth. The article draws attention to bullying and dating/relationship violence, not as new forms of violence-related behavior, but as behaviors with health outcomes that have received increased attention more recently.

ADOLESCENT VIOLENCE INVOLVEMENT: SCOPE OF THE PROBLEM

Despite increased awareness of the negative consequences of youth violence involve-ment over the past decade, violence-associated acts (including self-directed violence) remain among the leading causes of death for youth ages 10 to 24 years. In the United States in 2010, suicide and homicide were the third and fourth leading causes of death for youth ages 10 to 14 years, and the second and third leading causes of death for young people ages 20 to 24 years, respectively.[1] For youth ages 15 to 19 years, the order of cause was reversed, with homicide being the second leading cause of death and suicide a very close third.[1] In the United States, almost 5000 young people ages 10 to 24 years lost their lives due to homicide in 2010, an average of 13 individuals each day.[2] Overwhelmingly, the cause of these deaths involved the use of a firearm (71.3% among youth ages 10–14; 84.8% among youth ages 15–19; 82% among young people ages 20–24).[1] These numbers do not tell the whole story, as we know that homicide is experienced in greater numbers among some groups of youth. Among African Amer-ican youth ages 10 to 24 years, homicide is the leading cause of death; in this same age range, for Hispanic youth it is the second leading cause of death; and for American Indian and Alaska Native youth it is the third leading cause of death.[2]

Among youth taking the 2011 Youth Risk Behavior Survey (YRBS; youth grades 9–12), just more than 1 in 13 reported an attempt on their life at least once during the pre-vious year (1 in 10 females; 1 in 17 males).[3,4] In this same survey, more than 1 in 7 youth reported seriously considering suicide during the 12 months before survey administration (almost 1 in 5 female and 1 in 8 male youth).[3,4] For youth ages 10 to 24 years, firearms are the method used in 30% to 47% of suicides (male youth 37.8%–50.8%; female youth 13.8%–27.4%).[1]

Nonfatal injuries related to violence represent a significant source of poor health among adolescents. In 2012, assault-related injuries (physical assault by striking) top-ped the list for causes of nonfatal violence-related injuries among those 10 to 24 years old in the United States.[5] In this same year, more than 500,000 young people ages 10 to 24 years were treated in emergency departments for assault-related injuries.[5] The use of firearms resulted in nonfatal injuries requiring emergency department care for more than 26,000 10-year-olds to 24-year-olds in 2012.[5] For youth taking the 2011 YRBS, one-third reported being in a physical fight one or more times in the previous year[3]; approximately 4% reported being in a physical fight with injuries requiring med-ical attention from a doctor or nurse at least once during the same time period.[2] Just less than 10% of 2011 YRBS respondents reported being assaulted (eg, hit, slapped, or physically hurt on purpose) by a boyfriend or girlfriend in the previous year.[3] Earlier data from the 2005 National Survey of Adolescents estimates the overall prevalence of dating violence to be 1.6% (sexual assault 0.9%, physical assault 0.8%, alcohol-drug facilitated rape 0.1%).[6] Using 2005 Census data, this figure is equivalent to 400,000 US adolescents.[6]

Many behaviors contribute to youth violence. Among youth respondents for the 2011 YRBS, just more than 16% reported carrying a weapon (eg, gun, knife, or club) on at least 1 day during the previous month; 5% reported carrying a gun during the same time period.[3] Bully victimization occurred during the previous year for 1 in 5 to 1 in 6 respondents taking the 2011 YRBS (eg, 20.1% on school property; 16.2% electronically, including through e-mail, chat room, instant messaging, Web site, or texting).[3] In each type of bully victimization, the prevalence was higher among female than male youth (on school property 22.0% vs 18.2%; electronic 22.1% vs 10.8%).[2] Using data from a nationally representative group of 6th to 10th graders participating in the Health Behaviors in School-Aged Children Survey (2005–2006), Wang and colleagues[7] found the prevalence for bullying, being bullied, or both in the previous 2 months to vary according to type: 20.8% physical, 53.6% verbal, 51.4% relational (rumors to hurt reputation, relationships), and 13.6% cyber. The use of alcohol and other drugs presents another context in which violence may occur as a direct result of youth impairment in judgment and decisional capacity. For example, binge drinking (consuming 5 or more drinks in a row within a couple of hours) at least once in the previous month was reported by more than 1 in 5 2011 YRBS respondents (21.9%).[3]

For some youth, the school environment presents a context for vulnerability to violence involvement. In 2011, 5.9% of YRBS respondents reported skipping school at least once during the previous month because of concerns about safety at school or on the way to school.[3] Among students taking the same survey, 12.0% reported being in a physical fight on school property in the previous year and 7.4% reported being threatened or injured with a weapon at least once in the school setting during the previous year.[2] The Bureau of Justice estimates that 1,246,000 students ages 12 to 18 years experienced nonfatal victimizations at school in 2011, with 597,500 events related to simple assault (assault without a weapon, resulting in no, minor, or undetermined injury requiring <2 days hospitalization) and serious violence (including rape, sexual assault, robbery, and aggravated assault).[8]

RISK AND PROTECTIVE FACTORS FOR ADOLESCENT VIOLENCE INVOLVEMENT

Risk and protective factors for adolescent violence involvement are located in multiple contexts for adolescent development, including individual, familial/household, and community/environmental characteristics (**Table 1**). These contexts may be a target for interventions to reduce or prevent youth violence and its consequences.

Risk Factors for Adolescent Violence Involvement

In their early work exploring the impact of 3 contexts (individual, family, and school characteristics) on adolescent behaviors using data from Wave I of the National Longitudinal Study of Adolescent Health (Add Health), Resnick and colleagues[9] found that higher levels of adolescent violence involvement were associated with a number of factors, including household access to a gun, recent family history of suicidality (attempts or completion), having been a victim or witness to violence, carrying a weapon, involvement in deviant and antisocial behaviors, selling marijuana or other drugs, perceived risk of untimely death, and for younger adolescents (grades 7–8), lower grade point average. Follow-up studies using Add Health data confirm and build on the earlier findings. For example, using Add Health Wave I factors to predict Wave II violence perpetration, Resnick and colleagues[10] identified commonalities among males and females for risk of violence perpetration, including previous violence involvement and violent victimization, carrying a weapon to school, repeating a grade, alcohol and marijuana use, and self-reported learning problems. Additional risk factors for perpetration identified by the investigators include a history of treatment for emotional problems (boys), emotional distress (girls), and somatic complaints (girls).[10] Using the same data set and a similar study design, Borowsky and Ireland[11] found that factors predicting a future fight-related injury parallel those factors predicting violence

Table 1
Risk and protective factors for adolescent violence involvement

	Individual	Familial/Household	Community/ Environmental
Risk factors	Previous violent behavior Problem (antisocial) behavior Substance use Violence victimization; witnessing violence; history of fight-related injury Poor emotional health: depression, anxiety, hopelessness, anger, low self-esteem Hyperactivity Learning problems School failure	Family conflict Family violence Family socioeconomic disadvantage Adverse childhood experience (physical abuse, sexual abuse, witnessing violence, household dysfunction caused by parental substance use) Gun(s) in the home	Neighborhood violence Media violence Concentrated poverty Peer violence, involvement in gangs, antisocial groups Ready access to firearms, lethal weapons
Protective factors	Emotional health Spirituality Strong social skills School achievement Self-efficacy, self-esteem Sense of purpose, future	Parent-family caring/ connectedness Parental monitoring and supervision Parent expectations for school achievement, success Nonviolent disciplinary methods Open parent-child communication Good family problem-solving skills Authoritative parenting style	Neighborhood safety School connectedness Positive connection to an adult in the community Neighborhood social control (informal norms for behavior and adult monitoring of youth)

perpetration. Among boys and girls, witnessing or being a victim of violence, fighting, and fight-related injury predicted future fight-related injury requiring medical care.[11] Use of illicit drugs (boys) and increased depressive symptomatology (girls) also predicted future fight-related injury.[11]

As suggested by the aforementioned studies, adolescent emotional health has significant impact on adolescent violence perpetration. Several regional and population-based studies support this finding. For example, moderate-high levels of hopelessness, independent of a measure for poor affect, was significantly associated with delinquency, weapon carrying on school property, and all forms of self-directed violence across subgroups of youth participating in the 2007 Minnesota Student Survey.[12] Similarly, in a subsample of youth participating in the Mobile Youth Survey (a community-based, multiple cohort study of youth 10–19 years living in 13 extremely impoverished neighborhoods in Mobile, AL), Stoddard and colleagues[13] found that trajectories for hopelessness during middle adolescence portended engagement in serious violence in later adolescence, in particular violence with a weapon. Among youth participating in the Urban Indian Youth Health Survey 1995–1998, one of the strongest risk factors for violence perpetration was suicidal thoughts and behaviors.[14] In their study distinguishing profiles of violence perpetration among rural adolescents in North Carolina, Foshee and colleagues[15] report several factors associated with perpetration of violence against peers and dates, including higher levels of anger and anxiety.

Within the family context, being a direct victim and witness of physical violence is associated with greater risk of violent adolescent behavior than report of one of these types of victimization alone.[16] The increased risk for violent behavior includes attempted suicide, fighting, and gun-carrying.[16] Using data from the 2007 Minnesota Student Survey, Duke and colleagues[17] found that adverse childhood experiences (physical abuse, sexual abuse, witnessing violence, household dysfunction caused by family alcohol or other drug abuse) were significantly associated with adolescent interpersonal (delinquency, fighting, bullying, dating violence, weapon-carrying on school property) and self-directed (self-injury, suicidal ideation and attempt) violence perpetration. In this study, for each additional type of adverse experience, risk of adolescent violence perpetration increased by 35% to 144%.[17] In a study of youth and their parents attending 8 outpatient pediatric practices, youth report of corporal punishment as a means of discipline by their parent was significantly associated with a youth's intention to fight if hit or pushed by another, physical fighting in the last year, bullying, and violent victimization, and was negatively associated with a prosocial attitude toward peer violence.[18] Using data from the National Educational Longitudinal Survey, McNulty and Bellair[19] offer larger contextual explanations for differences in white-black, and white-Latino adolescent involvement in fighting, suggesting that concentrated poverty, including community and family disadvantage, should be targets for policy intervention.

Protective Factors Against Adolescent Violence Involvement

Connections, monitoring, and high expectations for young people, and positive social norms are protective against youth violence involvement. Parent-family connectedness, higher levels of school connectedness, and parent expectations for school achievement are associated with reduced likelihood of youth violence.[9,14] Positive peer social norms and parental norms against violence are negatively associated with physical fighting and other forms of violence perpetration, including shooting and stabbing.[14,18] In addition, for male adolescents, an ability to discuss problems with parents, higher grade point average, and a sense of connectedness to adults outside of the family are associated with reduced risk of violence involvement.[10,11] For female adolescents, higher grade point average and religiosity (valuing religious observance and personal prayer) are also protective against violence involvement.[10] Among rural adolescents in North Carolina, higher levels of individual social bonding (endorsement of conventional beliefs, commitment to prosocial values, degree of religiosity), parental monitoring, and neighborhood social control (adult monitoring of youth) were associated with reduced odds of perpetrating peer and dating violence.[15] Alternately, in a sample of middle school students living in urban, ethnically diverse, and economically disadvantaged neighborhoods, young adolescents' intentions to contribute to their neighborhoods were linked to lower levels of violence involvement.[20]

Resilience

In the context of violence, resilience may moderate the effects of vulnerabilities and environmental exposures. Resilience is the process of and capacity for adaptation and doing well in the context of challenging circumstances.[21] Resilience is not merely surviving, but it is thriving under conditions of adversity; it results in effective functioning, including meeting developmental tasks that are normal for a particular time period in life.[22] Resilience is evidenced when good outcomes for youth occur in vulnerable contexts, when there is sustained competence in settings of continued stress, and when there is recovery from trauma.[21] Critical components of resilience are instrumental in protection against violence involvement and include (1) strong verbal and communication skills, (2) easy temperament, (3) humor, (4) problem-solving capacities, (5) empathy, (6) perspective-taking skills, (7) spirituality,[22] (8) receipt of good and stable care and positive relationships with adults, (9) having capacity to engage others, and (10) having an area of competence or perceived efficacy that is valued by society, whether academic, artistic, athletic, or mechanical.[21]

TWO CONTEXTS OF ADOLESCENT VIOLENCE AND VIOLENCE-RELATED BEHAVIORS: BULLYING AND DATING
Adolescent Bullying Involvement

Definition of bullying
Broadly defined, bullying involves aggressive behavior perpetrated by one or more youth that is characterized by intimidation, harassment, and/or physical harm.[23,24] Bullying behavior is repetitious and there is a perceived power differential between perpetrator and victim.[23,24] Bullying involves 3 groups of youth: bullies and their followers, victims of bullying (youth who are targets of bullying by others), and bystanders, those who are aware of the bullying.[23] Some youth bully and are bullied by others, referred to as bully-victims. Direct and indirect forms of bullying most often occur in the 6th to 8th grades,[25] generally peaking in middle school[26]; however, verbal bullying remains high throughout adolescence.[26]

In general, there are 3 forms of bullying: direct (overt), indirect (covert, relational), and technology-based (cyber bullying). Direct bullying more commonly occurs in boys and includes all forms of physical and verbal aggression, including kicking, hitting, threatening, name calling, and insulting.[7,24,27] Covert and relational forms of bullying more commonly occur among girls and include social isolation, such as ignoring, excluding, backbiting, and starting rumors.[7,24,27] More recent attention has been given to cyber bullying, defined as intentional, repeated, and harmful acts of indirect aggression occurring via use of cellular telephone devices (eg, text messaging), personal digital assistants, computers (eg, e-mail and instant messaging), and social networking Internet sites.[7,23,26,28] This type of bullying frequently extends outside of the school environment; nevertheless, it seems to share common causal pathways with physical and verbal bullying, particularly verbal bullying (youth normative beliefs approving of bullying, negative school climate, negative peer support).[26] There is a unique emotional injury from cyber bullying that is related to 3 factors: (1) the seeming permanence of online messages; (2) ease in which a message of hate can be delivered, with the degree of malicious content facilitated for some by perceptions of anonymity; and (3) the invasive nature of the negative sentiment that can be transmitted at any time of day and night.[28,29]

Risk and protective factors for adolescent bullying involvement
Risk factors for bully perpetration, victimization, and combined bully-victim status are not dissimilar to risk factors for general violence involvement. Risk factors for bully perpetration and combined bully-victim status (**Table 2**) span contexts for mental and behavioral health, school expectations, involvement, and achievement, and communication, monitoring, and discipline in the home.[24,30–32] In addition to the factors listed in **Table 2**, risk of cyber bullying increases with increasing computer proficiency and spending more time online.[28] Risk factors for bully victimization (see

	Table 2	
	Risk factors, symptoms and long-term consequences of adolescent bullying	
Risk Factors	**Symptoms and Associated Behaviors**	**Long-Term Consequences**
Victimization • Depressive tendencies • Anxious tendencies • Insecurity • Low self-esteem • Submissive persona • Physical unattractiveness by arbitrary peer standards • Identification with marginalized groups (disability, sexual minority) • Difficult parent communication • Experience of caregiver maltreatment Bullying, bully-victim status • Generalized aggressive tendencies • Impulsivity, poor self-control • Low prosocial behavior • Lacking empathy • Teacher low expectations for academic achievement • Parent low academic expectations and school involvement • Poor school performance • Difficult parent communication • Lack of parent monitoring • Inconsistent parent discipline (use of aggression, disengagement) • Positive impressions of violence; parent tolerance for aggression	• Depressive symptomatology • Symptoms of anxiety • Oppositional behaviors • Disordered eating behaviors • Sleep disturbance • School avoidance, absenteeism • Multiple somatic complaints (abdominal pain, headache) • Negative change in academic achievement, low achievement • Low self-esteem • Poor problem-solving capacity • Poor relationships, loneliness • Fighting behaviors • Alcohol, other drug use	Victim • Depression • Anxiety • Posttraumatic stress disorder • Low self-esteem • Loneliness • Poor interpersonal function (poor relationship quality, trust difficulty) • Academic failure Bully, bully-victim • Criminal behaviors, thought patterns • Violence against partners, children • Alcohol and other drug use • Academic failure

Table 2) include contexts for mental and behavioral health, caregiver experiences and communication, and peer judgments and associations.[24,30–33]

There is limited evidence related to protective factors for adolescent bullying involvement. Higher parent support and positive, connective school environments are protective against bullying involvement.[7,26,33] Having more friends is associated with reduced risk of being victimized.[7]

Adolescent bullying involvement and other forms of adolescent violence

Bullying involvement is associated with more serious violent behaviors, including weapon carrying, frequent fighting, and fight-related injury[34]; suicidality[35]; and sexual harassment.[36] Using data from the 2001 Health Behaviors in School-Aged Children Survey, Nansel and colleagues[34] found that being bullied in school weekly was associated with 1.5 greater odds of weapon carrying in the past 30 days; being bullied away from school weekly was associated with 4.1 greater odds of weapon carrying in the past 30 days. In the same study, bullying in school weekly was associated with 2.6 greater odds of weapon carrying in the past 30 days; bullying away from school weekly was associated with 5.9 greater odds of weapon carrying in the past 30 days.[34] Using data from the 2010 Minnesota Student Survey, Borowsky and colleagues[35] found that among students involved in social and verbal bullying, suicidal thinking or suicide attempt in the past year was reported by 22% of perpetrators, 29% of victims, and 38% of bully-victims. Across all 3 groups, history of self-injury and emotional distress were risk factors for suicidality and parental connectedness was a protective factor against suicidality.[35] In a study of middle school students in grades 5 to 8 in a Midwestern state, the strongest predictor of future sexual harassment perpetration (making sexual comments, spreading rumors, and pulling at the clothing of another student) was previous bully perpetration (measurements about 6 months apart).[36]

Consequences of adolescent bullying involvement

Bullying involvement is associated with poor physical and psychosocial health and functioning in the immediate and later time periods (see **Table 2**). The poorest functioning is exhibited by youth who are both bullying and being bullied (bully-victims).[25,31] Being bullied is linked to poor emotional health, multiple somatic complaints, substance use, and impairment in forging healthy relationships.[24,30,31] Being a bully is associated with conduct disorder, oppositional and fighting behaviors, substance use, low academic achievement and school dropout, and current and future criminal behaviors.[24,25,30] Although traditional definitions for bullying focus on a repetitive component that is described as being particularly harmful (eg, frequency occurring once weekly or more often),[25] more recent research suggests that even infrequent bullying involvement is associated with significant consequence. Using data from the 2010 Minnesota Student Survey, Gower and Borowsky[37] found that infrequent bullies and victims of bullying (1–2 times in the past month) had greater odds of adjustment problems, including suicidality (victims and bullies), substance use (bullies), and physical fighting (bullies) when compared with youth with no bullying involvement.

Adolescent Dating/Relationship Violence

Definition of adolescent dating/relationship violence

More than half of adolescents report dating by age 16; relationships provide a means for achieving important goals of intimacy and identity development.[38] However, in the context of a close and intimate relationship, feelings of anger, jealousy, and inaccurate perceptions of protection and love may turn achievement of a healthy developmental milestone into a health threat. Adolescent relationship violence may be defined by the level of harm: (1) physical (hitting, punching, shoving, being hit with something hard, and being beaten up), (2) sexual (nonconsensual sex [rape or attempted rape], unwanted touching), and (3) psychological (isolating, name-calling, threats of harm, verbally coercive sexual aggression, and verbal threat of physical aggression).[38,39] There is some research to suggest that verbal-emotional, psychological, or nonphysical conflict escalation over time results in physical aggression and more severe forms of violence.[40]

    Gender differences in perpetration and victimization are not as distinct in adolescent relationships when compared with adult profiles; it is more common to find adolescent partners perpetrating and experiencing physical, sexual, and emotional violence within relationships.[38] The severity of physical violence may be gendered: girls experience more severe forms (when in context of opposite-sex partners), but perpetrate more moderate forms in general; boys experience more moderate forms (when in context of opposite-sex partners), but perpetrate more severe levels of physical violence in general.[41,42] Girls and boys most often identify anger as the reason for violence; boys more often report use of violence as a means of control and girls more often report use of violence as a means of self-defense.[43] Although limited, the research examining adolescent same-sex partnerships suggests comparable rates of perpetration[44] and victimization[44] (female victimization[45]). It is important to note that among individuals self-identifying as gay, lesbian, and bisexual, reports of dating/relationship violence are attributed to opposite-sex and same-sex partners.[42,44]

Risk and protective factors for adolescent dating/relationship violence

In general, dating/relationship violence is associated with negative family variables, such as history of child abuse and alcohol abuse, poor interpersonal adjustment (greater interpersonal sensitivity, hostility, insecurity), and poor personal resources (poor problem-solving, aggressive peer network, low positive peer support).[38] More specifically, victimization (**Table 3**) is associated with demographic characteristics, witnessing and experiencing violence in the home and other contexts, history of negative life events, and poor relationship quality.[6,41,43,46,47] Perpetration (physical abuse

Table 3
Risk factors, symptoms and long-term consequences of adolescent dating/relationship violence

Risk Factors	Symptoms and Associated Behaviors	Long-Term Consequences
Victimization	• Depressive symptomatology	Victim: intimate partner
• Female sex	• Symptoms of anxiety	violence general (all ages)
• Older age (15–17 y vs 12–14 y)	• Symptoms of posttraumatic stress disorder	• Depression
• Negative life events (trauma, recent stressors, maltreatment)	• Multiple somatic complaints	• Posttraumatic stress disorder
	• Unexplained injuries, bruising	• Chronic pain (headaches, back pain)
• Witness of victimization and perpetration (adults in home, interparental dating violence, friends)	• Isolation from previous friends	• Recurrent gynecologic complaints
	• Spending excessive amounts of time with a partner	• Gastrointestinal complaints (with disordered eating)
• Acceptance of violence as justified in certain contexts of relationship	• Abrupt change in friends	Victim: intimate partner violence sexual assault
	• Abrupt change in dress, activities	• Revictimization
• Communication difficulty in relationship		• Increased risk for sexual victimization during college
Perpetration		
• Interpersonal violence victimization		
• History of physical and/or sexual abuse		
• History of maltreatment (male adolescents)		
• Depressed mood		
• Witness of dating violence (friends)		
• Acceptance of violence as justified in certain contexts of relationship		
• Communication difficulty in relationship		

and threatening behavior) (see **Table 3**) is associated with previous victimization and abuse, poor emotional health, witness of dating violence in peer contexts, and poor relationship quality.[17,41,46-48]

As in the case of bullying involvement, there is limited research and evidence related to factors that are protective against dating/relationship violence involvement. However, given the multiple theories that have been put forth to explain partner violence, it is likely that there are many targets for protection and prevention. These theories include (1) social learning theory (witnessing violence or being a victim of violence in the family context has lasting impact on beliefs and attitudes related to violence as a potential problem-solving tactic), (2) conflict theory (use of coercion and power for social control), (3) attachment theory (children form mental images of relationships based on interactions with significant caregivers, which serve as a prototype for future relationships), and (4) feminist theory (focusing on gender-based norms, coercion, and power and control differentials that contribute to relationship violence).[38,42,49] Examples of protective factors could include familial and community contexts that affirm a youth's value, support good parent-child communication, use nonviolent strategies for conflict resolution and problem solving, and support development of efficacy and high self-esteem.

Adolescent dating/relationship violence and other forms of adolescent violence
Dating violence is associated with more serious violent behaviors, including peer violence and sexual aggression. In their study of 7th, 9th, 11th, and 12th graders in urban schools serving youth at high risk of violence involvement Swahn and colleagues,[50] found that youth reporting dating violence perpetration had more than 4 times the odds of also reporting peer violence perpetration, relative to those who did not report perpetration of dating violence. In a sample of male and female adolescent members of a large health maintenance organization, not identified as being at high risk for aggression and violence involvement, Ozer and colleagues[51] found that among boys, perpetration of dating violence was related to perpetration of peer violence and sexual aggression at follow-up 1 year later.

Consequences of adolescent dating/relationship violence
As in the case of bullying, adolescent dating/relationship violence has immediate and long-term health impact (see **Table 3**). Victimization is linked to poor emotional health, recurrent somatic complaint, and risk of revictimization.[39,52] For youth with a history of severe violence (physical assault, rape, alcohol-facilitated rape), the risk of posttraumatic stress disorder and major depression is increased fourfold over youth who do not experience dating violence.[6]

ADOLESCENT VIOLENCE INVOLVEMENT: IMPLICATIONS FOR PRIMARY OFFICE PRACTICE
Importance of Screening

Primary screening for violence involvement is recommended in the primary care office setting, and screening should include youth and parent components (**Tables 4** and **5**). Specific questions assessing youth risk of violence involvement should address a range of violence-related outcomes (**Box 1**). The FISTS(S) mnemonic may help to organize questions by violence type (fights, injuries, sexual and intimate partner violence, threats, self-defense, and suicidality). Questions screening youth for violence involvement should be part of a comprehensive assessment (see the article discussed, elsewhere in this issue, for review of HEADDSS[S] and SSHADESS mnemonics). For topics related to violence involvement, brief screening tools that are user-friendly

Table 4
Policies and recommendations related to screening for violence involvement

Institution, Medical Organization	Policies and Statements Related to Violence Screening, Prevention, and Intervention
American Academy of Family Physicians	Violence Position Paper: http://www.aafp.org/about/policies/all/violence.html Family and Intimate Partner Violence and Abuse: http://www.aafp.org/about/policies/all/family-abuse.html
American Academy of Pediatrics	Role of the Pediatrician in Youth Violence Prevention: http://pediatrics.aappublications.org/content/124/1/393.full.pdf+html Intimate Partner Violence: The Role of the Pediatrician: http://pediatrics.aappublications.org/content/125/5/1094.full.pdf+html Firearm-Related Injuries Affecting the Pediatric Population: http://pediatrics.aappublications.org/content/130/5/e1416.full.pdf+html Gun Violence Policy Recommendations: http://www.aap.org/en-us/advocacy-and-policy/federal-advocacy/Documents/AAPGunViolencePreventionPolicyRecommendations_Jan2013.pdf
American College of Obstetricians and Gynecologists	Intimate Partner Violence: https://www.acog.org/~/media/Committee%20Opinions/Committee%20on%20Health%20Care%20for%20Women/co518.pdf
American College of Physicians	Firearms: Safety and Regulation: http://www.acponline.org/acp_policy/policies/firearms_safety_and_regulation_2013.pdf
American Medical Association	H-60.943 Bullying Behaviors Among Children and Adolescents: http://www.ama-assn.org/ad-com/polfind/Hlth-Ethics.pdf Roadmaps for Clinical Practice Intimate Partner Violence: http://166.67.66.226/ofhs/Prevention/dsvp/projectradarva/documents/oldet/pdf/intpartvio_roadmap.pdf E-2.02 Physicians' Obligations in Preventing, Identifying and Treating Violence and Abuse: http://www.ama-assn.org/ad-com/polfind/Hlth-Ethics.pdf
Society for Adolescent Health and Medicine	Adolescent Firearm Violence: http://www.adolescenthealth.org/SAHM_Main/media/Advocacy/Positions/Aug-05-Firearms_and_Adolescents.pdf Bullying and Peer Victimization: http://www.adolescenthealth.org/SAHM_Main/media/Advocacy/Positions/Jan-05-Bullying_and_Peer_Victimization.pdf
US Department of Health and Human Services	Screening for Domestic Violence in Health Care Settings: http://aspe.hhs.gov/hsp/13/dv/pb_screeningDomestic.pdf
US Preventive Services Task Force	Screening for Intimate Partner Violence, Clinical Summary: http://www.uspreventiveservicestaskforce.org/uspstf12/ipvelder/ipveldersum.htm

Table 5
Screening and counseling related to adolescent violence involvement

Screening for Adolescent Violence Involvement	Counseling Related to Adolescent Violence Involvement
Youth	*Youth*
Routinely screen for violence involvement • Recognize the interrelatedness of violence involvement, finding impact from one type of violence should prompt screening and assessment for involvement in other forms of violence • Have separate questions that address bullying, dating violence, weapon carrying (access), weapon-related injury, physical fighting, and fight-related injury • Incorporate questions into a written questionnaire to facilitate screening and counseling • Include witnessing violence in screening: explore related feelings of stress and fear of becoming a target of violence	In general • Send clear messages that violence is not an answer to problems and conflict resolution • Support youth development of strategies that focus on communication skill building, conflict management, and brave bystander behavior • Counsel youth to notify an adult if witness violence Bullying involvement • Send a clear message that bullying is not normative • Include information about technology-based bullying: help youth distinguish neutral or positive experiences from abuse, coercion, and exploitation • For victims: counsel against retaliation behaviors; explore options for building key friendships (a buddy, older youth mentor to ease social isolation and loneliness); mental health referral (mindfulness skill-building, stress management and coping, ongoing evaluation) • For perpetrators: explore motivations for behavioral change; mental health referral (anger management, ongoing behavioral evaluation) Dating/relationship violence • Counsel youth about healthy dating relationships • Explore masculine norms that may impede prevention messages: toughness and dominance; male entitlement; power • Explore feminine norms that may impede prevention, abuse messages: vulnerability; submissiveness

Parent	Parent
• Screen parents for intimate partner violence during health supervision visits for youth • Screen for good parent communication and school involvement • Screen for presence and storage of weapons in the home	*In general* • Counsel on violence prevention and the importance of modeling behavior • Check-in on conflict resolution views and disciplinary practices; address nonviolent means of conflict resolution with child • Check-in on weapon access and storage in the home, other homes/places child visits *Youth bullying involvement* • For victims: provide supportive environment, recognize crisis, explore options for youth involvement in community activities, youth mental health referral • For perpetrators: disciplinary style (nonviolence; authoritative style: nurturing, responsive, having high expectations; setting clear rules and guidelines); monitor activities; have zero tolerance policy for aggression as a coping or problem-solving strategy; youth mental health referral *Youth dating/relationship violence* • Know child's friends and romantic partners • Set clear expectations for dating behavior • Discuss characteristics of healthy relationships • Review strategies for achieving safety if the youth feels threatened

Box 1
Example questions for assessing adolescent violence involvement

Fighting

Have you been in any fights during the past year? If yes, how many? Were weapons used?

Have you ever been injured or injured someone else in a fight?

Access, Carrying Weapons

Do you carry a weapon for any reason (even if for self-defense)? If yes, what weapon?

Do you have access to any weapons?

Bullying, Threatening Behavior

Have you ever been threatened, made fun of, or excluded from activities in school, in your neighborhood, through e-mail, texting, or online?

Have you ever threatened, made fun of, or excluded someone from activities in school, in your neighborhood, through e-mail, texting, or online?

Dating/Relationship Violence

Does the person you are seeing (people you hang out with)[a] shame you, make you feel stupid, or make you feel afraid?

Does the person you are seeing (people you hang out with)[a] pressure you to do things that you are not ready for?

Does the person you are seeing (people you hang out with)[a] want to know or try to control where you go, who you see, or what you wear?

Does the person you are seeing (people you hang out with)[a] yell at you, grab you, push you, or hit you?

[a] In early-middle adolescence, dating may more commonly start out in group form.

and applicable in the office setting are available (**Table 6**). Screening activities should be supported with counseling on strategies to facilitate healthy youth development and violence avoidance (see **Table 5**; **Table 7**). Counseling should address youth and parent needs (see **Tables 5** and **7**).

Table 6
Short, validated, clinically accessible screening tools on topics related to adolescent violence

Screen Name	Screen Characteristics	Screen Link
CRAFFT	• 6 items • Screen for high-risk alcohol and other drug use	http://www.ceasar-boston.org/CRAFFT/
Patient Health Questionnaire-9 Item (PHQ-9), Modified for Teens	• 13 items • Screen for major depression in adolescents	http://www.lfmp.com/Portals/8/PHQ-9%20(Depression%20Screener%20for%20Adolescents%2012-18).pdf
Pediatric Symptom Checklist-17 (PSC-17)	• 17 items • 3 psychosocial problem subscales (internalizing, attention, externalizing) • Youth and parent versions	http://www.massgeneral.org/psychiatry/services/psc_home.aspx
Rapid Assessment for Adolescent Preventive Services (RAAPS)	• 21 items • General risk assessment survey	https://www.raaps.org/. Accessible for clinical use with registration

Table 7
Online resources for the screening and management of adolescent violence involvement

Resource Name	Resource Components	Resource Link
Connected Kids: Safe, Strong, Secure (American Academy of Pediatrics)	• Provider focus on strength-based approach to anticipatory guidance • Reviews counseling schedule, with example questions for parents and youth according to early, middle, and late adolescence (and across age spectrum)	Connected Kids Materials: https://www2.aap.org/connectedkids/material.htm
Futures Without Violence	• Recommendations for discussing healthy relationships with adolescents (sample scripts) • Sample clinic protocol for adolescent relationship abuse prevention and intervention • Safety cards • Video case studies	Hanging Out or Hooking Up: Clinical guidelines on responding to adolescent relationship violence: http://www.futureswithoutviolence.org/userfiles/file/HealthCare/Hanging-Out-or-Hooking-Up_Low_Res_Cropped_FINAL.pdf
Massachusetts Medical Society Violence Prevention Project	• Clinical suggestions for violence screening, evaluation, anticipatory guidance, and documentation (across age spectrum) • Tools and tips for parents (adolescent examples): bullying, dating violence, street violence, gun violence	Violence Prevention and Intervention; Guidebook for Physicians: http://www.massmed.org/violence/
Department of Health and Human Services: Stop Bullying	• Parent, educator, community focus: bullying prevention training module • Youth engagement toolkit • Community engagement toolkit • State laws and policies	Stop Bullying: http://www.stopbullying.gov/index.html
Break the Cycle	• Youth, community focus on teen dating violence • State report cards	Break the Cycle: Empowering Youth to End Domestic Violence: http://www.breakthecycle.org/
Stop Bullying Now	• Focus on schools, parents, youth • Resources for building respect, resilience, relationships	Stop Bullying Now: http://www.stopbullyingnow.com/index.htm
Love is Respect	• Focus on youth, peer-led discussions on relationship abuse • Relationship quiz	Love is Respect: http://www.loveisrespect.org/

Preparing the Office Setting

Screening for violence involvement should occur in an office setting that is prepared to deal with a range of associated behavioral outcomes. It is important for providers to seek out and provide opportunities for training in screening for and management of adolescent violence involvement (see **Table 7**). If not already present, providers should work toward creating an office protocol for screening of domestic violence as well as other forms of violence. Protocols will facilitate identification of victims and assist in making appropriate referrals.[53,54] The importance of screening for intimate partner violence in the household setting cannot be overstated. Intimate partner violence in a household increases the risk of youth experiencing abuse and/or witnessing violence. Child abuse and witnessing violence are risk factors for youth violence involvement. As well, in-service training during staff and other clinic meetings may facilitate greater recognition of violence-related symptoms and create an environment of heightened surveillance. Staff skill-building should be supplemented with the development a repository of local resources and organizations that address youth violence involvement and violence-related conditions. These resources should include interventions found to be effective in violence prevention, including parent training programs, home visitation programs, family therapy, mental health counseling, and substance abuse/chemical dependency programing available to adolescents.[11,55] Research demonstrates that screening coupled with office-initiated referral may facilitate reductions in violence involvement. For example, in a study of 8 outpatient community and pediatric practices, psychosocial screening and the availability of a telephone-based parenting education program was associated with decreases in youth aggression, delinquent behavior, bullying, physical fighting, fight-related injury, and bullying involvement.[56]

Advocacy Outside of the Office

There also are opportunities for providers to advocate on behalf of adolescent patients in contexts reaching outside of the primary care office. Providers can meet the staff of community organizations that focus on youth development and engagement and establish referral mechanisms with them. Engagement with school staff (psychologist, social worker, school nurse, and administration) may serve to build a stronger system for communication and safety promotion.

SUMMARY

Adolescent interpersonal violence is preventable. Health care providers must be attentive to multiple levels of influence to identify youth at greatest risk for violence involvement and related poor health outcomes. Violence screening and counseling activities occurring in the context of periodic comprehensive health assessment represents one of our best opportunities for prevention, identification, and intervention on behalf of youth.

REFERENCES

1. National Center for Injury Prevention and Control, Web-based Injury Statistics Query & Reporting System (WISQARS). Leading causes of death reports, national and regional, 1999–2010. Available at: http://webappa.cdc.gov/sasweb/ncipc/leadcaus10_us.html. Accessed November 9, 2013.
2. National Center for Injury Prevention and Control. Youth violence: facts at a glance. 2012. Available at: http://www.cdc.gov/violenceprevention/pdf/yv-datasheet-a.pdf. Accessed November 9, 2013.
3. National Center for HIV/AIDS, Viral Hepatitis, STD, and TB Prevention, Division of Adolescent and School Health. Youth risk behavior surveillance system: 2011 national overview. Available at: http://www.cdc.gov/healthyyouth/yrbs/pdf/us_overview_yrbs.pdf. Accessed November 9, 2013.

4. National Center for HIV/AIDS, Viral Hepatitis, STD, and TB Prevention, Division of Adolescent and School Health. Youth risk behavior surveillance system: selected 2011 National Health Risk Behaviors and Health Outcomes by Sex. Available at: http://www.cdc.gov/healthyyouth/yrbs/pdf/us_disparitysex_yrbs. pdf. Accessed November 9, 2013.
5. National Center for Injury Prevention and Control, Web-based Injury Statistics Query & Reporting System (WISQARS). Leading Causes of Nonfatal Injury Reports, 2001-2012. Available at: http://webappa.cdc.gov/sasweb/ncipc/ nfilead2001.html. Accessed December 10, 2013.
6. Wolitzky KB, Ruggiero KJ, Danielson CK, et al. Prevalence and correlates of dating violence in national sample of adolescents. J Am Acad Child Adolesc Psychiatry 2008;47(7):755-62.
7. Wang J, Iannotti RJ, Nansel TR. School bullying among adolescents in the United States: physical, verbal, relational, and cyber. J Adolesc Health 2009;45:368-75.
8. Bureau of Justice. Indicators of School Crime and Safety 2012. Available at: http://nces.ed.gov/pubs2013/2013036.pdf. Accessed November 11, 2013.
9. Resnick MD, Bearman PS, Blum RW, et al. Protecting adolescents from harm: findings from the National Longitudinal Study of Adolescent Health. JAMA 1997;278:823-32.
10. Resnick MD, Ireland M, Borowsky IW. Youth violence perpetration: what protects? What predicts? Findings from the National Longitudinal Study of Adolescent Health. J Adolesc Health 2004;35:424.e1-10.
11. Borowsky IW, Ireland M. Predictors of future fight-related injury among adolescents. Pediatrics 2004;113:530-6.
12. Duke NN, Borowsky IW, Pettingell SL, et al. Examining youth hopelessness and an independent risk correlate for adolescent delinquency and violence. Matern Child Health J 2011;15:87-97.
13. Stoddard SA, Henly SJ, Sieving RE, et al. Social connections, trajectories of hopelessness, and serious violence in impoverished urban youth. J Youth Adolesc 2011;40:278-95.
14. Bearinger LH, Pettingell S, Resnick MD, et al. Violence perpetration among urban American Indian youth: can protection offset risk? Arch Pediatr Adolesc Med 2005;159:270-7.
15. Foshee VA, Reyes HL, Ennett ST, et al. Risk and protective factors distinguishing profiles of adolescent peer and dating violence perpetration. J Adolesc Health 2011;48:344-50.
16. Yexley M, Borowsky I, Ireland M. Correlation between different experiences of intrafamilial physical violence and violent adolescent behavior. J Interpers Violence 2002;17(7):707-20.
17. Duke NN, Pettingell SL, McMorris BJ, et al. Adolescent violence perpetration: associations with multiple types of adverse child experiences. Pediatrics 2010;125:e778-86.
18. Ohene S, Ireland M, McNeely C, et al. Parental expectations, physical punishment, and violence among adolescents who score positive on a psychosocial screening test in primary care. Pediatrics 2006;117:441-7.
19. McNulty TL, Bellair PE. Explaining racial and ethnic difference in adolescent violence: structural disadvantage, family well-being, and social capital. Justice Q 2003;20(1):1-31.
20. Widome R, Sieving RE, Harpin SA, et al. Measuring neighborhood connection and the association with violence in young adolescents. J Adolesc Health 2008;43:482-9.

21. Masten AS, Best KM, Garmezy N. Resilience and development: contributions from the study of children who overcame adversity. Dev Psychopathol 1990;2: 425–44.
22. Resnick MD. Protective factors, resiliency, and healthy youth development. Adolesc Med 2000;11:157–64.
23. American Academy of Pediatrics, Committee on Injury, Violence, and Poison Prevention. Policy statement: role of the pediatrician in youth violence prevention. Pediatrics 2009;124(1):393–402.
24. Olweus D. Bullying or peer abuse at school: facts and intervention. Curr Dir Psychol Sci 1995;4(6):196–200.
25. Nansel TR, Overpeck M, Pilla RS, et al. Bullying behaviors among US youth: prevalence and association with psychological adjustment. J Am Med Assoc 2001;285(16):2094–100.
26. Williams KR, Guerra NG. Prevalence and predictors of Internet bullying. J Adolesc Health 2007;41:S14–21.
27. Van der Wal MF, de Wit CA, Hirasing RA. Psychosocial health among young victims and offenders of direct and indirect bullying. Pediatrics 2003;111: 1312–7.
28. Hinduja S, Patchin JW. Offline consequences of online victimization. J Sch Violence 2007;6(3):89–112.
29. Mishna F, Saini M, Solomon S. Ongoing and online: children and youth's perceptions of cyber bullying. Child Youth Serv Rev 2009;31:1222–8.
30. Hensley V. Childhood bullying: a review and implications for health care professionals. Nurs Clin North Am 2013;48:203–13.
31. Smokowski PR, Kopasz KH. Bullying in school: an overview of types, effects, family characteristics, and intervention strategies. Child Schools 2005;27(2): 101–10.
32. Spriggs AL, Iannotti RJ, Nansel TR, et al. Adolescent bullying involvement and perceived family, peer, and school relations: commonalities and differences across race/ethnicity. J Adolesc Health 2007;41:283–93.
33. Swearer SM, Espelage DL, Vaillancourt T, et al. What can be done about school bullying? Linking research to education practice. Educational Researcher 2010; 39:8–47.
34. Nansel TR, Overpeck M, Haynie DL, et al. Relationships between bullying and violence among US youth. Arch Pediatr Adolesc Med 2003;157:348–53.
35. Borowsky IW, Taliaferro LA, McMorris BJ. Suicidal thinking and behavior among youth involved in verbal and social bullying: risk and protective factors. J Adolesc Health 2013;53:S4–12.
36. Espelage DL, Basile KC, Hamburger ME. Bullying perpetration and subsequent sexual violence perpetration among middle school students. J Adolesc Health 2012;50:60–5.
37. Gower AL, Borowsky IW. Associations between frequency of bullying involvement and adjustment in adolescence. Acad Pediatr 2013;13(3):214–21.
38. Wekerle C, Wolfe DA. Dating violence in mid-adolescence: theory, significance, and emerging prevention initiatives. Clin Psychol Rev 1999;19(4):435–56.
39. Smith PH, White JW, Holland LJ. A longitudinal perspective on dating violence among adolescent and college-age women. Am J Public Health 2003;93: 1104–9.
40. Noonan RK, Charles D. Developing teen dating violence prevention strategies: formative research with middle school youth. Violence Against Women 2009; 15(9):1087–105.

41. Arriaga XB, Foshee VA. Adolescent dating violence: do adolescents follow their friends', or their parents', footsteps? J Interpers Violence 2004;19(2):162–84.
42. Burke LK, Follingstad DR. Violence in lesbian and gay relationships: theory, prevalence, and correlational factors. Clin Psychol Rev 1999;19(5):487–512.
43. Hickman LJ, Jaycox LH, Aronoff J. Dating violence among adolescents: prevalence, gender distribution, and prevention program effectiveness. Trauma Violence Abuse 2004;5:123–42.
44. Freedner N, Freed LH, Yang W, et al. Dating violence among gay, lesbian, and bisexual adolescents: results from a community survey. J Adolesc Health 2002; 31(6):469–74.
45. Halpern CT, Young ML, Waller MW, et al. Prevalence of partner violence in same-sex romantic and sexual relationships in a national sample of adolescents. J Adolesc Health 2004;35(2):124–31.
46. Wolfe DA, Scott K, Wekerle C, et al. Child maltreatment: risk of adjustment problems and dating violence in adolescence. J Am Acad Child Adolesc Psychiatry 2001;40(3):282–9.
47. Sears HA, Byers ES, Whelan JJ, et al. "If it hurts, then it's not a joke": adolescents' ideas about girls' and boys' use and experience of abusive behavior in dating relationships. J Interpers Violence 2006;21(9):1191–207.
48. Banyard VL, Cross C, Modecki KL. Interpersonal violence in adolescence: ecological correlates of self-reported perpetration. J Interpers Violence 2006; 21(10):1314–32.
49. Whitaker DJ, Morrison S, Lindquist C, et al. A critical review of interventions for the primary prevention of perpetration of partner violence. Aggress Violent Behav 2006;11:151–66.
50. Swahn MH, Simon TR, Hertz MF, et al. Linking dating violence, peer violence, and suicidal behaviors among high-risk youth. Am J Prev Med 2008;31(1):30–8.
51. Ozer EJ, Tschann JM, Pasch LA, et al. Violence perpetration across peer and partner relationships: co-occurrence and longitudinal patterns among adolescents. J Adolesc Health 2004;34:64–71.
52. Campbell J. Health consequences of intimate partner violence. Lancet 2002; 359:1331–6.
53. Borowsky IW, Ireland M. Parental screening for intimate partner violence by pediatricians and family physicians. Pediatrics 2002;110:509–16.
54. Borowsky IW, Ireland M. National survey of pediatricians' violence prevention counseling. Arch Pediatr Adolesc Med 1999;153:1170–6.
55. Borowsky IW, Widome R, Resnick MD. Young people and violence. International Encyclopedia of Public Health 2008;6:675–84.
56. Borowsky IW, Mozayeny S, Stuenkel K, et al. Effect of a primary-care based intervention on violent behavior and injury in children. Pediatrics 2004;114: e392–9.

Health Care for Youth Involved with the Correctional System

Raymond C.W. Perry, MD, MS[a],*, Robert E. Morris, MD[b]

KEYWORDS

- Adolescents • Juvenile detention facilities • Correctional system

KEY POINTS

- Youth involved with the correctional system are disproportionately impacted by negative health outcomes, related to both physical and mental health.
- Detention settings allow time for providers to ensure that health issues for adolescents are addressed, but many challenges exist to providing care in these facilities.
- Community-based providers should be aware of adolescent patients who have a history of being detained and ensure that all necessary aspects of their health and well-being are followed closely after the youth is released home.

INTRODUCTION

Youth who are currently or who have been incarcerated represent a significant number of adolescents, a group that is often medically underserved and that has substantial physical and mental health needs.[1-3] In 2011, more than 60,000 youth in the United States spent time in correctional facilities.[4] Both the absolute numbers of youth who are detained and the rate of detention has steadily decreased over the past several years as a result of declining arrest rates and changing state and local legal policies regarding the management of youth who commit delinquent acts.[3,5,6] However, those who are detained often have the greatest need for physical and mental health care.

DEMOGRAPHICS

The demographics of youth in detention are important to consider because of health disparities that are related to gender, race, and ethnicity. Detained women account for

[a] Department of Health Services, Los Angeles County Juvenile Court Health Services, 1925 Daly Street, 1st Floor, Los Angeles, CA 90031, USA; [b] General Pediatrics, Department of Pediatrics, 12-460, University of California at Los Angeles, 10833 LeConte Avenue, Los Angeles, CA 90095-1752, USA
* Corresponding author.
E-mail address: rperry@dhs.lacounty.gov

Prim Care Clin Office Pract 41 (2014) 691–705
http://dx.doi.org/10.1016/j.pop.2014.05.007
0095-4543/14/$ – see front matter © 2014 Elsevier Inc. All rights reserved.

nearly 14% of all incarcerated youth, and tend to have more physical and mental health needs.[3,4,6] Youth of racial or ethnic minorities are overrepresented in correctional facilities: black youth represent 40% of detainees and Hispanic/Latino youth represent 23%. In comparison, white youth constitute 32% of detainees.[4] Another significant demographic consideration is that lower socioeconomic status is correlated with juvenile delinquency and is especially prevalent among the black and Hispanic youth who are detained.[3,6] These characteristics of incarcerated youth help define the health needs of these adolescents, because many of the social determinants of poor health are also associated with delinquency.[3]

JUVENILE JUSTICE PROCESS

Youth generally enter the juvenile justice system through law enforcement (ie, after an arrest). Other referrals to the juvenile courts may be made by parents, schools, victims, or probation officers. Fortunately, the rates of arrest and confinement for all crimes—violent crimes, person offenses, property offenses, drug offenses, public order offenses, technical violations, and status offenses (acts that are illegal based on the age of the offender, but not for adults)—have been steadily decreasing over the past decade.[5,7]

Youths arrested for an alleged infraction may be diverted to management outside of the court system (eg, to a community-based treatment program). According to the U.S. Department of Justice, in 2009 this accounted for 22% of police cases.[8] For other arrests, the police will determine if the youth can be safely released home with a date to return to court, or the police or judge may order the youth to stay in a secure detention facility until their court hearing (either because of the seriousness of the crime or because a stable place for release cannot be identified). After the court hearing, a youth who is found to be guilty (often referred to in juvenile courts as "the petition is sustained") may be released on house arrest or will be ordered to serve time in a residential treatment or rehabilitation facility. These residential facilities may be referred to as *placement homes*, *group homes*, *camps*, *ranches*, *halls*, or other names, depending on the jurisdiction. Residential placement accounted for 27% of adjudications in 2009.[8] After residential placement, youth will be released home and will remain on probation for a court-determined length of time, during which the youth remains under supervision of the court or the juvenile corrections department.

HEALTH CARE SERVICES IN DETENTION FACILITIES

Although the spectrum of services on-site varies widely between correctional facilities,[9] federal law requires that detention halls and residential treatment facilities offer health care services to all detained youth. Additionally, individual state case laws may mandate more specific provisions regarding the extent to which correctional health care services must be available. These laws dictate areas of care, including initial screening and evaluation, access to urgent care during detention, preventive care services, staff training, nutritional services, and several other areas.[10]

In addition to these laws, correctional facilities may voluntarily seek accreditation by the National Commission on Correctional Health Care (NCCHC), which sets standards for providing appropriate health care in all corrections facilities and has specific standards for juvenile facilities.[10] For example, NCCHC standards mandate a process for emergency care and a system of sick call in which youths' requests for care are assessed daily by a nurse and appropriate action is taken based on the urgency of the situation. They also require physical health, oral health, and mental health screenings on admission, and respective follow-up care by a trained professional within a specifically determined period.[10]

Various national provider organizations have policy statements that support the provision of comprehensive health care services to detained juveniles and offer guidelines for care. The American Academy of Pediatrics (AAP) Committee on Adolescence recently updated their extensive policy statement, "Health Care for Youth in the Juvenile Justice System," which reviews the health status of detained juveniles and suggests standards of appropriate care.[6] The Society for Adolescent Health and Medicine and the American Public Health Association also have policy statements supporting comprehensive health care in correctional settings.[11,12] The American Medical Association's Guidelines for Adolescent Preventive Services (GAPS) and the AAP's Bright Futures guidelines offer complete lists of all services that should be provided for adolescent health visits.[13,14] The NCCHC also publishes several clinical guidelines (available at http://www.ncchc.org/guidelines) specifically developed to address the needs of incarcerated youth.[15] All of these resources provide useful recommendations for providing optimal care to youth in correctional settings.

HEALTH OF DETAINED YOUTH AND GOALS FOR CARE IN DETENTION

Several studies and surveys have confirmed that youth involved in the juvenile justice system are disproportionately affected by poor health outcomes.[1,3,6,9,11,16–18] By the very nature of being involved in the juvenile justice system, these youth represent a group who are frequently involved in risky health behaviors related to substance use, sexual experiences, and delinquent activities.[1–3,6,11,16] Many of the physical, development, and mental health needs seen in juvenile detention settings are more prevalent than among the general adolescent population (**Box 1**). Furthermore, many enter detention facilities with medical or mental health issues that were previously undiagnosed or inadequately managed.[1,3,6,16]

Immunizations

In line with the standard guidelines for promoting adolescent health, immunizations are important for preventive care, and detention provides an opportunity to offer these services, particularly because many detained youth have not had a regular source of primary care before being incarcerated.[16] The Centers for Disease Control and

---

Box 1
Health disparities affecting incarcerated youth

- Sexually transmitted infections
- Teenage pregnancy and parenthood
- Chronic conditions affecting ethnic minorities and low socioeconomic status communities (eg, asthma, type II diabetes, sickle cell disease)
- Attention-deficit/hyperactivity disorder and learning disorders
- Behavioral problems (eg, conduct disorder, anger management)
- Posttraumatic stress disorder
- Mood disorders (eg, depression)
- Substance abuse
- Suicidality

Prevention (CDC) recommends that all adolescents older than 11 years receive tetanus, diphtheria, acellular pertussis (Tdap); meningococcal; and human papillomavirus vaccines. In addition, adolescents who are not up-to-date on other childhood vaccines (hepatitis A, hepatitis B, varicella, mumps, rubella, and polio) should receive vaccines according to the catch-up schedule.[19]

Chronic Illnesses

Chronic illnesses are very important health considerations in juvenile detention facilities. Regardless of whether the facility provides short-term detention while awaiting trial and disposition or longer-term residential custody, chronic conditions can be addressed and managed so that the health of the youth is stabilized. At a minimum, providing relevant health education and setting health goals for patients with chronic disease are important elements of care, and these recommendations are emphasized by the NCCHC Juvenile Standards.[10] Certain illnesses, such as seizure disorders, diabetes, sickle cell disease, and asthma, can have serious medical consequences if not managed adequately. Therefore, these conditions must be identified early on admission and managed appropriately.

Sexual and Reproductive Health Issues

Sexual and reproductive health issues are a significant area of morbidity among detained youth.[1,3,6,11,18] Compared with a general high school population, incarcerated youth report higher rates of sexual activity, a higher average number of lifetime partners, and lower use of contraception or condoms.[1,3,18] As a result, these youth are at a higher risk for sexually transmitted infections (STIs) and unplanned pregnancies. In 2011, the rate of chlamydia among women in juvenile correctional settings in 2011 was 13.5%, and was 6.7% for men entering juvenile detention facilities.[20] These rates, and those for gonorrhea, are significantly higher than STI rates in similar gender and age groups in the general population. Many incarcerated youth are also at higher risk for HIV and hepatitis C infection, particularly if they are involved in commercial sex work or injection drug use.[6] Education about STIs is important for this population. The U.S. Preventative Services Task Force (USPSTF) recommends high-intensity behavioral counseling to prevent STIs for all sexually active adolescents.[21] Furthermore, the CDC, in their 2010 Sexually Transmitted Disease Treatment Guidelines, recommends routine screening for sexually active adolescents, regardless of whether they are symptomatic (**Table 1**).[22] The common practice of only screening youth with symptoms misses many youth who are infected asymptomatically. Diagnosing and treating asymptomatic infections can prevent complications for individuals (eg, pelvic inflammatory disease) and may limit the spread of infections in the communities to which the detainees will be released. Despite the high prevalence of STIs among detained youth, less than one-quarter of juvenile detention facilities currently screen admitted youth for STIs or HIV.[9]

Parenthood and pregnancy status also impact incarcerated youth more than the general adolescent population, with 1 of 5 detained youth either having a child or expecting a child.[2,3,23] A 2009 survey found that 14% of incarcerated youth had children; 15% of men and 9% of women. In comparison, 2% of teenage men and 6% of teenage women in the general US population had children. Additionally, 12% of incarcerated youth were expecting a child while detained. More than one-third of detained women reported having ever been pregnant.[2] Less than one-fifth of all facilities test all entering women for pregnancy, although most offer testing when necessary or when requested by a youth.[23]

Table 1		
CDC recommendations for STI testing in detained adolescents		
	Women	**Men**
Chlamydia	Universal screening of all adolescents at intake in juvenile or jail facilities	All sexually active in adolescent clinics, correctional facilities, and sexually transmitted disease clinics on intake
Gonorrhea	Universal screening of all adolescents at intake in juvenile or jail facilities	Not recommended universally, but for men who have sex with men: urethral screening for insertive intercourse and anal screening for receptive intercourse Pharyngeal testing for receptive oral intercourse
Syphilis	Universal screening based on local area and institutional prevalence	Universal screening based on local area and institutional prevalence Screen all men who have sex with men
HIV	Screening for all sexually active and users of injection drugs	Screening for all sexually active and users of injection drugs Screening is especially important for men who have sex with men

Data from Workowski KA, Berman S, Centers for Disease Control and Prevention. Sexually transmitted diseases treatment guidelines. MMWR Recomm Rep 2010;59(RR-12):1–110.

General Health Complaints

General health complaints, although similar to those in nondetained youth, are more common in the juvenile justice population, because of the social determinants of health existent in the youths' lives before detention (eg, community-based health risks or exposures and a lack of access to medical care), and problems created by the institutional environment.[9] On admission to a detention center, the most common acute complaints include headache, abdominal pain, back or joint pain, and upper respiratory symptoms.[1,16] In long-term detention facilities, dental, dermatologic, musculoskeletal/trauma, and respiratory issues are among the more prevalent acute health needs, aside from psychiatric or behavioral issues.[1,16]

Mental Health Issues and Suicidality

Mental health issues represent some of the most predominant health needs of detained youth. Attention-deficit/hyperactivity disorder (ADHD), learning disorders, depression, anxiety, disruptive behaviors (eg, conduct disorder), posttraumatic stress, and substance abuse are among the most common diagnoses seen in this population, and are much more prevalent among detained youth than in the general population of adolescents.[1,3,6,11,17,18,24] In fact, although the prevalence of serious psychiatric conditions within the general pediatric and adolescent population is estimated to be 7% to 12%, the rate among detained youth is 60% to 80%, with rates generally higher for women.[1,24] Furthermore, many youth have more than one psychiatric diagnosis.[1,24] Diagnosing and treating these disorders during adolescence is crucial because of the associations with other mental health conditions later in life, such as the relation between disruptive disorders of adolescence and personality disorders in adulthood.[25] Early and effective management is also important to prevent worsening of the clinical or behavioral manifestations and to avoid the potential of more serious legal consequences as the youth enter adulthood. Screening for general mental health issues with validated tools, such as the Massachusetts Youth Screening Instrument, the Beck Depression Inventory, or the Patient Health Questionnaire, is offered to youth at many facilities, but not all.[1,17]

Histories of suicidal ideation, attempts, and completions are more than twice as frequent among youth in custody than among nondetained adolescents.[1-3,18,24,26] Even in the controlled setting of detention facilities, suicide attempts remain a significant concern. The stresses of being incarcerated, awaiting court decisions, and being separated from family and peers; a history of physical, sexual, or emotional abuse and/or substance use; and any preexisting mental health issues contribute to the risk of suicidality.[1,3,18,24,27] A study found that 52% of detained youth reported current suicidal ideation and more than one-third reported suicide attempts, with a direct relationship between suicidality and reported histories of abuse.[28] The rate of suicide completion among detained youth is more than 4 times higher than the rate for youth overall.[29] Additionally, even after release, youth with a history of incarceration have an ongoing substantial risk of suicidal attempts during their lifetime.[1,30] Effective suicide prevention programs that involve all staff who interact with youth are a vital part of correctional health services and should begin on a youth's admission to a facility.[6,27]

Substance Use and Abuse

Substance use or abuse is also common among detained youth and often exists comorbidly with other mental health issues.[1-3,6,18] The rates of tobacco, alcohol, and drug use among youth in custody are much higher than among the overall adolescent population (Table 2).[1,6,17,18] Despite high rates of substance use and abuse in association with psychiatric issues and delinquent behavior, not all facilities screen universally for substance use or offer individualized treatment plans for substance abuse.[6,17]

SPECIAL POPULATIONS
Girls

Girls in corrections are different from boys. Braverman and Morris outlined some of the medical differences, including a greater likelihood of having any psychiatric disorder, specifically anxiety and mood disorders.[3] Related to this is the common finding of physical, sexual, and emotional abuse in incarcerated girls that is associated with risky sexual behaviors and suicidality. Girls' substance abuse compared with boys is more likely to involve substances other than alcohol and marijuana.[3,31]

As a consequence of high exposure to all types of abuse, many girls are often in unequal power relationships with boys. This unequal relationship makes it difficult for delinquent girls to develop self-esteem or skills in self-protection. For this reason,

Table 2		
Lifetime substance use among detained youth and general adolescent population		
Substance	Detained Youth (%)	General Population of 12- to 20-Year Olds (%)
Alcohol	74	56
Marijuana or hashish	84	30
Cocaine or crack	30	6
Ecstasy	26	6
Crystal methamphetamine	22	2

Data from Sedlak AJ, McPherson KS. OJJDP Juvenile Justice Bulletin: youth's needs and services. 2010. Available at: https://www.ncjrs.gov/pdffiles1/ojjdp/227728.pdf. Accessed November 24, 2013.

it has been suggested that facilities for girls be staffed exclusively by women or, at minimum, that all staff are trained to help girls learn to be appropriately assertive in their relationships with both genders.[31] Health care providers should also understand these dynamics to avoid actions that may seem to be insensitive or domineering of female patients.

In 2002, Congress passed the Juvenile Justice and Delinquency Prevention Act mandating that states assess their services to girls and implement gender-specific services.[32] Other agencies have also documented the need for gender-specific services, including prenatal and postpartum health services, guidelines for overall treatment of pregnant detainees, and contraceptive options available during incarceration and on release.[10,31,33] Unfortunately, many of the recommendations have not been adopted by the various jurisdictions that govern coed and female juvenile justice facilities.[31]

Gay, Lesbian, Bisexual, or Transgender Youth

Gay, lesbian, bisexual, or transgender (LGBT) youth are particularly vulnerable while in correctional facilities, and constitute a significant proportion of the population, although they tend to remain "hidden."[34,35] In 2010, Irvine conducted a survey of 2100 youth in corrections and found that overall, 15% reported being LGBT, representing 11% of boys and 27% of girls, and with equal distribution among different races.[35] Most (80%) of these youth behave in a gender-conforming way and therefore are not immediately obvious to the staff.[36] As a result, most LGBT youth in corrections may not be identified unless they disclose this information.

Once in detention, LGBT youth often believe they must keep their sexual orientation a secret to avoid harassment, differential treatment, or sexual and physical assault from other detainees and staff.[36] In fact, they are significantly more likely to be sexually assaulted, with 12.5% of nonheterosexual youth reporting sexual victimization compared with 1.3% of heterosexual youth.[37] As a result of these fears, problems such as school troubles and family discord that are related to their sexuality may not be addressed, and LGBT youth may experience higher levels of stress than other detainees.[34]

Gender-nonconforming youth in the justice system are significantly more likely than heterosexual and gender-conforming LGBT youth to have experienced home removal, lived in foster homes, been homeless, been detained in a juvenile facility for running away, and been charged with nonviolent offense.[35] Because LGBT youth often have problems at school due to harassment by classmates, and problems at home due to rejection, they are more likely to be detained once arrested, because the authorities may judge their social situation as unstable and may assume that a detention facility is a safer setting. However, this results in incarceration that may be unnecessary and that may actually be more harmful to the youth because of the risks of assault or harassment in detention settings.[38] If the court deems home life undesirable, LGBT youth may be detained for long periods, further subjecting them to stress and interruption of their normal adolescent development.[38] On disposition, many LGBT youth will be placed on probation with stipulations, such as following parental dictates and attending school—requirements with which the youth may not be able to comply because they would be placed in unsafe situations.

The Juvenile Facility Standards of the Prison Rape Elimination Act issued by the U.S. Department of Justice in 2012 mandates national standards related to sexual assault and sensitivity toward LGBT inmates.[39] The promulgation of these regulations should bring a measure of uniformity to the appropriate management of LGBT youth in detention and allow for corrective action when the mandates are not met in a facility.

SELECTED RELEVANT BIOLOGICAL AND CONGENITAL GENETIC DISORDERS

A variety of biological issues are overrepresented in delinquent youth, although none of them are reliably predictive of criminal behavior. Shonkoff and colleagues[40] published a review of 114 studies in 2009 that argued that the roots of maladaptive behaviors that may lead to incarceration are associated with fetal and neonatal toxic stresses, such as nutritional deficiencies, obesity in the mother, drug/alcohol exposure, postnatal child abuse/neglect, extreme poverty, and family violence. These stresses can modify epigenes, which determine how genes are read and expressed. The epigenes can ultimately act to induce a negative health status and behavior difficulties. These transformed epigenes are then passed to the next offspring, amplifying the bad effects from generation to generation. Given the poor social structures many incarcerated youth experienced in childhood, this work provides a theoretic framework to understand the genesis of much delinquent behavior.[40]

Klinefelter Syndrome

Klinefelter syndrome is a genetic disorder (47,XXY) that affects boys and can led to gonadal dysfunction and in some cases social and/or cognitive problems. The physical findings include very firm small testes approximately the size of shelled peanut. A patient with Klinefelter syndrome may be tall and lack typical secondary characteristics associated with testosterone effects; they may have scant facial hair, gynecomastia, and features of a female habitus. Although most of these boys are sterile, they may otherwise have normal sexual function. Laboratory tests will show low or low normal testosterone and elevated follicle-stimulating and luteinizing hormones. Shortly after puberty, the testosterone level may be normal, but will eventually decrease to low levels. Testosterone replacement therapy will cause appropriate androgenization for the boy and may ameliorate some of the various social/cognitive problems. The phenotype of these patients varies from obvious to near-normal, except for the small testicles. Therefore, they are often not diagnosed until adulthood when their sterility is discovered.[41]

If this diagnosis is made in a detained youth, a provider may opt to discuss the possible need for testosterone replacement therapy, but should avoid discussing the possibility of sterility because this might cause additional stress to the patient. A better course of action might be to reassure the youth that on release he will have continuing management by a pediatric endocrinologist who is knowledgeable about Klinefelter syndrome.

Some youth with Klinefelter syndrome may have a propensity to offend, including fire setting,[42] although most never offend. Furthermore, this increased crime rate is not seen when socioeconomic status is taken into account.[41] The increased fire-setting propensity is controversial, and some authors do not believe it exists.[43]

Fetal Alcohol Spectrum Disorders

Ethyl alcohol ingestion during pregnancy causes a series of facial anomalies, growth failure, and variable levels of cognitive dysfunction, including ADHD.[44] As the child grows, some of the classic facial stigmata associated with fetal alcohol syndrome may lessen, making diagnosis more difficult.[45] Some evidence suggests that nutritional deficiencies during pregnancy magnify the deleterious effects of alcohol on the brain.[46,47] These children have substantial problems with memory and a poor understanding of the consequences of behavior, and they tend to be easily influenced by peers and make poor decisions in life.[48,49] For these reasons, youth with fetal alcohol spectrum disorders (FASDs) may be more likely to commit offenses and be detained.

However, their underlying medical condition may not be diagnosed by facility staff.[49] A recent study highlighted the implications of FASDs as important precursors to delinquency and discussed the relevance to law enforcement, the correctional system, and the judicial system.[49]

Recent experimental work with animals exposed to alcohol during gestation found that a combination of postnatal choline, folate, and vitamin A reversed many of the learning problems in the animals even if they were adults when treatment began.[50,51] One-fifth of school age children and adults with FASD are diagnosed with anxiety, and many receive neuroleptic drugs for this.[51] Other evidence-based interventions include "Math Interactive Learning Experience," "Good Buddies," "Language to Literacy Program," and "USFA Kids." Additionally, "Parents and Children Together" and "Families Moving Forward" provide positive parenting interventions for children 4 to 12 years of age.[51] Details of some of these programs are available at http://www.aap.org/en-us/advocacy-and-policy/aap-health-initiatives/fetal-alcohol-spectrum-disorders-toolkit/Pages/default.aspx.

CHALLENGES TO CARE

Correctional facilities are particularly unique settings for providing health care. Although the basic responsibilities of providers are similar to those in any clinical setting, many considerations are distinctive to youth detention facilities (**Box 2**). When youth are detained, their daily schedules are usually strict and structured. Although health care services are mandated for detention facilities, they must compete with several other required services for all youth. For example, correctional departments are responsible for ensuring educational periods that meet state and federal requirements, providing time and resources for daily physical activity, serving 3 meals per day, and administering other rehabilitative programs. Therefore, clinical visits must fit within the other daily activities. Court hearings may also interfere with scheduling clinical visits. Court processes generally take precedence over all other activities for youth. However, if the health care professional finds that a youth is not medically stable for a court appearance, the provider can engage the court and correctional departments in a discussion about balancing health needs with legal priorities.

Youth must be escorted to the detention facility clinic by correctional officers; therefore, appointments must be coordinated with correctional staff. Low staffing available within the correctional department may create a challenge. The safety and security of

---

Box 2
Challenges to providing health care in youth detention facilities

- Daily schedules/conflicting priorities (eg, school, court)
- Security concerns
- Transportation considerations
- Lack of parental presence during visit
- Youths' perceptions of the association between health care providers and the correctional/penal system
- Availability or proximity of emergency or subspecialty care
- Recruitment of health care providers

Data from Morris RE. Health care for incarcerated adolescents: significant needs with considerable obstacles. Virtual Mentor 2005;7:1.

the youth and staff are important, and therefore there may be a limit to the number of youth held in the clinical area at any given time. Additionally, the needs for gender separation and avoidance of rival gang problems may prevent certain youth from being allowed in the clinic at the same time.

During detention, youth will receive health care in clinic without the presence of their parents or guardians. State laws vary in the extent of health services to which minors can consent for themselves.[52,53] The rights remain applicable in detention facilities and are listed for each state and the District of Columbia at https://www.guttmacher.org/statecenter/spibs/spib_OMCL.pdf.[53] Additionally, some correctional systems attempt to obtain a general consent for medical care from the parents or guardians at the time of admission to the detention facility. States and local jurisdictions have varying statutory codes that confer legal authority to the correctional health care staff to provide routine and medically necessary care whenever indicated, although parental/guardian or court consent is usually required for surgery or other invasive procedures. An example detailing the nuances of consent specifically within the juvenile detention setting of California is available at http://www.teenhealthlaw.org/fileadmin/teenhealth/teenhealthrights/ca/Juv._Justice_Consent_Manual_11-09.pdf.[54]

Many youth are not accustomed to seeking care, receiving care, or answering health questions without the guidance or assistance of parents, which can result in incomplete past medical or family histories. Parents may be reached by phone to obtain more information when necessary, but the delay between the clinic appointment and the phone conversation with a parent is less optimal than real-time access to parents in community-based health clinics and offices. For nonbasic primary care needs, the policies of the detention facility will specify when parental consent is needed for vaccinations, procedures, or access to previous medical information. Challenges in obtaining consent from parents or guardians (eg, unknown contact information, inaccurate phone numbers provided by the youth, language barriers) can lead to delays in care.

Youth who are detained may understandably associate the doctors, nurses, and other providers with the correctional/penal system, although health care staff may not answer directly to the corrections administration.[55] For this reason, some youth are reluctant to cooperate with health care staff because they view them as part of the detention system that may further penalize them. In particular, youth may think that disclosure to health care providers about risky behaviors (eg, drug use, past violence) will affect their legal charges. Helping youth understand the separation between health services and the correctional/penal system and explaining the health-focused reasons why providers may inquire about risky behaviors will facilitate gathering important health information from the youth, especially their histories of substance use and other risk behaviors. Arrest and detention are upsetting experiences and can result in uncooperative behaviors, even when the youth is ill. Considerate providers can play an important role in helping youth cope with their situation, and can lead to acceptance of health care during detention.

When youth require a higher acuity of medical care than the level of resources available in a detention facility, the youth can be referred to a local comprehensive medical facility, emergency care center, or subspecialty clinic. In making arrangements for access to outside care, the aforementioned challenges of time priorities, security, and transportation may present difficulties. Providers must convey the medical necessity clearly to correctional staff so that youth can be transported to outside care in a timely manner. Depending on the location of the detention facility (eg, proximity to a tertiary care facility, availability of pediatric subspecialties), certain medical resources may not be easily accessible.[55] Providers in detention facilities must balance the medical need with the availability of resources to develop the most feasible management plan for each youth.

Lastly, but not insignificantly, the challenges of providing adequate care in detention facilities may be amplified by the problems of inadequate health services staffing and difficulty recruiting providers.[55] Physicians may not be on-site regularly, which may limit the extent of care that can be provided in a timely manner.[9] This issue is even more significant because youth who are detained are at high risk for significant medical needs at the time of admission to the facility.[1,3,6,16]

FOLLOW-UP CARE CONSIDERATIONS

When youth are released from a detention facility, they must receive follow-up care by a community-based primary care provider so that they can continue to receive treatment for any ongoing health care issues, including monitoring their health status and health risk behaviors (**Box 3**). When seeing patients after they have been released from a detention facility, it is not essential to know the reasons for incarceration or to be concerned about innocence or guilt. Many youth involved with the correctional system have committed low-level offenses or may have been detained primarily because of poor home or social situations. However, it is important to know how long they were detained, whether they had any acute health issues while detained (eg, injuries during a fight, appendicitis, scabies), what immunizations and treatments they received in the facility, and whether any ongoing care was recommended. Community-based providers can contact correctional facilities to request copies of the health records with consent from the youth's parent. This exchange of information can help to ensure continuity of care, limit redundancy of medical workups, and prevent unnecessary changes to successful treatment plans. Providers should also ask the parent or guardian about whether any medical, mental health, or substance abuse therapy has been recommended or is required for the probation period.

Underlying factors that may have contributed to the reasons for being detained should also be investigated and managed by providers to help prevent repeated incarceration. For example, providing support and resources for a parent of an LGBT youth may help families manage related difficulties at home and school, thus avoiding behavioral problems that may lead to legal infractions. Likewise, working with a youth's school to ensure a safe environment or providing assistance to youth with learning difficulties may promote academic success and fewer behavioral troubles in school.

Box 3
Key points for community providers caring for formerly detained youth

- Request medical records or discharge summaries from detention facility
- Determine if patient needs subspecialty, mental health, or substance abuse treatment referrals
- Ask youth about current risk behaviors
- Communicate with youth's assigned probation officer as needed
- Understand requirements of probation
- Continue regular screenings for sexually transmitted diseases and mental health issues
- Assist family with academic needs (eg, request Individualized Education Program from school)

Many youth have histories of drug or alcohol abuse. To preserve an optimal patient-provider relationship, clinicians should avoid becoming involved in court or mandated drug testing, because these proceedings might result in reincarceration or other sanctions being placed on the youth. However, clinicians can work with youth to encourage them to remain in substance abuse treatment. As with all teens, clinicians should continue ongoing regular risk assessment and refer youth for drug abuse treatment as needed.

When ongoing follow-up appointments are required, providers must be aware of the youth's other priorities and responsibilities after release from the detention facility. The terms of probation are often strict, and they must be followed so that youth are not detained again. Youth may be released on house arrest, in which they are not permitted to be anywhere except home or school. Therefore, providers should be aware of this when suggesting follow-up appointments, and must be willing to call or write to probation officers or courts about the importance of medical visits. Similarly, scheduling of appointments during daytime hours may be challenging for recently released youth, because school attendance may be a monitored requirement of the probation period.

Physicians caring for youth should ideally monitor all aspects of well-being, not just physical health. Therefore, the physician must ask about a youth's sexual activity, substance use, school performance, home safety, and involvement in behaviors that may have legal consequences. The same social factors that led to the youth's arrest are also risk factors for poor health outcomes. Therefore, if any risky behaviors are identified, the provider should provide needed care and connect the youth with resources to prevent repeated arrests and negative health consequences.

It is wise to follow these youth regularly, at least twice per year, especially to assess their mental health status, because youth in the detention system have a much higher prevalence of mental health issues, including depression and suicidality. For further guidance in managing these youth, the AAP and AMA have publications that provide guidance to practitioners dealing with children involved in the juvenile justice system.[55,56]

SUMMARY

Although several challenges exist to providing optimal care for adolescents in correctional facilities, their medical and mental health needs are high, and it is critical to ensure that health care during detention is a priority. These needs also require attention once youth have been released from detention and are receiving health care in community-based settings. Providing well-rounded and sensitive care to these adolescents during and after incarceration has a great effect for each youth, and a positive impact on their families and communities.

REFERENCES

1. Golzari M, Hunt SJ, Anoshiravani A. The health status of youth in juvenile detention facilities. J Adolesc Health 2006;38:776–82.
2. Sedlak AJ, Bruce C. Youth's characteristics and backgrounds: findings from the Survey of Youth in Residential Placement. Available at: https://www.ncjrs.gov/pdffiles1/ojjdp/227730.pdf. Accessed November 13, 2013.
3. Braverman P, Morris R. The health of youth in the juvenile justice system. In: Sherman FT, Jacobs FH, editors. Juvenile justice- advancing research, policy, and practice. Hoboken (NJ): Wiley; 2011. p. 44–67.

4. Sickmund M, Sladky TJ, Kang W, et al. Easy access to the census of juveniles in residential placement. Available at: http://www.ojjdp.gov/ojstatbb/ezacjrp/. Accessed November 24, 2013.
5. Statistical Briefing Book: Law Enforcement & Juvenile Crime. Office of Juvenile Justice and Delinquency Prevention Web site. Available at: http://www.ojjdp.gov/ojstatbb/crime/JAR.asp. Accessed November 24, 2013.
6. Committee on Adolescence, American Academy of Pediatrics. Health care for youth in the juvenile justice system. Pediatrics 2011;128:1219–35.
7. KIDS count data snapshot: youth incarceration in the United States. Annie E. Casey Foundation Web site. Available at: http://www.aecf.org. Accessed November 13, 2013.
8. Statistical Briefing Book: Juvenile Justice System Structure & Process. Office of Juvenile Justice and Delinquency Prevention Web site. Available at: http://www.ojjdp.gov/ojstatbb/structure_process/case.html. Accessed November 24, 2013.
9. Gallagher C, Dobrin A. Can the juvenile detention facilities meet the call of the American Academy of Pediatrics and the National Commission on Correctional Health Care? A national analysis of current practices. Pediatrics 2007;119: e991–1001.
10. National Commission on Correctional Heath Care. Standards for health services in juvenile detention and confinement facilities. Chicago: National Commission on Correctional Health Care; 2011.
11. Ad Hoc Committee Juvenile Justice Special Interest Group of the Society of Adolescent Health and Medicine. Health Care for incarcerated youth: position paper of the Society for Adolescent Medicine. J Adolesc Health 2000;27: 73–5.
12. Correctional heath care standards and accreditation. American Public Health Association Web site. Available at: http://www.apha.org/advocacy/policy/policysearch/default.htm?id=1291. Accessed November 11, 2013.
13. Elster A, Kuznets N. AMA guidelines for adolescent preventive services (GAPS). Baltimore (MD): William & Wilkins; 1994.
14. Hagan JF, Shaw JS, Duncan PM, editors. Bright futures: guidelines for health supervision of infants, children, and adolescents. 3rd edition. Elk Grove Village (IL): American Academy of Pediatrics; 2008.
15. Guidelines for disease management in correctional settings. National Commission on Correctional Health Care Web site. Available at: http://www.ncchc.org. Accessed November 24, 2013.
16. Feinstein RA, Lampkin A, Lorish CD, et al. Medical status of adolescents at time of admission to a juvenile detention center. J Adolesc Health 1998;22:190–6.
17. Sedlak AJ, McPherson KS. OJJDP Juvenile Justice Bulletin: Youth's Needs and Services. Available at: https://www.ncjrs.gov/pdffiles1/ojjdp/227728.pdf. Accessed November 24, 2013.
18. Morris RE, Harrison EA, Know GW, et al. Health risk behavioral survey from 39 juvenile correctional facilities in the United States. J Adolesc Health 1995;17: 334–44.
19. Centers for Disease Control and Prevention. Advisory Committee on Immunization Practices (ACIP) recommended immunization schedules for persons aged 0 through 18 years and adults aged 19 years and older: United States, 2013. MMWR Surveill Summ 2013;62(Suppl 1):1–19.
20. Centers for Disease Control and Prevention. Sexually transmitted disease surveillance 2011. Atlanta (GA): US Department of Health and Human Services; 2012.

21. U.S. Preventive Services Task Force. Behavioral counseling to prevent sexually transmitted infections: recommendations statement. Ann Intern Med 2008;149: 491–6.

22. Workowski KA, Berman S, Centers for Disease Control and Prevention. Sexually transmitted diseases treatment guidelines. MMWR Recomm Rep 2010; 59(RR-12):1–110.

23. Gallagher CA, Dobrin A, Douds AS. A national overview of reproductive heath care services for girls in juvenile justice residential facilties. Womens Health Issues 2007;17:217–26.

24. Teplin LA, Abram KM, McClelland GM, et al. Psychiatric disorders in youth in juvenile detention. Arch Gen Psychiatry 2002;59:1133–43.

25. Rey J, Morris-Yates A, Singh M, et al. Continuities between psychiatric disorders in adolescents and personality disorders in young adults. Am J Psychiatry 1995; 152:895–900.

26. Abram KM, Choe JY, Washburn JJ, et al. Suicidal ideation and behaviors among youths in juvenile detention. J Am Acad Child Adolesc Psychiatry 2008;47:291–9.

27. Hayes L. Juvenile suicide in confinement: findings from the first national survey. Suicide Life Threat Behav 2009;39:353–63.

28. Esposito CL, Clum GA. Social support and problem-solving as moderators of the relationship between childhood abuse and suicidality: applications to a delinquent population. J Trauma Stress 2002;15:137–46.

29. Memory J. Juvenile suicides in secure detention facilities: correction of published rates. Death Stud 1989;13:455–63.

30. Thompson MP, Ho CH, Kingree JB. Prospective associations between delinquency and suicidal behaviors in a nationally representative sample. J Adolesc Health 2007;40:232–7.

31. Watson L, Edelman P. Improving the juvenile justice system for girls. Georgetown Center on Poverty, Inequality and Public Policy. Available at: http://www. law.georgetown.edu/academics/centers-institutes/poverty-inequality/upload/ jds_v1r4_web_singles.pdf. Accessed December 7, 2013.

32. The Juvenile Justice and Delinquency Prevention Act. 42 USC §5633(a)(7)(B)(i-ii).

33. Greene, Peters and Associates, editor. Guiding principles for promising female programming: an inventory of best practices. Washington, DC: Office for Juvenile Justice and Delinquency Prevention; 1998.

34. Recommendations for Promoting the Health and Well-Being of Lesbian. Gay, bisexual, and transgender adolescents: a position paper of the society for adolescent health and medicine. J Adolesc Health 2013;52:506–10.

35. Irvine A. "We've had three of them": addressing the invisibility of lesbian, gay, bisexual, and transgender youth in the juvenile justice system. Columbia J Gend Law 2010;19:675–701.

36. Majd K, Marksamer J, Reyes C. Hidden injustice: lesbian, gay, bisexual, and transgender youth in juvenile courts. San Francisco (CA): Legal Services for Children, National Juvenile Defender Center and National Center for Lesbian Rights; 2009.

37. Beck AJ, Harrison PM, Guerino P. Sexual victimization in juvenile facilities reported by youth. United States Department of Justice Programs, Bureau of Justice Statistics, NCH 228416. Available at: http://bjs.ojp.usdoj.gov/index.cfm? ty=pbdetail&ciid=2113. Accessed December 7, 2013.

38. Garnette L, Irvine A, Reyes I, et al. Lesbian, gay, bisexual and transgender (LGBT) youth and the juvenile justice system. In: Sherman FT, Jacobs FH,

editors. Juvenile justice advancing research, policy, and practice. Hoboken (NJ): John Wiley & Sons, Inc; 2011. p. 156–73.

39. National Standards to Prevent, Detect, and Respond to Prison Rape. Final Rule. Fed Regist 2012;77(119):37105–37232. To be codified at 28 CFR §115.

40. Shonkoff JP, Boyce WT, McEwen BS. Neuroscience, molecular biology, and the childhood roots of health disparities. JAMA 2009;301:2252–9.

41. Aksglaede L, Link K, Giwercman A, et al. 47,XXY Klinefelter syndrome: clinical characteristics and age-specific recommendations for medical management. Am J Med Genet C Semin Med Genet 2013;163C:55–63.

42. Miller M, Sulkes S. Fire-setting behavior in individuals with Klinefelter syndrome. Pediatrics 1988;82:115–7.

43. Hecht F, Hecht BK. Behavior in Klinefelter Syndrome, or where there is smoke there may not be a fire [letter to the editor]. Pediatrics 1990;86:1001.

44. Keuhn D, Aros S, Cassorla F, et al. A prospective cohort study of the prevalence of growth, facial, and central nervous system abnormalities in children with heavy prenatal alcohol exposure. Alcohol Clin Exp Res 2012;36:1811–9.

45. Foroud T, Wetherill L, Vinci-Booher S, et al. Relation over time between facial measurements and cognitive outcomes in fetal alcohol-exposed children. Alcohol Clin Exp Res 2012;36:1634–46.

46. Keen CL, Uriu-Adams JY, Skalny A, et al. The plausibility of maternal nutritional status being a contributing factor to the risk for fetal alcohol spectrum disorders: the potential influence of zinc status as an example. Biofactors 2010;36:125–35.

47. Rufer ES, Tran TD, Attridge MM, et al. Adequacy of maternal iron status protects against behavioral, neuroanatomical, and growth deficits in fetal alcohol spectrum disorders. PLoS One 2012;7:e474–99.

48. Gagnier KR, Moore TE, Green M, et al. A need for closer examinations of FASD by the criminal justice system: has the call been answered? J Popul Ther Clin Pharmacol 2011;18:e426–39.

49. Fast DK, Conry J. Fetal alcohol spectrum disorders and the criminal justice system. Dev Disabil Res Rev 2009;15:250–7.

50. Ballard M, Sun M, Ko J. Vitamin A, folate, and choline as a possible preventive intervention for fetal alcohol syndrome. Med Hypotheses 2012;78:489–93.

51. Fetal Alcohol Spectrum Disorders Program: Toolkit. American Academy of Pediatrics Web site. Available at: http://www.aap.org/en-us/advocacy-and-policy/aap-health-initiatives/fetal-alcohol-spectrum-disorders-toolkit/Pages/default.aspx. Accessed December 7, 2013.

52. English A, Bass L, Boyle AD, et al. State minor consent laws: a summary. 3rd edition. Chapel Hill (NC): Center for Adolescent Health & the Law; 2010.

53. Guttmacher Institute. State policies in brief: an overview of minors' consent law. Available at: https://www.guttmacher.org/statecenter/spibs/spib_OMCL.pdf. Accessed January 7, 2014.

54. Gudeman R. Consent to medical treatment for youth in the juvenile justice system: California law: a guide for health care providers. National Center for Youth Law Web site. Available at: http://www.teenhealthlaw.org/fileadmin/teenhealth/teenhealthrights/ca/Juv._Justice_Consent_Manual_11-09.pdf. Accessed January 7, 2014.

55. Morris RE. Health care for incarcerated adolescents: significant needs with considerable obstacles. Virtual Mentor 2005;7:1.

56. Morris RE. Contributor to: addressing mental health concerns in primary care: a clinician's toolkit. Elk Grove Village (IL): Juvenile Justice TIPPS; 2010.

Index

Note: Page numbers of article titles are in **boldface** type.

Prim Care Clin Office Pract 41 (2014) 707–718
http://dx.doi.org/10.1016/S0095-4543(14)00055-4
0095-4543/14/$ – see front matter © 2014 Elsevier Inc. All rights reserved.

primarycare.theclinics.com

Moving?

Make sure your subscription moves with you!

To notify us of your new address, find your **Clinics Account Number** (located on your mailing label above your name), and contact customer service at:

Email: journalscustomerservice-usa@elsevier.com

800-654-2452 (subscribers in the U.S. & Canada)
314-447-8871 (subscribers outside of the U.S. & Canada)

Fax number: 314-447-8029

Elsevier Health Sciences Division
Subscription Customer Service
3251 Riverport Lane
Maryland Heights, MO 63043

*To ensure uninterrupted delivery of your subscription, please notify us at least 4 weeks in advance of move.

Printed and bound by CPI Group (UK) Ltd, Croydon, CR0 4YY

03/10/2024

01040488-0010